Practical Guide to Musculoskeletal Disorders

Practical Guide to Musculoskeletal Disorders: Diagnosis and Rehabilitation

Second Edition

Edited by

Ralph M. Buschbacher, M.D.

Clinical Associate Professor and Interim Chair, Department of Physical
Medicine and Rehabilitation, Indiana University School of Medicine,
Indianapolis; Community Health Network, Indianapolis

Foreword by

Randall L. Braddom, M.D., M.S.

Professor, Department of Physical Medicine and Rehabilitation, Indiana
University School of Medicine, Indianapolis

with 22 contributing authors

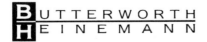

BUTTERWORTH
HEINEMANN

Boston   Oxford   Auckland   Johannesburg   Melbourne   New Delhi

Library of Congress Cataloging-in-Publication Data
Practical guide to musculoskeletal disorders : diagnosis and rehabilitation / [edited by] Ralph M. Buschbacher ; with a foreword by Randall L. Braddom.—2nd ed.
    p. ; cm.
  Rev. ed. of: Musculoskeletal disorders. c1994.
  Includes bibliographical references and index.
  ISBN 0-7506-7357-5
   1. Musculoskeletal system—Diseases. 2. Musculoskeletal
system—Diseases—Patients—Rehabilitation. I. Buschbacher, Ralph M. II.
Musculoskeletal disorders.
   [DNLM: 1. Musculoskeletal Diseases—diagnosis. 2. Musculoskeletal
Diseases—rehabilitation. 3. Musculoskeletal System—physiopathology. WE 140 P895 2002]
  RC925 .M853 2002
  616.7—dc21

                                                                          2001052907

British Library Cataloguing-in-Publication Data
A catalogue record for this book is available from the British Library.

The publisher offers special discounts on bulk orders of this book.
For information, please contact:

Manager of Special Sales
Butterworth–Heinemann
225 Wildwood Avenue
Woburn, MA 01801-2041
Tel: 781-904-2500
Fax: 781-904-2620

For information on all Butterworth–Heinemann publications available,
contact our World Wide Web home page at: http://www.bh.com

10 9 8 7 6 5 4 3 2 1

Printed in the United States of America

To Lois, Michael, Peter, John, and Walter

Contents

I Principles of Musculoskeletal Rehabilitation

II Management of Specific Anatomic Regions

III Special Issues

Contributing Authors

Joanne B. (Anne) Allen, M.D.
Private practice, Physical Medicine and Rehabilitation, SailSportMed, Inc., Atlanta

William J. Barrish, M.D.
Physiatrist, Orthopedic Associates of Southern Delaware, Loewes

J. Greg Bentley, M.D.
Co-Chief Resident, Department of Physical Medicine and Rehabilitation, Indiana University Medical Center, Indianapolis

Michael E. Berend, M.D.
Orthopedic Surgeon, Center for Hip and Knee Surgery and St. Francis Hospital, Mooresville, Indiana

Rina M. Bloch, M.D.
Assistant Professor, Department of Rehabilitation Medicine, Tufts University School of Medicine, Boston; Department of Rehabilitation Medicine, New England Medical Center, Boston

Randall L. Braddom, M.D., M.S.
Professor, Department of Physical Medicine and Rehabilitation, Indiana University School of Medicine, Indianapolis

Steven E. Braverman, M.D.
Assistant Professor, Departments of Neurology and Physical Medicine and Rehabilitation, Uniformed Services University of the Health Sciences, F. Edward Hebert School of Medicine, Bethesda, Maryland; Deputy Commander for Clinical Services, Montcrief Army Community Hospital, Fort Jackson, South Carolina

Ralph M. Buschbacher, M.D.
Clinical Associate Professor and Interim Chair, Department of Physical Medicine and Rehabilitation, Indiana University School of Medicine, Indianapolis; Community Health Network, Indianapolis

Angela T. Carbone, M.D.
Clinical Assistant Professor, Department of Physical Medicine and Rehabilitation, Indiana University Medical Center, Indianapolis

Denise L. Carpenter, M.D.
Clinical Assistant Professor, Departments of Pediatrics and Physical Medicine and Rehabilitation, Riley Children's Hospital, Clarian Health, Indiana University School of Medicine, Indianapolis; Medical Director, Department of Pediatric Physical Medicine and Rehabilitation, Clarian Health, Methodist Hospital, Indianapolis

Rayden C. Cody
Assistant Professor of Physical Medicine and Rehabilitation, University of Vermont College of Medicine, Burlington

Andrea R. Conti, D.O.
Assistant Professor, Department of Physical Medicine and Rehabilitation, Indiana University School of Medicine, Indianapolis; Chief, Physical Medicine and Rehabilitation Services, Roudebush Veterans Administration Medical Center, Indianapolis

Katherine L. Dec, M.D.
Medical Director, Mind-Body Medical Institute, Bon Secours Hospital, Richmond, Virginia; Private practice, Integrated Musculoskeletal Medicine Institute, Richmond

Van Evanoff, Jr., M.D.
Resident Physician, Department of Physical Medicine and Rehabilitation, Indiana University Medical Center, Indianapolis

David R. O'Brien, Jr., M.D.
Adjunct Clinical Associate Professor, Department of Physical Medicine and Rehabilitation, University of North Carolina at Chapel Hill School of Medicine; Director of Physiatry, Interventional Pain Management and Rehabilitation Services, Orthopedic Specialists of the Carolinas, Winston-Salem, North Carolina

Binduben A. Patel, M.D.
Co-Chief Resident Physician, Department of Physical Medicine and Rehabilitation, Indiana University Medical Center, Indianapolis

Nathan D. Prahlow, M.D.
Resident Physician, Department of Physical Medicine and Rehabilitation, Indiana University Medical Center, Indianapolis

Mark S. Randall, Psy.D, D.R.P.H., M.A.
Department of Physical Medicine and Rehabilitation, Indiana University School of Medicine, Indianapolis; Clinical Director of Pain Medicine Center, Department of Rehabilitation, Community Hospital of Indianapolis

Matthew W. Smuck, M.D.
Fellow, Department of Physical Medicine and Rehabilitation, Stanford University School of Medicine, Stanford, California

Michael J. Stonnington, M.D.
Orthopaedic Surgeon, Southern Bone and Joint Specialists, P.A., Hattiesburg, Mississippi

Mary J. Wells, Ph.D.
Rehabilitation Psychologist, Department of Medical Psychology, Sheltering Arms Physical Rehabilitation Centers, Richmond, Virginia

Robert P. Wilder, M.D.
Assistant Professor, Department of Physical Medicine and Rehabilitation, University of Virginia School of Medicine, Charlottesville

Foreword

In the first edition, Dr. Buschbacher and his contributors created a user-friendly book about the musculoskeletal system and its disorders that was immediately popular with medical students, residents, and practicing physicians. Physicians of all specialties embraced it, as no specialty of medicine can totally avoid caring for problems of the musculoskeletal system. Readers noticed that they could go from an introductory level of understanding of the musculoskeletal system and its problems to a remarkably sophisticated level quickly and with great learner efficiency.

With the second edition, Dr. Buschbacher and his contributors have made the book even better. This is one of those rare instances in which the "sequel" is actually better than the original. The second edition contains even more concise and carefully selected information on a large group of common musculoskeletal disorders. New chapters and many new illustrations add to its value. It would be hard to find a book with more up-to-date information about the musculoskeletal conditions that are frequently encountered in clinical practice.

If you are a neophyte in regards to the musculoskeletal system, this book will get you up to speed quickly. If you are an experienced musculoskeletal clinician, the book will help you update your approach to these clinical problems. For those who want an even more in-depth view of a specific aspect of the musculoskeletal system, an outstanding list of references and suggested readings is provided at the end of each chapter. These references were selected by the experts and are much more valuable than a cold, computerized keyword search.

The second edition will help bring you to a new level of competence and confidence in treating musculoskeletal problems and will whet your appetite for further study. Bon appétit!

Randall L. Braddom

Preface

As an author, I have been extremely flattered that people have spent their hard-earned money to buy one of my books. It has been even more gratifying when I have run into people who have purchased and read the previous edition of this book, and they tell me that they have enjoyed it, learned from it, and found it clinically useful. It is for these people that I undertook the task of putting together a second edition.

For this second edition, I have tried to update each chapter and provide cutting-edge knowledge whenever possible. I have tried to make each chapter even more clinically useful and practical and have expanded the range of conditions that are discussed. I have recruited an excellent group of clinicians and have instructed them to keep their individual chapters as clear, straightforward, and readable as possible. I think they have succeeded. I certainly have learned a wealth of new information in reading their work, and I hope that the readers will appreciate this effort as much as I have.

My goal in putting together this book has been to create a clear and concise source of knowledge for musculoskeletal medicine. A text of this size cannot, obviously, provide the definitive, in-depth approach to each individual condition; however, it certainly can provide a clinically useful and practical overview that encompasses most of what is known in the field. My goal has been to make sure that this book covers 95% of the musculoskeletal problems that would be seen in a clinical setting.

In this second edition, I have continued to provide an anatomic and therapeutic background sufficient to lay the groundwork for the specific conditions that are covered. I have also tried to include the more useful physical examination tests, especially if those tests have proven diagnostic benefits. I have expanded on the diagnosis and treatment of specific conditions, including even more practical information and protocols for treatment.

I have also added quite a bit of new, original artwork, which I think works very well in complementing the written text.

This book is organized into three sections. The first includes the principles of musculoskeletal rehabilitation. It contains chapters on the basics of the treatment and testing armamentarium. The second section includes the management of specific body parts, and the third section includes chapters on various diseases that require more elaboration, as well as on special patient populations, such as pediatrics, geriatrics, women, and persons with disability. I close the book with a chapter on the role of exercise in treating and preventing illness.

I hope that the readers find this book to be relevant to their practices and a readable reference source.

R. M. B.

Acknowledgments

I wish to thank Judy Smith for her support in helping me prepare this manuscript, Sharon Teal for her artwork, and each of the contributors for the excellent work that they have done.

Practical Guide to Musculoskeletal Disorders

I **Principles of Musculoskeletal Rehabilitation**

1 Tissue Injury and Healing: Maximizing Outcomes with the Sports Medicine Approach

Matthew W. Smuck and Ralph M. Buschbacher

Types of Musculoskeletal Injuries

Macrotrauma

Tissue injury can be classified by etiology as resulting from either macrotrauma or microtrauma. Macrotrauma is acute damage due to a strong force. It is seen in injuries due to collisions, falls, or other accidents. Patients are usually immediately aware of the injury and its cause. Macrotrauma can be due to either direct trauma to the injured area or indirect trauma resulting from a transmission of forces. Older age, inactivity, osteoporosis, and a history of previous injury increase the risk of macrotraumatic injury.

Repetitive Microtrauma

Microtrauma is an overuse condition caused by repetitive motion. After any injury the body needs time to heal. If the damaged tissues are overstressed and re-injured, the natural healing process can become pathologic. Chronic inflammation occurs, leading to further tissue weakness and injury such as tendon and ligament rupture, stress fracture, and abnormal calcification of soft tissues. At the microscopic level collagen fiber failure is seen.

Stages of Healing

After injury there are three stages of healing: inflammation, repair, and remodeling.

Inflammation

When body tissues are injured there may be bleeding, clot formation, swelling, and a cellular reaction. The initial cellular reaction consists of an influx of macrophages and other mediators of inflammation. They ingest particulate matter and excrete chemicals that promote the inflammatory response and increase local blood flow.

Repair

Between days 3 and 5 after injury, fibroblast proliferation begins the next stage of healing. Fibroblasts produce collagen that, in early repair, takes the place of the fibrin clot that is being broken down and resorbed. Initially the collagen is oriented at random and has very little structural strength.

Remodeling

Beginning approximately 1–2 weeks after injury, the collagen scar begins to remodel. The randomly oriented fibers are gradually broken down and replaced with longitudinally arranged fibers. Thus, the collagen is reoriented in the direction it is needed, and the tissue slowly regains its structural strength. This entire process requires months to years to complete.

Maximizing Repair Success

In macrotraumatic injuries, such as acute fractures or sprains, there is a tissue defect that needs to be filled. If it is filled with disorganized collagen fibers it will not have adequate strength to resume normal function. If the tissue is immobilized for a prolonged period of time, only disorganized tissue will form.[1] When light stress is applied to the healing area, the collagen fibers align longitudinally and heal to form a stronger structural and functional support (Figure 1.1). Thus it is clear that prolonged immobilization is contraindicated after injury.

Repetitive microtrauma is an overuse cycle in which tissue repair is outpaced by recurring injury. The tissue becomes chronically engaged in the inflammatory stage of healing. Inflammation alone can weaken connective tissues by up to 50% of their original strength. Thus, inflammation added to cumulative microtrauma often leads to rupture or failure of the involved tissues. Therefore, to maximize healing, adequate rest and control of inflammation are essential.

Inflammation is a necessary part of the early healing process; however, prolonged inflammation is detrimental. Therefore, control of inflammation is desirable in the subacute stages of healing. Nonsteroidal anti-inflammatory medications are helpful, and occasionally steroid medications are used to reduce inflammation. However, steroids actually inhibit healing if given too early, such as in the first days of inflammation, or if given for prolonged periods.

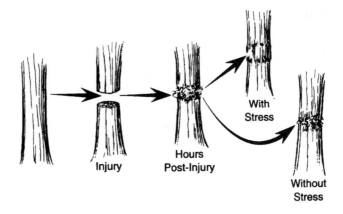

With
Stress

Hours
Post-Injury

Injury

Without
Stress

FIGURE 1.1 *Normal recovery progression of a tendon after being lacerated. If the tendon is not stressed, the collagen scar is unorganized instead of being arranged as parallel fibers.*

Other factors are known to impact healing. Some of these are not correctable, such as older age and poor vascular supply. Other factors, such as nutrition, health, and compliance with treatments, should be optimized to promote maximal healing.

Specific Tissue Injury

Tendon and Ligament Injury

Tendons and ligaments are mostly made of parallel collagen fibers. If they are not mobilized soon after injury (or surgery) they develop adhesions to the surrounding tissues. The loose connective tissues that ordinarily allow these structures free movement become denser. They may bind to the tendons or ligaments and further limit their motion. Without stress from active motion, the collagen fibers remain disorganized, with poor strength.[1-4]

Some ligaments, such as those in the back, must stretch to allow proper body movements. They contain elastin fibers. If these ligaments are immobilized, elastin is lost and the ligaments shorten and lose strength and flexibility. This process predisposes these tissues to re-injury and places undue stress on neighboring tissues.

Ligamentous sprains are often classified by severity into grades I, II, or III. Grade I injury is a microscopic tear of the ligament that causes pain. Joint stability is normal but ligamentous stress testing reproduces pain. Grade II sprains involve tearing of enough fibers to result in ligamentous laxity in addition to pain. Stability testing reveals the laxity with abnormal joint motion, but a firm end point remains. Grade III sprains are a complete disruption of the ligament. Joint laxity with abnormal motion and a loose end feel are characteristic findings.

Muscle Injury

When muscles are torn, it is called a *strain*. In conditions of muscle strain or laceration, a scar forms between the disrupted ends similar to tendon and ligament injuries. The scar may interrupt the contractile fibers of the muscle, but usually such injuries heal well, with little residual dysfunction.

Muscles may also become contused or develop hematomas. This type of injury involves a crush or stretch injury to muscle cells, with local bleeding. Sometimes abnormal islands of calcification occur in the injured muscle. These form in a similar manner to normal bone, with calcification of a fibro-cartilaginous matrix. This condition is called *myositis ossificans* and may lead to muscle contracture or joint immobility, depending on the extent and location of the ossifications. Surgical excision may be required in such severe cases; however, it should be delayed until the new bone islands have fully calcified.

When a contused muscle is stressed too soon after injury, the healing process can be interrupted, edema exacerbated, and the condition worsened. Therefore, such traumatic injuries should be rested until pain and acute inflammation have mostly resolved. Compression and ice are used acutely to decrease edema and inflammation, and to prevent worsening of the damage.

Joint Injury

Cartilage may be fractured along with bone in macrotraumatic injuries. When this occurs in a joint, surgical fixation is usually required. The normal hyaline cartilage in a joint cannot be replaced after injury, so a fibrocartilaginous scar forms to fill the defect. This fibrocartilage is not as well suited to the repeated stress of joint function as is normal hyaline cartilage, and future pain and degeneration may occur.

When the cartilage of the epiphyseal growth plate is injured in a growing child, future growth abnormalities may result. Such an injury should always be suspected and ruled out in a child with painful bone or joint trauma. Assessment by an orthopedist is essential.

Degenerative joint disease is primarily due to degeneration of hyaline joint cartilage. The cause is unknown, but previous injury to a joint and a genetic predisposition increase an individual's risk. The condition is sometimes viewed as "normal wear and tear" on joints, especially in older individuals. It is more common with advanced age, obesity, and in weight-bearing joints. It remains unclear why this condition is painful for some patients and not for others. As the hyaline cartilage degenerates, the normal healing response causes a mild inflammation of the involved joint. This inflammation may become chronic due to persistent stress on the joint cartilage. Hallmark features are nonuniform cartilage destruction and "spurring" (bony proliferation) of the surrounding bones. These findings are classically seen in the hips, knees, and spine, but may also be present elsewhere.

Cartilage is also destroyed in connective tissue diseases such as rheumatoid arthritis. In these conditions, the synovial membrane becomes inflamed and releases enzymes that destroy the cartilage. Uniform cartilage degeneration and painful swollen joints are the hallmark features. Range-of-motion exercise, even when done passively, can aggravate the inflammation of acutely inflamed arthritic joints.[5] Therefore, it should be avoided in the acutely inflamed stages. This needs to be balanced with the concern over development of contractures. Patients with acutely inflamed joints tend to hold them in the position creating the least intra-articular pressure. If held in this position too long, they may develop permanent loss of range of motion. The inflammation of joints in connective tissue disease may weaken adjacent tendons and ligaments. Ruptures of these structures may occur; however, this can be avoided by not placing undue stress on the affected areas.

Bone Injury

Bone, as all other connective tissue, can be injured by macrotrauma or repetitive microtrauma. When macrotrauma causes a fracture, osteoblasts within the periosteum lay down new bone in what is termed a *callus*. The callus is formed and remodeled by a combination of osteoblastic and osteoclastic activity. In osteoporosis, bones have lost overall density and are more likely to fracture; however, fracture healing occurs at the same rate as in normal bones.

According to Wolf's Law, bone grows or remodels in response to the force placed on it. When greater than average stress is placed on a bone, it responds by initial resorption (osteoclastic activity) and weakening. This is followed by bone regeneration (osteoblastic activity) and strengthening. Thus regular weight-bearing exercise causes bone density and strength to increase. But when stressors are excessive and repeated, the initial resorption is not allowed to heal. Additional resorption outpaces the bone's regenerative capabilities and fracture lines appear. This is the scenario in so-called *stress fractures*. Stress fractures are common, for example, in runners who have recently increased their mileage or changed their footwear or terrain.[6,7]

Nerve Injury

Peripheral nerves can be injured by a direct blow, laceration, stretch, or chronic compression. Damage may be isolated to the Schwann cells of the myelin sheath. This leads to slowing of the nerve conduction but does not cause weakness. If the involved segment is large enough, normal saltatory conduction is interrupted, resulting in a conduction block and potential clinical weakness. If the injury only involves the myelin, identification and removal of the insulting factor allows myelin regeneration, and complete functional recovery normally occurs over time. Such injuries to myelin are seen in the early stages of compression neuropathies like carpal tunnel syndrome.

If the compression is not relieved, the axon inside the myelin sheath may die. The segment of the axon distal to the site of injury deteriorates by a process called *Wallerian degeneration*. The more proximal segment is sustained by its connection to the cell body. If the myelin sheath or other supportive connective tissue structures remain intact, then removal of the compression allows the intact proximal axon segment to attempt to regenerate down the tube it previously inhabited. Such axon regeneration occurs at a rate of approximately

1 in. per month. In the meantime, denervated muscle fibers begin to atrophy. If not re-innervated before complete fibrosis, between 12 and 18 months after denervation, muscle recovery is not possible. Intact nerve axons may create distal "sprouts" to help innervate orphaned muscle fibers. Therefore, recovery is variable depending on the amount of axons involved and the distance the axons must regenerate.

When a nerve is cut, the axon distal to the lesion undergoes Wallerian degeneration. The intact proximal segment attempts to regrow by sending out "sprouts," which may contact the opposite end and begin to regenerate as described above. But because the connective tissue tube is disrupted, this is often unsuccessful. Nerve sprouts may form a small bulb on the end of the severed nerve. This bulb, called a *neuroma*, can be painful. Painful neuromas may be seen after injury or surgical amputations. Microsurgery may help to reattach the ends of cut nerves.[8] Outcome is not usually optimal, but may be better than with no intervention. Electrodiagnostic studies such as electromyography and nerve conduction studies can help identify which lesions are better suited for surgery and which may heal better if left alone. These studies are also useful to help differentiate muscle weakness caused by conduction block verses axonal loss.

Principles of Rehabilitation: The Sports Medicine Approach

Musculoskeletal medicine owes a lot to the pioneering efforts of sports medicine physicians, athletes, and trainers, who have helped revolutionize treatment in the field. The unproven dogma of medical treatment in the past consisted of prolonged periods of rest, immobilization, or casting—often for minor injuries. This treatment was used after childbirth and surgery as well as for musculoskeletal injuries. We now know that excessive pampering of the body is one of the worst things we can do to it. Although sports medicine developed many ideas that were initially controversial, many are now considered mainstream musculoskeletal medicine.

Early Mobilization

As described earlier, prolonged immobilization causes connective tissues to shorten and stiffen, creating contractures and mechanical dysfunction. Cartilage nutrition suffers, bone density decreases, muscles atrophy, neural coordination decreases, and cardiorespiratory fitness deteriorates.[2–4,9–11] These conditions should be prevented when possible. Correcting them after they have occurred is time-consuming and frustrating. It takes at least twice as long for muscle strength and cardiac fitness to recover as it takes for them to deteriorate.[9,11] Cartilage function may never completely recover, and bone density may require years to return to its premorbid level.[11]

As a rule of thumb, injured areas should be mobilized as soon as acute inflammation is under control. Motion may be passive or active as long as the condition is not aggravated. Isometric strengthening exercises are useful to prevent muscle deterioration when full range of motion is not possible. It is also important that other noninjured areas not be allowed to deteriorate.

When treating musculoskeletal disorders, immobilization is sometimes required. At other times, relative rest is prescribed. When possible, relative rest is the preferred option. Immobilization is, of course, necessary after some fractures and tendon ruptures. It is also useful in acutely inflamed joint conditions, ligament sprains, and tendonitis. It should not usually be prescribed for more than a few days for the latter two conditions. It may be necessary for up to 2 weeks in inflamed joints, and up to 6 weeks or more for fractures and tendon ruptures.

Relative rest is intended to allow the damaged tissue to maintain at least some level of function. Aggravating motions are specifically restricted. For instance, relative rest in rotator-cuff tendonitis might require refraining only from overhead activities. Other motions are allowed and even encouraged. Determining when to prescribe relative rest or immobilization is not always easy. In general, if a joint is stable and not acutely inflamed, it is safe to prescribe rest.

One of the most impressive arguments for early mobilization has been described by Deyo et al. in the treatment of acute low back pain.[12] They randomized patients into treatment groups that were instructed to remain on bed rest for 2 days or 7 days. Both groups actually stayed in bed for a shorter period than recommended and outcome in both was essentially the same.

Proprioceptive Exercises

In 1965, Freeman et al. first postulated and provided evidence that a proprioceptive defect after ankle sprain caused functional instability of the joint.[10] They explained that ligaments contain nerve endings that inform the brain of joint position. If the ligaments are disrupted, proprioception is impaired. This has been demonstrated by multiple subsequent studies, not only regarding injury to the ankle, but in other joints as well. Immobilization of the joint results in further deterioration of proprioceptive function. When activity is resumed, the patient is more likely to re-injure the tissues due to poor sensory feedback.

It is now clear that proprioception plays an important role in preventing re-injury. Exercises that stress proprioceptive awareness, such as balance boards and backward walking, help to improve joint recovery from injury.

Rehabilitation Progression

Early after injury it is particularly important to control pain and inflammation. The RICE (rest, ice, compression, elevation) protocol is used after sports injuries and can be modified for just about any musculoskeletal condition. In addition, nonsteroidal anti-inflammatory medications may reduce inflammation and pain. They are especially useful in overuse conditions such as tendonitis and bursitis. Ice is a helpful adjunct to treatment, reducing pain and edema. It is especially useful in the acute postinjury period, until swelling subsides, as well as for overuse conditions and before or after exercise to avoid aggravation of swelling. Heat is generally used in the subacute period (after 1–2 days). It is also especially helpful in overuse syndromes.

While controlling pain and inflammation and resting the affected area, it is important not to neglect fitness of the rest of the body. In upper extremity injury, exercise bicycles help maintain cardiorespiratory and lower body fitness. In lower extremity injury, arm crank ergometry may be performed. Other modified activities, such as kickboard swimming, can be done if the patient wishes. Regardless of injury, some type of exercise should be encouraged to maintain overall fitness.

After pain and inflammation are under control, it is important to maintain or regain adequate mobility. When a body part hurts, it is natural to try to protect it. This type of splinting is helpful during acute recovery, but if prolonged may result in contracture, reduced strength and function, and ultimately, more pain. As soon as inflammation is controlled, the patient must work on restoring and maintaining normal range of motion.

When the patient has near normal range of motion and can tolerate more activity, a strengthening exercise program is initiated. Without proper strength and flexibility, re-injury is more likely. Later, as tolerated, activity- or sports-specific training is indicated. It is not good enough for patients to achieve good recovery of flexibility and strength in the therapy gym; functional tasks similar to those that are to be resumed must be practiced before return to activity. Proper biomechanics and technique should be taught before return to activity, and preferably even before the first injury occurs.

Points of Summary

1. The two primary types of musculoskeletal injury are macrotrauma and repetitive microtrauma.
2. There are three stages of connective tissue healing: inflammation, repair, and remodeling.
3. Following injury, ligaments and tendons must be stressed to achieve proper alignment of the collagen fibers and to maximize healing.
4. Myositis ossificans is the abnormal formation of bone within muscle after injury.
5. When hyaline cartilage is injured a fibrocartilaginous scar forms.
6. Stress fractures occur when bone resorption outpaces bone regeneration in response to repeated stress.
7. Peripheral nerve dysfunction may be due to demyelination, axon damage, or both. Electrodiagnostic studies help differentiate the type of nerve injury. Recovery depends on the type and degree of injury.
8. Prolonged immobility causes deterioration of the cardiorespiratory system, cartilage, muscle, bones, and coordination.
9. Relative rest is preferred to immobilization when possible.
10. Ligament injury may impair proprioception.
11. Rehabilitation should encompass control of inflammation and pain, restoration of mobility, restoration of strength, and functional reconditioning, with progression to normal activity.

References

1. Hyman J, Rodeo SA. Injury and repair of tendons and ligaments. Phys Med Rehabil Clin N Am 2000;11:267–288.

2. Tipton CM, Matthes RD, Maynard JA, et al. The influence of physical activity on ligaments and tendons. Med Sci Sports Exerc 1975;7:165–175.
3. Pneumaticos SG, McGarvey WC, Mody DR, Trevino SG. The effects of early mobilization in the healing of Achilles tendon repair. Foot Ankle Int 2000;21:551–557.
4. Noyes FR. Functional properties of knee ligaments and alterations induced by immobilization: a correlative biomechanical and histological study in primates. Clin Orthop 1977;123:210–242.
5. Merritt JL, Hunder GG. Passive range of motion, not isometric exercise, amplifies acute urate synovitis. Arch Phys Med Rehabil 1983;64:130–131.
6. Fredericson M. Common injuries in runners. Diagnosis, rehabilitation and prevention. Sports Med 1996;21:49–72.
7. Bergman AG, Fredericson M. MR imaging of stress reactions, muscle injuries, and other overuse injuries in runners. Magn Reson Imaging Clin N Am 1999;7:151–174.
8. Lee SK, Wolfe SW. Peripheral nerve injury and repair. J Am Acad Orthop Surg 2000;8:243–252.
9. Perhonen MA, Zuckerman JH, Levine BD. Deterioration of left ventricular chamber performance after bed rest: "cardiovascular deconditioning" or hypovolemia? Circulation 2001(Apr 10);103:1851–1857.
10. Freeman MAR, Dean MRE, Hanham IWF. The etiology and prevention of functional instability of the foot. J Bone Joint Surg 1965;47B:678–685.
11. Saltin B, Blomquist G, Mitchell JH, et al. Response to exercise after bedrest and after training: A longitudinal study of adaptive changes in oxygen transport and body composition. Circulation 1968;38(Suppl 7):VII1–VII78.
12. Deyo RA, Diehl AK, Rosenthal M. How many days of bed rest for acute low back pain? A randomized clinical trial. N Engl J Med 1986;315:1064–1070.

Suggested Readings

Best TM. Soft tissue injuries and muscle tears. Clin Sports Med 1997;16:419–434.

Kibler WB, Herring SA, Press JM (eds). Functional Rehabilitation of Sports and Musculoskeletal Injuries. Gaithersburg, MD: Aspen, 1998.

Nicholas JA, Hershman EB. The Lower Extremity and Spine in Sports Medicine (2nd ed). St. Louis: Mosby, 1995.

2   Therapeutic Modalities

J. Greg Bentley

Medicine is often thought of as a "high-tech" profession. Yet when it comes to therapeutic modalities, the most commonly used treatments are decidedly "un-tech." Heat and cold are the most widely used modalities, both historically and today. Their pain-relieving effects have been known for some time, although the exact mechanism is still controversial (Table 2.1).[1-5] In addition to relieving pain, these modalities have other actions, including effects on flexibility, joint stiffness, blood flow, and inflammation. To take advantage of these properties, for treating pain and other conditions, numerous heating and cooling devices have been developed. This chapter describes the characteristics of several such devices and also explains the use of electrical stimulation, massage, and traction.

Heat

Heating modalities create local and reflex effects. The local response is an increase in tissue temperature and metabolic rate.

The reflex effects include regional and generalized responses. The regional responses include increased blood flow to the treated area and muscle relaxation (Figure 2.1). The generalized responses include increased blood flow to the contralateral limb, sedation and relaxation, sweating, and body thermo-regulation.

Heating modalities can be classified by their mechanism of heating, namely conduction, convection, or conversion. They can also be classified as causing superficial or deep heating. Table 2.2 lists the common modalities using each of these mechanisms.

Conduction

Conduction is the simplest heating modality (Figure 2.2). It occurs whenever two objects of differing temperatures come in contact with each other. Heat flows from the warmer to the cooler object. This occurs because the molecules in the warmer material vibrate faster and stimulate the cooler molecules to move faster as well. The temperature of the object being warmed rises most at the surface in

TABLE 2.1 Hypotheses of mechanism of reduction of pain by heat and cold

Decreased pain-spasm cycle

Vasodilation, resulting in an increased clearing of cell waste products (heat only)

Inhibition of pain fibers

Increased level of endorphins

Vasodilation, resulting in decreased ischemic pain (heat only)

Counterirritant effect

Equalized temperature gradient between injured and noninjured tissues

Decreased inflammation and swelling (cold only)

Direct block of pain transmission (cold only)

General relaxation and sedation (heat only)

contact with the heating source, and drops off rapidly in a gradient from that point on. Similarly, the heating agent is warmest at its center and gets cooler closer to its surface of contact with the surroundings, also a temperature gradient. Because of this, heating by conduction is relatively inefficient. Unless the conducting material has a way of replenishing its own heat content, it will quickly cool off and lose its effect.

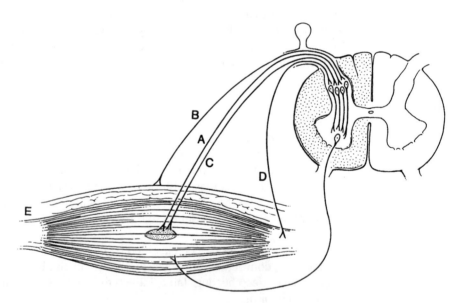

FIGURE 2.1   *The effects of heat and cold on decreasing muscle tension. A. Heating certain afferent muscle spindle fibers causes them to have a decreased rate of firing, thus relaxing tonic muscle activity. B. Cooling the skin facilitates the alpha-motor neurons, thus increasing spasticity and muscle stretch reflexes. C. Cooling the afferent muscle spindle fibers (deep cooling) causes a direct effect of inhibiting their firing, thus relaxing muscle spasticity. D. Heating the Golgi tendon organ increases its firing, which inhibits the alpha motor neuron and decreases spasticity. E. Direct effect of heat increases collagen extensibility.*

TABLE 2.2   Common heating modalities by category

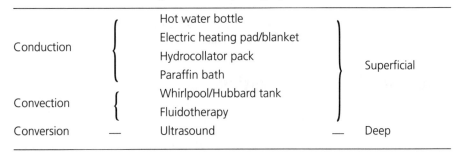

Conduction	Hot water bottle	
	Electric heating pad/blanket	
	Hydrocollator pack	Superficial
	Paraffin bath	
Convection	Whirlpool/Hubbard tank	
	Fluidotherapy	
Conversion	Ultrasound	Deep

Convection

Convection is the exchange of heat from a moving liquid (e.g., a whirlpool). As described above, in conduction there is a temperature gradient such that the surface of the warming object is cooler than the rest of that object. This slows down effective heat transfer. Convection eliminates this gradient by constantly moving the fluid (see Figure 2.2). Thus the heating fluid's temperature at the surface of the skin is constant and is not reduced by a temperature gradient.

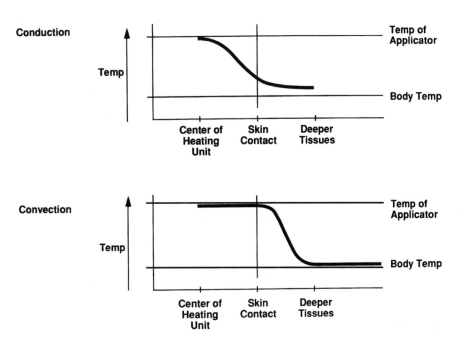

FIGURE 2.2   *Temperature gradients for conductive and convective heating. In convection, the temperature of the surface of the skin is the same as that of the rest of the heating element. This creates a more effective heating of the tissues.*

Conversion

This type of heating involves the conversion of one type of energy, usually sound waves, into thermal energy.

Superficial Heat Modalities

When prescribing heating modalities, a fundamental knowledge of the forms of heat transfer, as well as depth of penetration, is needed. Heating modalities are generally prescribed based on their ability to heat the body tissues either superficially or more deeply (see Table 2.2).

Superficial heating agents cause the greatest temperature rise to occur at the surface of the skin. The warming effect rapidly drops off, and is generally not appreciable deeper than 3–5 mm below the surface level of the skin. Deeper heating with such modalities is not practical because the temperature of the surface would have to be so high that it would burn the skin.

Superficial heat causes a reflex increase in blood flow to the skin and muscles below the heat, as well as an increase in blood flow in the skin of the limb distal to the site of the heating. In conditions of painful muscle splinting, such as acute neck or back strain, the superficial heat may provide significant relief of pain.

Superficial heat also causes a reflex generalized sedation and relaxation and a mild increase in blood flow to the contralateral limb in an area corresponding to the body part being heated. If applied over the abdomen, it decreases gastric acid production, gastrointestinal motility, and uterine menstrual cramping.

The main contraindication to using superficial heat is the risk of thermal burns (Figure 2.3). Electric heating pads and blankets may actually become hotter over the course of 30–60 minutes. This, coupled with decreased pain perception because of the heat, increases the risk of burns. When used chronically, heat treatment may cause a discoloration of the skin called *erythema ab igne*. Because superficial heat increases the metabolic rate and oxygen requirements of the tissues being warmed, it should not be applied in patients with ischemic ulcers or arterial insufficiency. Table 2.3 lists the characteristics of a number of different superficial heating devices.

Deep Heating

In conditions such as tendonitis, bursitis, and myofascial pain,[6] heat is needed at a deeper level than is possible with the superficial heating agents. Deep heat can be used for hard-to-reach anatomic regions (ex facet joints) and some of the larger joints of the body. It can help loosen contractures from tight joint capsules. There are three types of deep heating modalities, but only one, ultrasound, will be discussed here, due to the relative obscurity of the other two.

Ultrasound

Ultrasound was first developed for sonar in World War II, and has been used therapeutically for the past 50 years. Ultrasound machines create sound

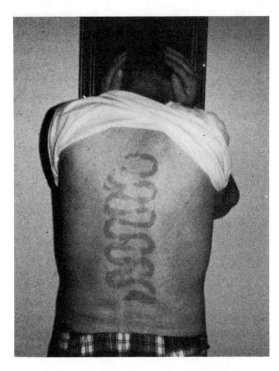

FIGURE 2.3   *Superficial burn caused in a patient who fell asleep on a heating pad.*

waves that are transmitted through the skin and deep into the tissues, down to the bone. The waves have a frequency of 0.8–1.0 MHz and cause the tissues to vibrate rapidly so that they generate heat. This effect is most evident at tissue interfaces—mainly muscle-bone, but also at fat-muscle, skin-fat, and applicator-skin.

To be effective, the ultrasound applicator must be pressed firmly to the skin. A coupling agent, such as ultrasound gel or degassed water, is placed between the applicator and the skin. This gel reduces the contrast in material at the surface of the skin and allows heat to travel deeper. When the ultrasound waves hit bone they heat the surface of the bone and reflect back to the muscle.[7] This creates the maximal heating effect right next to the bone, where joint capsules are often tight. At clinically used intensities ultrasound cannot pass through bone.

There are two techniques of ultrasound application, stroking and stationary. In the stationary technique, the applicator is not moved. This technique is usually discouraged because small variations in the ultrasound energy can create local hot spots, which can burn the deep tissues. The stroking technique does not allow hot spots to form. The stroking technique should be confined to a relatively small area so that the tissues do not cool down between passes.

Ultrasound—especially when used as a stationary technique—can cause "cavitation" of gasses. This occurs when gasses come out of solution and actually form small bubbles. These bubbles can cause tissue damage and are more likely to occur over fluid-filled organs.

TABLE 2.3   Common superficial heating modalities

Hot water bottle
  Simple and easy to use
  Loses its warming effect rapidly
Electric heating pad/blanket
  Relatively constant heating source
  Actually gets hotter over 30–60 minutes
Hydrocollator packs
  Silicate gel holds large amount of water
  Release heat slowly over the course of 20–30 minutes
  Applied over layers of towels to prevent burns
Paraffin bath
  Warmed liquid: wax mixed with mineral oil
  Usually used in heating distal extremities
  Can be applied directly to skin because of low specific heat
  Can be applied by repeated dipping (like candle dipping), immersion, or painting
    liquid onto skin with a brush
Whirlpool baths/Hubbard tanks
  Isolated body part or whole body may receive treatment
  Useful in patients with open sores and burns—but tank must be drained, cleaned,
    and disinfected after use
  Space consuming
  Form of heating by convection
  Limb being treated is in a dependent position, which may promote edema
  Warming of large part of body may raise core body temperature
Fluidotherapy
  Dry heating modality that transfers heat via convection in a cabinet filled with finely
    divided cellulose particles or glass beads. Heated air is circulated through the parti-
    cles to create a mixture that behaves as a "fluid."
  Particles can be sterilized by heat.
  Cabinet may have portals to allow treatment by a therapist.
  Patient may exercise (i.e., small ball) while receiving treatment.

Ultrasound is usually prescribed at a dosage of 0.5–4.0 W/cm^2 (2.5 W/cm^2 aver-age), with the lower dose being used over small joints with the stationary or stroking technique. Generally, 2.5 W/cm^2 is safe for most forms of tendonitis or contracture. The higher dose is rarely used except in deep structures such as the hip joint or in obese patients, and is always performed with the stroking tech-nique. Treatment is for 5–10 minutes once or twice a day, followed by stretching. It is usually done for 5–10 days. When a large joint is treated it must be heated from multiple directions, because bone blocks the passage of the waves.

One advantage of ultrasound over the other deep heating modalities is that it can be applied to limbs with metallic implants, as long as these implants are not secured with cement. It can also be applied to a limb immersed in a bucket of degassed water; for example, to heat the small joints of the hand.

Phonophoresis

Some clinicians prescribe a variant of ultrasound called *phonophoresis*. This (in theory) uses ultrasound to facilitate movement of surface creams or solutions into the tissues. Medications such as steroids or analgesics are commonly used. The problem with phonophoresis is that blood "washes out" the transmitted medications rapidly and that fairly small amounts, if any, of the solutions actually make it through the skin. It is a time-consuming procedure, and with other options such as oral medication or local injection available, there is almost never a good reason to use phonophoresis.

Guidelines for Use of Therapeutic Heat

The effects of and contraindications to using heat therapy are listed in Tables 2.4 and 2.5.[3,4] What follows are some general guidelines to help in using and prescribing heat.

1. When using superficial heating modalities, the patient should not lie on top of the heating source. This is more likely to cause skin burns because the pressure from the body weight masks the pain and prevents capillary blood flow from dissipating the heat.
2. When using heat to help increase flexibility, it should be accompanied and followed by prolonged gentle stretching. When collagen is warmed to a proper temperature (42–45°C) it will slowly elongate with this stretching. Heat alone, without the stretching, does not increase flexibility. As a rule, the highest dose of heat that can be tolerated without producing tissue damage is required to have an effect on flexibility. This technique is mainly used to treat contractures.

TABLE 2.4   Effects of therapeutic heat

Increases collagen extensibility

Decreases joint stiffness

Increases inflammation

Reduces sensation of pain

General relaxation and sedation

Increases local blood flow

Reduces spasticity

Increases core body temperature

TABLE 2.5 Contraindications to the use of heat

Anesthetic area

Obtunded or uncommunicative patient

Impaired vascular flow to the limb

Acute injury

Acutely inflamed joints

Hemorrhagic conditions

Over the pregnant uterus

Over the testes

Over cemented metallic implants (ultrasound)

Over cancers

When used for multiple sessions over a child's epiphyseal growth plate

Over the eyes

Over the spinal column after laminectomy (deep heat)

Over the heart (deep heat)

Over sites of infection (except over some superficial skin infections)

---

3. Heat increases blood flow to the tissues being warmed. This increase in blood flow may help to resolve inflammation in some cases. In others it will aggravate the inflammation. It may be followed by massage to reduce edema.
4. The increase in blood flow will "wash out" the heat. Thus, after a certain amount of time, prolonging the heating session is no longer useful. For most superficial heating sessions 20–30 minutes of heat application is useful. For deep heating, 5–10 minutes per field is used.
5. Let the patient's sensation of warmth guide treatment. For ultrasound, a useful technique to achieve optimal heating is to go right up to the point of pain and then back off slightly on the intensity. For superficial heat, pain to the patient is reduced by putting an extra towel or more distance between the skin and the heat source. This technique is reliable only if the patient is alert, mentally competent, and has normal sensation.
6. Heat can be used as a counterirritant to raise the pain threshold. This may be therapeutic in states of pain, but can also mask a skin burn from the heating source.
7. Heat should not be used in peripheral vascular disease because it increases the metabolic demands of the tissues even more than it increases the blood flow.
8. Vigorous heating generally is not indicated in acute injury or in inflamed joints because it may worsen the inflammation.
9. When possible, heat should be avoided in dependent limbs. The dependent (hanging down) position may generate edema worsened by heat application.

Cryotherapy

Cryotherapy, or cold application, in essence removes heat from the body, with a resultant decrease in body tissue temperature. The result is a myriad of influences on the hemodynamic, neuromuscular, and metabolic processes.

Cold therapy is commonly used in musculoskeletal conditions, especially after acute injury. It helps decrease tissue inflammation and swelling. It also helps to decrease pain sensation, either by acting as a counterirritant or by blocking pain transmission directly.

Cold produces a vasoconstriction, which decreases blood flow to the area being treated. Thus the cooling effect is not "washed out" as quickly as with heat, and the effects are more long lasting. When the tissues are cooled enough to cause damage, there is an axonal-reflex mediated vasodilation that increases blood flow to prevent frostbite. This level of cooling should not be approached in a clinical setting.

Cryotherapy is used in the first 1–2 days after injury. It is commonly applied for 20–30 minutes every 1–2 hours as tolerated. It can also be used before or after exercise to decrease inflammation. In states of painful muscle splinting it can reduce pain and relax the muscle. It is also used to treat spasticity. Because of its effect on skin temperature receptors, cold may make spasticity slightly worse when first applied, but as the deeper muscles and muscle spindle are cooled, the spasticity decreases (see Figure 2.1).[3,8]

When cryotherapy is used to cool the muscles, the actual cooling that takes place is primarily related to the length of time that the cooling agent is applied. The cooling does not plateau even up to 30 minutes of cooling. Adipose thickness retards deep cooling.[9]

Table 2.6 lists some commonly used applications of cold therapy.

TABLE 2.6 Common forms of cryotherapy

Immersion/ice pack/ice slush/ice chips

    Simple, easy to use

    Separate ice and skin with a moist towel

    Use with compression and elevation in acute injury to decrease swelling

Ice massage

    Direct stroking application of ice to skin

    Follow with stretching

Vapocoolant spray

    Evaporative cooling

    Follow with stretching for myofascial pain

Cryotherapy-compression unit

    Sleeve, cuff, or bag that alternately pumps cold water or air around limb

    Used after acute injury or surgery

Cold whirlpool

    Commonly used after acute injury

Guidelines for Cryotherapy

Tables 2.7 and 2.8 list the effects of and contraindications to cryotherapy. As a general rule, cold therapy should be used in conjunction with other therapies, such as exercise and stretching. It is often not as well tolerated initially as heat, but once patients get accustomed to it they experience significant relief of pain, splinting, spasticity, and inflammation. Cold is usually applied for 20–30 minutes, 2–3 times a day, or before and after exercise in conditions of tendonitis or overuse. Care must be taken not to cause frostbite with cold application.

Electrical Stimulation

There are two main uses of electrical stimulation as therapeutic modalities for pain. These are transcutaneous electrical nerve stimulation (TENS), and electrical stimulation (ES). Electrical treatment can also be used to help heal nonunions of fractured bones.

TABLE 2.7   Effects of cryotherapy

Decreases pain
Decreases spasticity
Decreases blood flow
Decreases edema
Increases joint stiffness
Decreases joint inflammation
Decreases metabolic activity
Decreases nerve conduction velocity

TABLE 2.8   Contraindications to cryotherapy

Anesthetic areas
Obtunded or unresponsive patient
Cold allergy
Cryoglobulinemia
Raynaud's phenomenon
Paroxysmal cold hemoglobinuria
Prolonged use over superficial nerves
Paramyotonia congenita
Delayed application after burns

Transcutaneous Electrical Nerve Stimulation

TENS units are small battery-powered sources of electrical current used to treat pain. With the attachment of wires and electrodes, the current can be used to superficially stimulate the skin over various parts of the body. This is believed to act as a counterirritant.

TENS units are used to treat the symptom of pain. They do not affect the underlying disease. Which type of TENS to use and where to place the electrodes involves some educated guesswork. In general, for neurogenic or dermatomal pain, the electrodes are placed in the painful skin distribution or over more proximal nerves supplying that skin. They are also sometimes placed over acupuncture points with good results.

TENS units are not for everyone, but in some patients they result in significant pain relief. Patients must be taught to properly apply and adjust them. They should initially be prescribed for a trial period to see whether the particular patients in question will benefit from them.

TENS units are fairly safe; however, they should not be used over the pregnant uterus, over the neck, or over the chest of a patient with a pacemaker. Occasionally the stimulating pads cause superficial skin burns or local skin irritation.

Electrical Stimulation

ES can also be applied directly to muscles to reduce pain or spasticity, or to retard atrophy. Unlike TENS, in which the object is to stimulate the skin, ES causes actual muscle movement. This can improve pain in myofascial pain states or can give prolonged relief of spasticity. In nerve damage that is expected to heal, ES can slow down muscle atrophy so that when the nerve does heal, the muscle will achieve better function and further recovery. Contraindications to use include active hemorrhage, cardiac arrhythmia or pacemaker, phlebitis, and fracture sites in which movement will stress weakened bones.

Iontophoresis

Iontophoresis is another electrical treatment that involves applying an electrical current to the skin to help drive charged particles of various medications, such as corticosteroids, through the skin and into the tissues. Conceptually, it has the same drawback as phonophoresis, in that the medication is washed away as it crosses the subcutaneous blood vessels. It is generally more precise, and easier, to apply medication through injection.

Massage

Therapeutic massage mobilizes the soft tissues, either manually or mechanically. It is believed to have psychological, mechanical, physiologic, and reflexive effects. Potential psychological benefits include sedation, improved relaxation, and a higher pain threshold. Mechanical or physiologic effects include reduction or prevention of venous stasis and edema, mobilization of scar tissue, and improved removal of products of metabolism. Obligate edema, however, cannot be reduced with massage. Additional physiologic effects may include a counter-irritant phenomenon, sensory inhibition or excitation, a reflex increase in muscle tone, and arteriolar constriction or dilation. Massage cannot decrease obesity or increase strength.

Traction

Traction is a stretching force directed along a longitudinal axis. This pull can be performed manually, with weights and a pulley system, or with a motorized device. Newer cervical traction devices use an air bladder placed between the patient's head and shoulders. Inflating the bladder stretches the neck. Traction is generally limited to use in the neck and lumbar spine regions. Its purpose is to provide a separation of the vertebrae, especially posteriorly. It may relieve pain due to compressed spinal nerves. It may also relieve pressure on painful facet joints or relax the neck muscles.

Traction of the cervical and lumbar spine is generally prescribed for individuals with radicular symptoms attributable to nerve root injury, usually due to a herniated disk. X-ray should be considered before ordering traction.

Traction is contraindicated in a number of cases. Relative contraindications include elderly or overly anxious patients. In individuals with respiratory compromise, the use of a chest harness in lumbar traction may create further respiratory distress. Traction is unequivocally contraindicated when either the therapist or patient (if a home cervical traction unit is used) is inexperienced with regard to the proper angle of pull, optimal body position, and appropriate range of traction force. Other contraindications include cervical ligamentous instability (may cause atlantoaxial subluxation and secondary spinal cord injury), existing vertebrobasilar artery disease, signs or symptoms of myelopathy, suspected or known spinal column tumors, significant osteoporosis, infection of the spine or paravertebral soft tissue, and diskitis. Lumbar traction is also contraindicated in pregnant patients. If traction is applied too soon after acute neck or back injury, it may exacerbate rather than alleviate the patient's discomfort (Table 2.9).

TABLE 2.9   Contraindications to traction

Spinal instability
Spinal cord compromise
Vertebrobasilar artery disease
Myelopathy
Osteoporosis
Tumor
Spinal infection
Pregnancy (lumbar traction)
Acute soft tissue injury

Conclusion

The key to successful use of physical modalities is not to expect too much from them. Rarely do they "cure" any problems. Their real benefit comes in allowing the patient to move around more comfortably, feel better, and participate more fully in the rest of the rehabilitation exercise program.

Points of Summary

1. Heat and cold both reduce pain and spasticity, but have opposite effects on inflammation, blood flow, and joint stiffness.
2. Heat can be applied deeply or superficially.
3. Ultrasound is the most commonly used deep heating modality. It can heat down to the surface of the bone.
4. Vapocoolant sprays are useful in myofascial pain syndromes.
5. TENS units block pain, but do not affect the underlying condition.
6. ES may retard muscle atrophy and is used only if the damaged nerve is expected to recover.
7. Iontophoresis and phonophoresis are rarely indicated as methods of applying medications under the surface of the skin.
8. Traction may be useful in cases of radiculopathy; it causes vertebral body separation and intervertebral foraminal enlargement.

References

1. Whitney SL. Physical agents: Heat and cold modalities. In RM Scully, MR Barnes (eds), Physical Therapy. Philadelphia: JB Lippincott, 1989;844–874.
2. On AY, Colakoglu Z, et al. Local heat effect on sympathetic skin responses after pain of electrical stimulus. Arch Phys Med Rehabil 1997;78:1196–1199.
3. Weber DC, Brown AW. Physical agent modalities. In RL Braddom (ed), Physical Medicine and Rehabilitation. Philadelphia: Saunders, 2000;440–458.
4. Lehmann JF, deLateur BJ. Therapeutic Heat. In JF Lehmann (ed), Therapeutic Heat and Cold (4th ed). Baltimore: Williams and Wilkins, 1990.
5. Wells HS. Temperature equalization for the relief of pain. Arch Phys Med Rehabil 1947;28:135–139.
6. Esenyel M, Caglar N, Aldemir T. Treatment of myofascial pain. Am J Phys Med Rehabil 2000;79:48–52.
7. Lin WL, Liauh CT, Chen YY, et al. Theoretical study of temperature elevation at muscle/bone interface during ultrasound hyperthermia. Med Phys 2000;27:1131–1140.
8. Bell KR, Lehmann JF. Effects of cooling on H- and T-reflexes in normal subjects. Arch Phys Med Rehabil 1987;68:490–493.

9. Jutte LS, Merrick MA, Ingersoll CD, Edwards JE. The relationship between intramuscular temperature, skin temperature, and adipose thickness during cryotherapy and rewarming. Arch Phys Med Rehabil 2001;82:845–850.

Suggested Readings

Cameron MH. Physical Agents in Rehabilitation. Philadelphia: Saunders, 1999.

Weber DC, Brown AW. Physical agent modalities. In RL Braddom (ed), Physical Medicine and Rehabilitation. Philadelphia: Saunders, 2000;440–458.

3 Exercise: Principles, Methods, and Prescription

Steven E. Braverman

Exercise is a necessary component of any fitness and conditioning program, whether for rehabilitation, decreasing weight, or increasing general well-being. This chapter summarizes the physiologic response to exercise, describes the several types of exercise used in rehabilitation and conditioning of the musculoskeletal system, and provides a rationale for prescribing particular exercises when rehabilitating musculoskeletal injuries.

Physiologic Response to Exercise

The human body adapts to the demands placed on it. Muscles, bones, and ligaments all gain strength when they are regularly stressed. Similarly, cardiovascular and neural adaptations take place to provide for more efficient energy delivery and improved coordination. The body senses the demands placed on it and, within certain constraints, alters its structure and metabolism on a cellular level to meet those demands. Thus, the body (or its component parts) must be stressed or overloaded beyond its current level of activity or ability in order to adapt and enhance function. This is known as the *overload principle*.

The ability to adapt is somewhat specific. Certain types, durations, intensities, and frequencies of exercise preferentially lead to certain results. Exercises that improve strength may not improve endurance, and vice versa. However, recent research suggests that although specificity is important, exercise types may not be as mutually exclusive in achieving specific results as was once believed.[1-3] One should think of specificity as a continuum in which specific exercise types maximally improve some tasks with less improvement for other tasks.

Strengthening Exercise

Strength gains from exercise stem from two components: the extent and synchrony of motor unit recruitment and muscle hypertrophy. In the initial stages of strengthening (3–6 weeks), neural factors account for most of the increase in force capability.[4] Simply put, subjects learn to activate their muscles more completely and efficiently.

As repetitive overloads are imposed on the muscles they develop hypertrophy, which leads to even greater strength gains. Hypertrophy is an increase in the size of the muscle fibers along with an increase in cellular components and enzyme activity. An increase in the actual number of muscle fibers, termed *hyperplasia*, has been documented by some researchers, but remains controversial.[5]

Both type I (slow twitch) and type II (fast twitch) muscle fibers develop hypertrophy with strengthening exercise, but type II fibers exhibit a greater degree of change.

Endurance Exercise

Fuel Use

The immediate source of energy at the initiation of exercise is adenosine triphosphate (ATP) (see Figure 3.1). Primary ATP stores in the muscle are used within 3–4 seconds. Other local sources of ATP, creatinine phosphate and adenosine diphosphate, are then converted to ATP. These sources are depleted within approximately 20 seconds of maximal exercise. By 20–30 seconds, carbohydrate stores (glycogen) are broken down into ATP and by-products through anaerobic glycolysis. This energy supply peaks at 40–50 seconds and then declines.

For high-intensity activity to continue, aerobic (oxidative) processes must then take over. By-products of the glycolytic pathway just described are routed to the mitochondria and produce ATP through the Krebs cycle. This aerobic metabolism takes a minimum of 2–3 minutes to reach its maximum level of energy production. Later on, triglycerides (fats) and, to a smaller extent, proteins are also broken down.

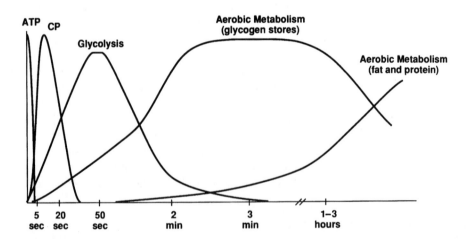

FIGURE 3.1   *Sources of energy during muscle contraction. (ATP = adenosine triphosphate; CP = creatine phosphate.)*

Regular endurance exercise increases the number of mitochondria and mitochondrial enzymes in the muscle fibers, thus raising the efficiency of oxidative metabolism. Utilization of fat is enhanced and postpones glycogen depletion in prolonged exercise.

When energy requirements surpass the availability of oxygen, the by-products of glycolysis can no longer be shunted into the oxidative pathways, and anaerobic energy production once again becomes important. However, this mode of energy production cannot be sustained for long. By-products such as lactate accumulate and herald the onset of this "anaerobic threshold." Regular aerobic exercise raises the level of exertion at which this threshold is reached (primarily through the cardiovascular adaptations described next).[6]

Cardiovascular and Respiratory Response

During exercise the cardiovascular system must supply oxygen to and remove metabolic waste and heat from the active muscles.

The rate of total body consumption of oxygen at peak exercise ($\dot{V}O_2$max) is a good correlate of work capacity. It is a measure of the maximal amount of oxygen that the body can possibly consume and therefore gives an indication of one's maximal aerobic potential. It is limited by the amount of blood the heart can pump (cardiac output) and by the ability of the body to extract oxygen from this blood. Cardiac output (CO) is the product of the heart rate (HR) and the stroke volume (SV). During exercise, HR increases, CO increases, and venous compliance decreases. Blood flow to the muscles is enhanced. The active muscles in turn help to push blood back to the heart, which increases SV and CO even further. Vasoconstriction of blood vessels feeding the internal organs also helps to shunt blood to the active muscles.

Over time and with regular exercise, SV may be improved by more efficient cardiac contractility, enhanced ejection fraction, and most important, by increased end diastolic volume of the heart. Myocardial hypertrophy is variable and usually global, with little change in relative wall thickness versus end diastolic volume. Enhanced parasympathetic tone at rest results in a resting bradycardia. The increased CO and peripheral extraction of oxygen allow for a smaller rise in HR with submaximal exercise. Maximal HR is not changed by endurance exercise. Table 3.1 shows some of the physiologic adaptations to endurance exercise training.

TABLE 3.1 Adaptations to endurance exercise training at rest and at maximal exercise

	Rest	Maximal exercise
Oxygen uptake	No change	Increased
Heart rate	Decreased	No change
Stroke volume	Increased	Increased
Cardiac output	No change	Increased
Ventilation	No change	Increased
Muscle blood flow	No change	Increased
Blood pressure	Decreased	No change

Flexibility

Flexibility is essential to allow for the greatest efficiency of the musculoskeletal system. It is a measure of the degree of normal motion of a joint and is limited by the extensibility of the periarticular tissues. It must be differentiated from joint laxity, which is due to a failure of the joint-supporting structures and implies a degree of abnormal motion of the joint.

Connective Tissue

Increased flexibility results primarily from stretching the connective tissues within and around the muscle and tendon rather than the contractile elements of muscle. Connective tissues are composed fundamentally of collagen enmeshed in a ground substance made of glycosaminoglycans.

Connective tissues progressively shorten when not opposed by a stretching force and elongate when challenged with a constant stress. Stretching occurs when there is a linear deformation of the fibers that leads to an increase in length. There are two types of elongation. Elastic stretch occurs when the elongation produced by loading is followed by a recovery to resting length when the load is removed. Plastic stretch or creep is when the elongation is maintained after removing the load.

Plastic elongation is the type necessary to improve the flexibility of connective tissue. It is maximized by applying a prolonged static stretch with the tissues warmed to 42–45°C.[7]

Neural Factors

Neural factors play a role in muscle relaxation and flexibility. Muscle spindles are muscle stretch receptors that respond to the rate of muscle length change and absolute length change by reflex contraction of the muscle. Golgi tendon organs, via the spinal cord, cause relaxation of the agonist muscles and contraction of the antagonist to enhance the ability to stretch. Prolonged stretching enhances Golgi tendon organ response and inhibits muscle spindle response to increase flexibility.[8]

Exercise Methods

The theoretical basis for exercise has led to several methods to accomplish improvements in strength, flexibility, general conditioning, and endurance (Table 3.2). Each method may be appropriate in a specific setting, based on the goals of the exercise program.

Any exercise prescription is founded on four variables, which can be manipulated: mode, intensity, frequency, and duration. Mode is the type of exercise to be undertaken. Intensity is the percent of the individual's maximum capacity, whether measured in weight lifted, percent $\dot{V}O_2$max, or percent maximum HR achieved. Frequency refers to the number of workouts per unit of time (usually per week), and duration is the length of each workout. General guidelines for prescribing an exercise program are included in Table 3.3.

TABLE 3.2 Types of exercise training

Strength
  Isometric
  Isotonic
     Concentric
     Eccentric
  Isokinetic
     Concentric
     Eccentric
  Plyometric
Endurance
Flexibility
  Static
  Passive
  Proprioceptive neuromuscular facilitation
Rehabilitation protocols and exercise regimens
  Proprioception and coordination
  Closed kinetic chain
Activity specific

TABLE 3.3 Guidelines for prescribing an exercise program

The needs, goals, and limitations of the individual must be addressed and defined before prescribing exercise.

The patient's introduction to exercise training should be at a low to moderate intensity with slow to moderate progression to allow gradual adaptation.

Adequate medical information, including medical history, physical examination, and, when appropriate, laboratory and radiographic tests, should be obtained before embarking on a rigorous exercise program. This allows for the prescription of a safe and effective program.

Realistic long- and short-term goals should be set.

The individual should be educated in the principles of exercise, including the prescription and methods of monitoring and recording progress.

Progress should be evaluated with timely follow-up visits.

When possible, exercise should approximate the specific movements or activities being trained for.

The exercise program should allow time for warm up and cool down to prevent injuries.

Strengthening Exercises

Techniques for building muscle strength employ high resistance loads against which a muscle must work. Resistance to motion can be applied manually by a therapist, by using weights, or through various types of equipment. Strengthening exercises take one of three forms: isometric, isotonic, or isokinetic. They can be varied in velocity of movement or contraction type (concentric versus eccentric). A *concentric contraction* is a shortening contraction, as when lifting a weight. An *eccentric contraction* is a lengthening contraction, as when lowering a weight. Positioned between these two are *isometric contractions*, which involve neither shortening nor lengthening of a muscle, such as when holding a suitcase or pushing against a wall. Eccentric contractions have the potential to generate a greater muscle tension than do concentric contractions. This may seem counterintuitive at first, but actually makes sense; we can lower a heavier weight than we can lift. We can lift a heavier weight more slowly than a lighter weight.

Clinically this suggests that eccentric contraction strength is greater than concentric contraction strength, but eccentric exercises carry a higher risk of injury.[9] Postexercise muscle soreness and damage to type II muscle fibers is most prevalent with eccentric exercises. Many daily activities use eccentric contractions.

Isometric Exercises

An isometric contraction is a muscle contraction that does not produce movement of the joint. This exercise may be performed by exertion against an immovable object or by holding an object in a static position. Isometric contractions can generate a large amount of force, and daily isometric exercise at 50% of maximal strength may retard disuse atrophy.[10]

One drawback to isometric exercise is that strength gains are made primarily at the joint angle at which the muscle is exercised, with little transference of strength to other activities. In addition, these exercises cause a rise in blood pressure and may therefore be contraindicated in persons with cardiac disease. However, the lack of joint motion makes isometric exercises useful for maintaining strength and muscle mass in the immobilized limb and when joint motion is painful or otherwise contraindicated (e.g., acute inflammatory phase of rheumatoid arthritis).

Isotonic Exercises

Isotonic exercises involve moving a constant load through a full range of motion with or without changing the velocity of movement. Lighter weights can be lifted through more repetitions than heavier weights. Lifting heavy weights is generally considered to be a strengthening exercise, whereas lifting lesser loads (or performing other activities that require relatively little strength) is considered endurance exercise.

DeLorme is credited with establishing resistive exercises as a rehabilitative tool to increase strength.[11] His program involved the use of progressive resistance exercises with increasing loads. Each individual determined the maximal weight he could lift 10 times with each muscle group to be strengthened. This was called the *10 repetition maximum* (10RM). Subjects would then perform three sets of 10 repetitions daily at 50%, 75%, and 100% of the 10RM with 2 minutes of rest between sets. Each week a new 10RM would be determined. The drawbacks to this exercise included difficulty in completing the final set of exercises due to fatigue and the fact that full motor unit recruitment was only accomplished during the last set.

The Oxford technique[12] reversed the DeLorme regimen by ordering the exercise sets with 100% 10RM first, followed by 75% and then 50%. With this regimen, fatigue caused by the 100% 10RM set is offset by lower loads on the second and third sets.

One problem with isotonic exercise is that maximal muscle torque varies with the length of the muscle. The muscle can contract at its maximum capacity at only one point in the full range of motion, a point slightly longer than resting length. However, lifting a weight through a full range of motion requires that the muscle be able to lift it even at its weakest point. Thus, true isotonic exercise is inefficient, because it does not cause muscle overload throughout the whole contraction. The use of cams and pulleys, as in Nautilus exercise equipment, attempts to circumvent this problem by varying the resistance of the load to match the average torque curve for specific muscle groups. The advantages of isotonic training are its effectiveness and its universal availability.

Isokinetic Exercises

Isokinetic exercises employ special machines with lever arms that rotate around fixed axes. The person pushes or pulls the lever arm through a set range of motion at a preset speed. The speed remains constant, no matter how hard the subject pushes. By maintaining the speed (velocity), the person can generate maximal force (torque) at all angles of the range. The chosen velocity of concentric isokinetic exercise may be important in strengthening muscles. Training at slow velocities generates the greatest torque, and strength gains are related to the maximal torque generated during training.[13] However, it must be stressed that activity- or sport-specific training may require different training velocities than those designed just to build strength. Activities involving fast musculoskeletal movements may require training at fast velocities. Training at slower velocities will lead to relatively larger strength gains; however, these may not be completely transferable to faster activities.[1]

The biggest drawback to isokinetic exercise is the reliance on special equipment. These machines may be unavailable to the general public. The newer isokinetic machines allow training with eccentric as well as concentric resistance.

Plyometric Exercises

Plyometric exercises are designed to increase power by linking sheer strength with speed of movement to produce an explosive-reactive movement.[14] These exercises train the neuromuscular system to react quickly and forcefully by applying a quick stretch just before contracting the muscle. Plyometrics are used primarily by the athlete to train in specific activities required of a sport (e.g., football linemen). Other individuals whose jobs may require these explosive types of movements may also benefit from this type of training.

These high intensity bouncing/ballistic type drills are believed to use the muscle stretch reflex to augment normal muscle contraction to produce an explosive reaction (although possibly it is just the eccentric training that is helping to increase strength). The force of the concentric contraction is enhanced by the immediately preceding rapid eccentric contraction. The ability to rapidly switch from an eccentric to a concentric contraction determines the power. Squat jumps, drop push-ups, catch and throws, and hops are examples of plyometrics. The action should try to duplicate any rapid movement with an intensity that is equal to or greater than that which is normally occurring.

Obviously, these rapid eccentric and concentric contractions may cause injury if the individual does not have adequate flexibility and agility. These exercises are only used after complete healing of any injury and after proper warm-up and flexibility exercises.

Endurance Exercises

Endurance exercises may cause selective hypertrophy of type I muscle fibers while increasing the oxidative capacity of some type II fibers. For cardiovascular fitness, the American College of Sports Medicine recommends aerobic exercise using large muscle groups that causes an elevation of training heart rate to 60–90% of the maximum HR, or that reaches 50–85% of $\dot{V}O_2max$, for 20–60 minutes 3–5 times per week.[15] Training heart rate is calculated by taking 60–90% of predicted maximum heart rate, which is approximately 220 minus age in years (Figure 3.2). Treadmill running and walking are the most effective indoor aerobic training methods to increase $\dot{V}O_2max$, followed by rowing, stair stepping, and cycling.[16]

When starting an endurance training program one should start with low-intensity sessions to allow the exercise novice to maintain an appropriate training HR for the minimal length of time required to cause cardiovascular adaptation. Such a program results in improved cardiovascular fitness, aids in weight control, and improves the person's sense of well-being. Regular aerobic exercise is also an important adjunct to the treatment of myofascial pain and chronic pain states.

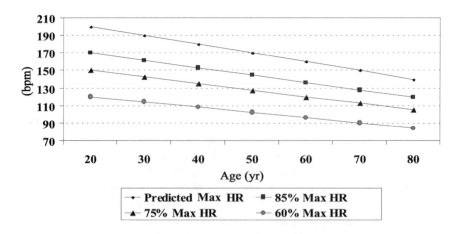

FIGURE 3.2   *Recommended heart rate (HR) based on age and training intensity.*

Flexibility Training

A program to improve flexibility can be beneficial in a number of ways. It can lessen the likelihood of injury, minimize postexercise soreness, reduce contractures, decrease joint pain, and alleviate myofascial pain. Techniques for stretching include ballistic stretching, static stretching, passive stretching, and proprioceptive neuromuscular facilitation.

Ballistic stretching involves repeated, rapid, forceful stretching maneuvers such as bouncing or twisting. This technique is no longer recommended for routine stretching due to the high risk of injury caused by the rapid generation of force. The rapid movement creates a muscle stretch reflex response, which actually makes it harder to achieve tissue lengthening. Athletes with good flexibility may use this technique after proper warm up as part of plyometric exercises.

In static stretching, the body part is positioned to provide a gradual stretch over a duration of at least 15 seconds. The stretch is usually repeated several times. It is the easiest stretch to perform and is widely used for pre-exercise stretching (after a warm up). It also helps reduce muscular soreness following exercise. The best results are obtained when stretching is combined with an increase in tissue temperature into the therapeutic range (42–45°C, 104–115°F). This may be accomplished by using heating modalities or warm-up exercises.[8]

Passive stretching is performed by a partner applying stretch to a relaxed muscle or extremity. Trainers and physical therapists commonly apply this method. Expertise and good communication between partners are essential to prevent injury from overstretching.

Proprioceptive neuromuscular facilitation techniques were described by Knott and Voss.[17] They take advantage of the (theoretical) neural factors described earlier. For example, the hamstring muscles may be stretched to their limit. Then, while maintaining the stretch, they are contracted isometrically against resistance for 5 seconds, followed again by slow duration passive or static stretching. The isometric contraction may relax the muscle by affecting the neural elements, or it may help stretch the fascia and tendons within the muscle. Partners are often used for this technique. Vibration applied to the limb during stretching may increase effectiveness through similar neural pathways.[18]

When stretching to correct connective tissue contractures, temperature elevation should be accomplished through heating modalities. The choice of modality depends on the depth of the tissue to be heated. Deep joint capsules with surrounding tendons, such as the hip or shoulder, require ultrasound diathermy. More superficial tissues such as the finger flexors or Achilles tendon are adequately heated by superficial modalities such as moist heat. Concomitant, gentle, prolonged stretching should be applied across the joint once elevated temperatures are attained. Passive or static stretch is used depending on partner availability and the ability of the individual to participate in therapy.

When improving or maintaining flexibility in uninjured individuals, elevated tissue temperatures are achieved during the exercise warm-up period. Static stretching is done after the warm up. Pre-activity stretching without warm up is of dubious benefit and may lead to injury. Holding the stretch until the muscle cools may help to maintain length deformation changes.

Rehabilitation Protocols and Exercise Regimens

When it comes to the rehabilitation of musculoskeletal injuries or advanced training for sports activities, the exercise methods listed previously are rarely used exclusively from one another. Rather, they are combined into various exercise protocols or regimens consisting of a combination of strength training, endurance training, and flexibility training that include some additional specialized techniques, which are described in the section Activity-Specific Training. Rehabilitation exercise protocols are designed with specific injuries in mind and often call for a daily or weekly schedule of progressive exercises.

Many musculoskeletal injuries result in impaired joint position sense, called *proprioception*. This may be a common factor in re-injury, even after the static integrity of the muscles and ligaments has been restored. Proprioception is trainable through exercises that target joint stability and movement recognition. Exercises are most commonly used for ankle, knee, and back injuries. An example of an ankle proprioception exercise consists of using a balance board for standing. The various ankle positions activate the neuromuscular reflex arcs to retrain the position sense.[19] Coordination exercises, such as running in place, running backwards, running in figure-of-eight patterns, running stairs, or various hand-motion or ball-catching exercises, also help to improve proprioception.

Another commonly used group of exercises are closed kinetic chain exercises. A closed kinetic chain condition occurs when the arm or leg is fixed in place at both ends, with the feet or hands meeting enough resistance to prohibit or restrain their free motion.

Biomechanically, these techniques place little or no translation, shear, or distraction loads on the damaged tissues, and thus minimize injury.[20] In closed kinetic chain exercises single muscles are rarely isolated and often work in patterns requiring less tension than during open kinetic chain exercises. A wall squat is an example of a closed kinetic chain exercise for the knee. The foot and the back are fixed in place. Knee extension is aided by hamstring and gastrocnemius contraction in this closed system. In an open kinetic chain exercise, such as leg extensions with ankle weights, the distal limb is not fixed in place. This results in less stabilization and coordination by the hamstrings and gastrocnemius.

Activity-Specific Training

Although the exercises described thus far offer a great base on which to build, they cannot surpass activity-specific training to develop proper technique. In sports or work, the final exercises need to at least resemble the activity for which one is training. If the activity is complex, it can be broken down and practiced in component parts that are easier to master. All types of exercise; for strengthening, endurance, flexibility, proprioception, coordination, and activity-specific training; address specific deficits that may have occurred from disease of injury to the musculoskeletal system. Commonly, all of these exercises must be integrated into a rational, comprehensive, and well-managed conservative rehabilitation program.

Points of Summary

1. All exercise follows the overload principle of performing an activity that stresses the body beyond its baseline, leading to adaptation and enhanced function.
2. Strength, endurance, and flexibility may all be improved with specific exercises.
3. Specificity of exercise is important. The exercise should simulate the activity being trained for.
4. Early strength gains are due to neural factors; later, hypertrophy takes place.
5. Eccentric exercise can generate greater muscle tension, and has a greater potential for injury, than concentric exercise.
6. Plyometric exercises use stretching followed by contraction to enhance the contraction.
7. Proprioception is often impaired after injury and should be retrained.
8. Closed kinetic chain exercises cause less stress on the joints than open kinetic chain exercises.
9. All exercise prescriptions should include the mode, intensity, frequency, and duration of each exercise, as well as precautions.
10. Close monitoring is essential to prevent injury and to assure safe progression of training.
11. Exercise should be used in concert with other therapeutic interventions such as medications and modalities for a comprehensive integrated rehabilitation program.

References

1. Delecluse C. Influence of strength training on sprint running performance. Current findings and implications for training. Sports Med 1997;24:147–156.
2. Mayhew TP, Rothstein JM, Finucane SD, et al. Muscular adaptation to concentric and eccentric exercise at equal power levels. Med Sci Sports Exerc 1995;27:868–873.
3. Petersen S, Wessel J, Bagnall K, et al. Influence of concentric resistance training on concentric and eccentric strength. Arch Phys Med Rehabil 1990;71:101–105.
4. Moritani T, DeVries AH. Neural factors versus hypertrophy in the time course of muscle strength gain. Am J Phys Med Rehabil 1979;58:115–130.
5. Antonio J, Gonyea WJ. Skeletal muscle fiber hyperplasia. Med Sci Sports Exerc 1993;256:1333–1345.

6. Pierce EFA, Weltman A, Seip RL, et al. Effects of training specificity on the lactate threshold and O$_2$ peak. Int J Sports Med 1990;11:267–272.
7. Taylor DC, Dalton JD, Seaber AV, et al. Viscoelastic properties of muscle-tendon units: the biomechanical effects of stretching. Am J Sports Med 1990;18:300–309.
8. Krivickas L. Training flexibility. In WR Frontera, DM Dawson, DM Slovik (eds), Exercise in Rehabilitation Medicine. Champaign, IL: Human Kinetics, 1999.
9. Ploutz-Snyder LL, Tesch PA, Dudley GA. Increased vulnerability to eccentric-induced dysfunctional muscle injury after concentric training. Arch Phys Med Rehabil 1998;79:58–61.
10. Muller EA. Influence of training and of inactivity on muscle strength. Arch Phys Med Rehabil 1970;51:449–462.
11. DeLorme TL, Watkins AL. Techniques of progressive resistance exercise. Arch Phys Med Rehabil 1948;29:263–273.
12. Zinovieff AM. Heavy resistive exercise. The Oxford technique. Br J Phys Med 1951;14:6.
13. Esselman PC, DeLateur BJ, Alquist AD, et al. Torque development in isokinetic training. Arch Phys Med Rehabil 1991;72:723–728.
14. Fleck SJ, Kraemer WJ (eds). Designing Resistance Training Programs (2nd ed). Champaign, IL: Human Kinetics, 1997.
15. American College of Sports Medicine. Guidelines for Exercise Testing and Prescription (6th ed). Philadelphia: Lea and Febiger, 2000.
16. Zeni A, Hoffman M, Clifford P. Energy expenditure with indoor exercise machines. JAMA 1996;275:1426.
17. Knott M, Voss DE. Proprioceptive Neuromuscular Facilitation. New York: Harper & Row, 1968.
18. Issurin VB, Lieberman DG, Tenenbaum G. Effect of vibratory stimulation training on maximal force and flexibility. J Sports Sci 1994;12:561–566.
19. Laskowski ED, Newcomer-Aney K, Smith J. Proprioception. Phys Med Rehabil Clin N Am 2000;11:347–358.
20. Kibler WB. Closed kinetic chain rehabilitation for sports injuries. Phys Med Rehabil Clin N Am 2000;11:369–384.

Suggested Readings

American College of Sports Medicine. Guidelines for Exercise Testing and Prescription (6th ed). Philadelphia: Lea and Febiger, 2000.

Fleck SJ, Kraemer WJ (eds). Designing Resistance Training Programs (2nd ed). Champaign, IL: Human Kinetics, 1997.

Frontera WR, Dawson DM, Slivik DM (eds). Exercise in Rehabilitation Medicine. Champaign, IL: Human Kinetics, 1999.

Laskowski ED, Newcomer-Aney K, Smith J. Proprioception. Phys Med Rehabil Clin N Am 2000;11:347–358.

4   Electrodiagnosis, Imaging, and Diagnostic/Therapeutic Injections for the Evaluation and Treatment of Spinal and Musculoskeletal Pain

David R. O'Brien, Jr.

Electrodiagnostic Medicine

Electrodiagnostic medicine is the practice of using electrodiagnostic studies to diagnose abnormalities of the central nervous system or peripheral nervous system. The studies reviewed in this chapter include nerve conduction studies (NCS), electromyography (EMG), somatosensory evoked potentials, and surface electromyography. Other diagnostic tests, such as electroencephalography and electrocardiography, are based on the same principles, but are not relevant to our discussion.

The cell membranes of nerve and muscle tissue are electrically polarized. Depolarization of these cell membranes results in an electrical current. This current can be detected by recording electrodes that are placed on the skin overlying a nerve or muscle or by a needle placed into the muscle tissue (needle EMG). Abnormalities or diseases affecting muscles, peripheral nerves, or the neuromuscular junction (NMJ) are commonly diagnosed and subsequently classified using the tests presented here.

Electromyography and Nerve Conduction Studies

The term *electromyography* specifically refers to needle examination of muscles. However, in everyday practice, it is commonly understood that when patients are referred for EMG testing they are being referred for NCS and EMG examinations. A variant of this type of testing known as *surface EMG* has many diagnostic limitations and is described later in this chapter.

Nerve Conduction Studies

Nerve conduction study basically refers to the study of nerves that comprise the peripheral nervous system (not central nervous system). This commonly involves testing motor nerves and sensory nerves. Normal voluntary muscle contraction begins with stimulation of the anterior horn cells in the spinal cord, resulting in nerve root and subsequent nerve depolarization. The depolarization wave travels down the nerve axon and terminates at the NMJ. The subsequent release of acetylcholine from the nerve ending crosses the NMJ and attaches to its receptors on the muscle end plate. This subsequently leads to muscle depolarization and contraction. A motor unit, by definition, includes a motor neuron (originating in the anterior horn cell of the spinal cord), the NMJ, and the muscle fibers it innervates.

Sensory nerves work in the same way, but the direction is opposite. A stimulus at the nerve ending, such as a pinprick, results in an impulse that travels proximally up the nerve to the spinal cord and subsequently the brain, which perceives this as a sensation. Nerves can be thought of as analogous to telephone wires. The speed of conduction depends on the cell diameter (i.e., size of the wire), amount of myelin (insulation), and body or limb temperature (conduction slows as temperature decreases).

NCS involve stimulating a nerve at some point with an electrical current (shock), which causes the nerve to depolarize at that point. The resulting impulse travels along the nerve and can be detected at a distal site by recording electrodes placed over the nerve or muscle it innervates. The electrical impulse detected by the recording electrodes is converted to a waveform, which is displayed on an oscilloscope or television-like screen. The waveform generated by recording electrodes placed over a sensory nerve is called a *sensory nerve action potential*. If a motor nerve is stimulated, the recording electrodes will pick up the electrical activity generated by depolarization and contraction of the underlying muscle, and the subsequent waveform generated on the EMG machine is referred to as a *compound muscle action potential*. The time it takes for an impulse to travel along the nerve from point of stimulation to the recording electrode can be measured and the nerve conduction velocity can be calculated between the two points along the nerve (Figure 4.1).

The waveforms generated on the EMG equipment have characteristic shapes, amplitudes, and speeds that can be measured and recorded. These results can be compared to databases of "normal" asymptomatic volunteers. The electromyographer establishes an accurate diagnosis by analyzing significant deviations from established normal values. For example, in sensory nerve studies, the amplitude of the sensory nerve action potential is an indirect measure of the amount of axons present within the nerve. If the amplitude of the waveform generated is significantly below normal range, it indirectly indicates axonal loss. If the myelin (insulation) around the nerve becomes significantly disrupted (demyelination) by disease or pressure, the nerve impulse or conduction across that segment is blocked or slowed. These measurements can then be used to diagnose and subsequently classify neuropathies into axonal versus demyelinating, focal versus diffuse. Carpal tunnel syndrome would be an example of a focal neuropathy, whereas a diabetic peripheral polyneuropathy is a diffuse neuropathy.

Sensory NCS are obviously important in the evaluation of patients with sensory complaints. In some cases, abnormal sensory NCS may be the first finding in patients with illnesses as serious as an underlying carcinoma presenting as a paraneoplastic syndrome, or something as simple as an early carpal tunnel

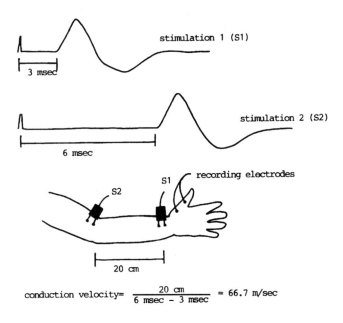

$$\text{conduction velocity} = \frac{20 \text{ cm}}{6 \text{ msec} - 3 \text{ msec}} = 66.7 \text{ m/sec}$$

FIGURE 4.1   *Calculation of nerve conduction velocity.*

syndrome. Motor nerve conduction studies are obviously useful, but should be compared to findings noted on needle EMG in establishing an accurate diagnosis because the results noted on motor NCS rely on the integrity of the muscle stimulated in addition to the nerve.

Needle Electromyography
Needle EMG involves placing a small gauge needle into muscle tissue. These specialized needles have small recording electrodes at their tips that can detect the electrical current generated by depolarization of individual muscle fibers or motor units. This can provide more specific information regarding the health and state of the muscle tissue. Findings on needle EMG can be compared to abnormalities noted on motor NCS. Abnormalities noted on needle EMG testing alert the examining physician as to whether the abnormalities seen on motor NCS are acute or chronic, and help give an indication as to the severity of the neuropathy (i.e., if denervation is occurring). In some myopathic diseases, a patient may present clinically weak despite normal nerve conduction studies. Needle EMG is useful in evaluating this patient population.

After an acute nerve injury, such as a radiculopathy, it usually takes 2–3 weeks to see changes on EMG testing. Therefore, if testing is done within the first 2 weeks, abnormalities (and the diagnosis) may be missed. Abnormalities noted within the first 2 weeks of an injury more likely indicate a pre-existing injury or disease (which is also often helpful information). This factor needs to be recognized when deciding when to order EMG testing. Waiting too long (months to years) is also not a good idea, as findings may change over time. Generally, a 2–6 week window after onset of symptoms is reasonable.

Surface Electromyography

Surface EMG involves placing electrodes on the skin overlying particular muscles. The electrical activity generated by muscle depolarization and contraction can be detected by these electrodes. It can then be transformed into a visual waveform or amplified into some form of audio feedback. This information can be perceived by the investigator or patient, and can be used in biofeedback to help the patient perceive underlying muscle activity. Clinically, this can re-educate a patient who suffers from functional weakness due to a spinal cord or peripheral nerve injury. Biofeedback can also be used to strengthen or re-educate remaining muscle groups. This technique has been used for research purposes in analyzing muscle-firing patterns in gait analysis and lumbar function in patients complaining of back pain. With subsequent computer analysis, one can classify muscle-firing patterns into normal and abnormal patterns by comparing them to those of asymptomatic, "normal" patient populations. Therapies such as strengthening and stabilization exercises can then be focused toward the deficits noted on surface EMG testing in an attempt to restore normal lumbar function. However, this technique is very limited from a diagnostic standpoint and, in the author's experience, has been abused as a substitute for true diagnostic needle EMG and NCS.

Somatosensory Evoked Potentials

Cutaneous stimulation of nerves in the skin results in signals being sent to the spinal cord and subsequently to the somatosensory cortex of the brain. These signals can be detected by recording electrodes placed over the spine and scalp. The waveforms seen, called *somatosensory evoked potentials* (SEPs), can then be analyzed. If there is an abnormality located along this pathway, such as a brain stem lesion, it can be detected by SEP testing. SEP testing can be used to check the integrity of specific cutaneous nerves and to evaluate isolated nerve root function and peripheral sensory conduction velocity. It may detect subclinical disease such as might exist in early multiple sclerosis (however, magnetic resonance imaging [MRI] is probably equally as sensitive and more specific than SEPs in diagnosing multiple sclerosis). Variations of this procedure, such as visual and auditory evoked potential tests, can be used to assess vision and hearing impairments. The rather complex technicalities involved with performing and interpreting SEP tests make SEP testing clinically limited when compared to other tests such as MRI and EMG.

Summary

Electrodiagnostic tests are helpful in the evaluation of patients with a variety of neuromuscular disorders, as noted in Table 4.1. Patients who present with

TABLE 4.1 Conditions commonly diagnosed with the help of electrodiagnosis

Carpal tunnel syndrome
Ulnar neuropathy/cubital tunnel syndrome
Radiculopathy
Peripheral neuropathy
Amyotrophic lateral sclerosis/motor neuron disease
Bell's palsy
Muscular dystrophies
Myasthenia gravis

complaints such as numbness, tingling, limb pain, or weakness are appropriate candidates for electrodiagnostic testing. Patients with radiculopathy, myopathy, NMJ disorder, or neuropathy often present with such complaints. Electrodiagnostic tests are useful in evaluating these patients and can often diagnose the patient's problem accurately, determine whether it is an acute or chronic condition, provide insight into the severity of the illness, and assist in directing appropriate workup and treatment. Patients should be informed that the procedure is somewhat uncomfortable but extremely safe.

Radiographic and Imaging Studies

Plain Radiographs

Radiographs (x-rays) are common and necessary in the evaluation of musculoskeletal injuries. They are relatively inexpensive, safe, and easy to obtain. X-ray beams pass through soft tissues easily while largely being blocked by bone, thereby resulting in excellent views of skeletal structures. X-rays are useful in the evaluation of fractures, arthritic changes, bony tumors, and joints. They can indirectly evaluate certain soft tissues and cartilaginous structures. However, x-rays do have limitations, and the findings noted (or lack thereof) may not necessarily correlate with clinical findings or symptoms. The radiation exposure can also be quite significant and needs to be taken into account, especially if gonadal exposure is possible. For these reasons, and because information obtained from x-rays is often limited and only a precursor to more definitive tests such as MRI, their use should be prudent.

Computed Tomography

An x-ray source can be used to produce a computerized cross sectional image (computed tomography [CT] image) that represents tissues of varied x-ray attenuation. Spatial and contrast resolution depends on the thickness of the slice, the size of the area to be studied, and the scanning matrix, or field of view. High-resolution, multiplanar CT images are produced by acquiring a series of axial images from which computerized-reformatted sagittal and coronal images are then generated. Because it uses x-rays, CT is an excellent test for depicting osseous structures and abnormalities. With the advent of MRI, the use of intravenous contrast with CT is infrequent. However, intrathecal contrast with CT (CT myelogram) can be useful, and in many cases is more sensitive at detecting nerve root impingement or stenosis than MRI. It is also helpful in the evaluation of patients in whom MRI is not practical or not an option due to the presence of instrumentation or pacemakers. CT can be combined with diskography (described later) in evaluating patients with low back pain due to internal disk disruption (Figure 4.2). These annular tears are often undetected by MRI and other imaging studies. CT scans are excellent in evaluating fractures and other osseous lesions, such as tumors. Newer scans can produce three-dimensional reconstructed images that are useful in evaluation of more complex fractures (i.e., cranial) and help guide surgical interventions. Unfortunately, CT does expose the patient to fairly high doses of radiation.

Magnetic Resonance Imaging

In contrast to the x-rays used with CT, MRI images are generated by placing the patient in a static external magnetic field, which is then subjected to repeated bursts of radio waves of a specific radiofrequency (RF). This excites and polarizes hydrogen protons within the body. With termination of the RF, these protons "relax" or release the RF energy they absorbed, which is then detected by receiver coils within the unit. The "relaxation" is then characterized by two independent time constants, T1 and T2. T1 is referred to as longitudinal relaxation time and T2 as transverse relaxation time. T1 and T2 values are intrinsic physical properties of tissue. The MR signal intensity displayed on the images is

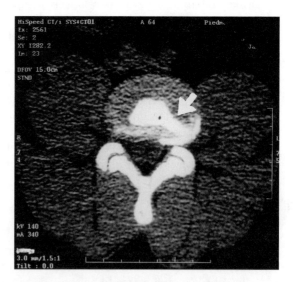

FIGURE 4.2 *Postdiskography computed tomography depicting a left, posterior-lateral radial fissure (arrow) extending into an outer, circumferential annular fissure.*

mainly dependent on T1, T2, and the proton density of the tissue being evaluated. Tissues that are rich in hydrogen (water and fat) are preferentially depicted.

MRI, like CT, can produce various axial, sagittal, or coronal images. MRI is better than CT at evaluating soft tissue such as lumbar disks, muscle, ligaments, and tendons. MRI is also good at evaluating herniated lumbar disks (Figure 4.3), rotator cuff tears, and other soft tissue abnormalities. When combined with intravenous contrast, it can evaluate various neoplastic and infectious abnormalities and differentiate postoperative scar tissue from recurrent disk herniations in patients who have had prior back surgery. MRI combined with arthrography is useful in detecting subtle, intra-articular defects such as labral tears of the shoulder or hip. MRI and radionucleotide bone scans are excellent in identifying cancer in the bony portions of the spine and skeletal structures. MRI is confined to tight spaces, which makes it difficult for patients who are claustrophobic, although many scanners are "open" and therefore better tolerated by patients. Also, MRI cannot be performed in patients who have certain types of heart valves, pacemakers, or other surgically implanted metal.

Diagnostic and Therapeutic Injections

Although x-rays, CT scans, and MRI evaluations can provide good information regarding anatomic defects, it is important to recognize that such defects are not always clinically important. The patient's symptoms may be inappropriately attributed to an abnormality seen on x-ray or other imaging studies. The uses of diagnostic and therapeutic injections often fill the gap in determining the actual etiology of the patient's pain or problem by providing anatomic and

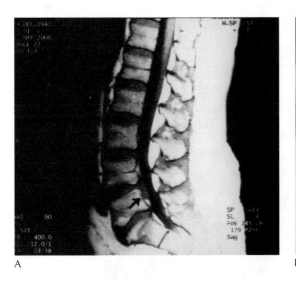
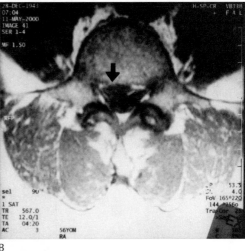

A   B

FIGURE 4.3 *Magnetic resonance imaging of the lumbar spine.* **A.** *Sagittal view demonstrates an L4–5 disk herniation extending along the posterior L4 vertebral body* (arrow). **B.** *Axial view of the same disk herniation* (arrow).

physiological information that imaging studies alone cannot provide. Diagnostic injections are performed under fluoroscopic or occasionally CT guidance, and involve injecting contrast dye and possibly anesthetics into areas of the spine, into a joint, or onto a nerve. Anatomic information may relate to the integrity of a particular joint, as with rotator cuff tears in the shoulder (Figure 4.4), or include whether a spinal nerve root is being compressed, as with a radiculopathy. By injecting anesthetic agents into joints or onto specific nerves, the subsequent elimination of pain (or lack thereof) can provide important information as to the location or etiology of a patient's pain problem (Figure 4.5). Conversely, some injections, such as diskography, are used in an attempt to provoke or reproduce a patient's pain to diagnose the source (Figure 4.6). Examples of diagnostic and therapeutic injection procedures are noted in Table 4.2. In addition to providing diagnostic information about the source of a patient's pain, these procedures, in combination with corticosteroids, can provide substantial therapeutic improvement in the patient's underlying condition, thereby alleviating the need for subsequent surgery or other interventions. This has been demonstrated by studies showing the effectiveness of fluoroscopically administered epidural injections in the nonsurgical treatment of herniated lumbar disks and radiculopathy, resulting in a 70–90% success rate (depending on the study reviewed).[1-4]

Diagnostic and therapeutic injection procedures also can be used to confirm a specific diagnosis, thereby guiding subsequent treatment, rehabilitation, or surgery. For example, an elderly patient who presents with hip and thigh pain and imaging evidence of degenerative arthritis of the hip and spine may have pain referred from either the hip joint or spine (due to nerve root irritation). A diagnostic hip arthrogram or spinal nerve block may clarify exactly where the patient's pain is coming from and thus determine the most appropriate treatment or surgical intervention. Procedures such as sympathetic blocks not only provide diagnostic information as to whether a patient suffers from sympathetically mediated pain, but also help in pain management and rehabilitation (see Chapter 15).

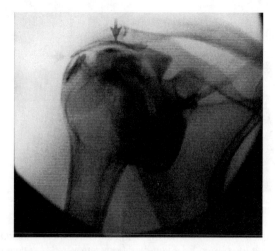

FIGURE 4.4   *Right shoulder arthrogram, 1 minute postexercise. Arrow demonstrates leakage of contrast into the subacromial bursa consistent with a full-thickness tear of the rotator cuff.*

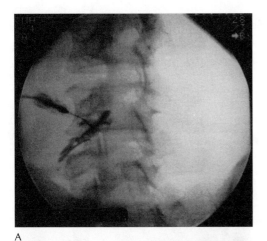

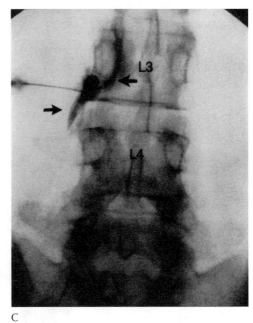

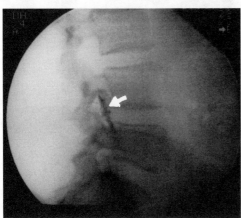

FIGURE 4.5 *A. Oblique view of a selective, left L4 spinal nerve block. **B.** Lateral view of the same left L4 spinal nerve block, arrow indicating the L4 nerve. **C.** Demonstrates a left L3–4 transforaminal epidural injection as noted by contrast tracking along the left L3 nerve root (arrows).*

Arthrography is usually performed and viewed under fluoroscopic guidance. It involves injecting contrast dye into a joint, often with anesthetic (and perhaps corticosteroids). It can help detect joint pathology such as a ruptured ligament, rotator cuff tear, or joint capsule tears (Figures 4.4 and 4.7). Post-arthrography CT or MRI imaging can provide even greater anatomic detail in the evaluation for potential intra-articular pathology.

Patients with chronic low back pain often experience internal disk disruption, resulting in chronic, discogenic pain. Plain x-rays and other imaging studies may not correlate well with the patient's symptoms. Figure 4.6 depicts a diskogram that demonstrates a posterior annular tear. The patient's symptoms were reproduced by the injection, thereby confirming the patient's diagnosis. Prior work up and MRI had been unable to detect this lesion.

Ultrasound

Diagnostic ultrasound uses high-frequency sound waves to form images of internal body structures. It has somewhat limited usefulness in musculoskeletal

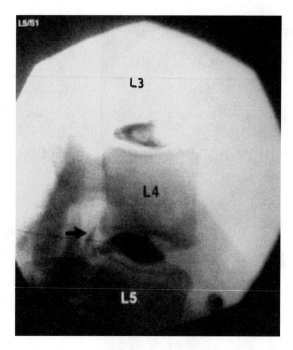

FIGURE 4.6   *An asymptomatic, normal-appearing diskogram at L3–4 and a posterior annular tear seen as extravasation of contrast into the outer, posterior annular wall that reproduced the patient's pain during injection of the L4–5 disk (arrow).*

injuries, but can detect soft tissue abnormalities such as torn ligaments and tendinopathies. Still, it does not appear to be as useful as MRI or CT at this time. One advantage is that it can evaluate functional movements of skeletal tissues and joints in real time. However, this requires an extensive amount of training on the part of the examiner, thereby making this type of evaluation unavailable in most cities.

TABLE 4.2   Examples of diagnostic and therapeutic injections

Interlaminar epidural injection[a]

Transforaminal epidural injection[a]

Caudal epidural injection[a]

Spinal nerve block[a,b]

Sympathetic block[a,b]

Zygapophysial joint injection[a]

Medial branch and dorsal ramus block[b]

Provocative diskography[b]

Sacroiliac joint injection/arthrogram[a,b]

[a]*Indicates procedure can be therapeutic.*
[b]*Indicates procedure can be diagnostic.*

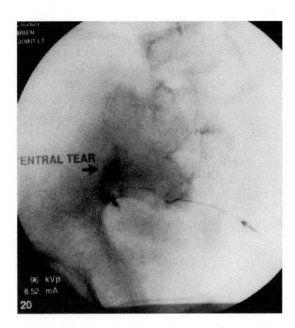

FIGURE 4.7   *Oblique view of a sacroiliac arthrogram showing leakage of contrast material, indicating a ventral tear of the left sacroiliac joint.*

Bone Scan

Radioactive compounds that are preferentially drawn to regions of active bone turnover can be injected into the bloodstream, where they then can then be detected by a scanner. Abnormal concentrations of the radioactive compounds are seen in a variety of disorders and diseases. This can be used to help diagnose stress fractures, osteomyelitis, and, to a limited degree, reflex sympathetic dystrophy. Clinically suspicious findings and abnormalities detected on x-ray films can be compared to bone scan results to help determine whether the injury is acute or old. Bone scans are often helpful in evaluating underlying metastatic disease affecting bone. It should be noted, however, specifically in the evaluation of multiple myeloma, that bone scans can be falsely negative. It is important to remember that although bone scans are very sensitive, they are not specific at detecting osseous injuries and abnormalities.

Bone Densitometry

Osteoporosis, which affects 25 million Americans, is a substantial cause of morbidity and mortality. The National Osteoporosis Foundation (NOF) estimates the annual direct and indirect costs associated with osteoporosis to be $18 billion, with $7 billion related to hip fractures alone in the United States. Osteoporosis is the cause of more than 1.5 million fractures annually, including more than 500,000 vertebral fractures, 300,000 hip fractures, and 250,000 wrist fractures. The NOF estimates that up to half of all women older than age 50 will have an osteoporotic fracture in their lifetimes.[5]

Bone densitometry tests use either sound waves or x-ray beams to determine the density of bones. The tests are safe, painless, and noninvasive. Measurements are often taken of the spine, wrists, or hips. The results, reported as T-scores, are determined by comparing a patient's bone density to that of a young adult. The NOF recommends testing all women older than age 65, as well as those younger than age 65 with positive risk factors (see Chapter 23).[6] Patients with T-scores below −2.0 in the absence of other risk factors, or below −1.5 with positive risk factors, should be considered for treatment. The NOF recommends following Health Care Financing Administration guidelines for repeat bone mineral density testing in response to therapy.[7] At this time, the Health Care Financing Administration covers follow-up bone density measurements every two years, or even more frequently when determined to be medically necessary (such as when monitoring patients on long-term glucocorticoid therapy).[8] The results of bone density testing can be used to assess a patient's risk for an osteoporotic fracture and help in determining appropriate treatment.

Points of Summary

1. NCS and EMG testing can provide objective information in patients with complaints of numbness, tingling, limb pain, or weakness. These tests can help differentiate, classify, and evaluate the severity of radiculopathies, neuropathies, and myopathies.
2. X-rays and CT imaging are useful in the evaluation of osseous injuries.
3. MRI is superior to x-rays and CT imaging in the evaluation of soft tissue injuries such as rotator cuff tears, herniated lumbar disks, and anterior cruciate ligament tears.
4. Diagnostic injections can provide both anatomic and physiological information. These injections are useful in verifying the location and etiology of a patient's pain problem, can help correlate findings on imaging tests to the patients' complaints and examination, and can often provide a therapeutic benefit in treating the underlying problem, thereby eliminating the need for more invasive surgical procedures.

References

1. Riew DK, et al. Can nerve root injections obviate the need for operative treatment of lumbar radicular pain? A prospective, randomized, controlled, double-blinded study. Chicago: 14th Annual Meeting of the North American Spine Society, 1999.
2. Saal JA, Saal JS. Nonoperative treatment of herniated lumbar intervertebral disk with radiculopathy: an outcome study. Spine 1989;14:431–437.
3. Lutz GE, Vad VB, Wiseneski RJ. Fluoroscopic transforaminal lumbar epidural steroids: an outcome study. Arch Phys Med Rehabil 1998;79: 18–22.
4. Maigne J-Y, Rime B, Deligne B. Computed tomographic follow-up study of 48 cases of nonoperatively treated lumbar intervertebral disk herniation. Spine 1992;17:1071–1074.

5. Black DM. Bone density, bone quality, and fracture risk. Toronto, Canada: 22nd Annual Meeting of the American Society for Bone and Mineral Research, 2000.
6. Watts NB. Understanding the Bone Mass Measurement Act. J Clin Densitom 1999;2(3):211.
7. Bone Mass Measurements. Medical Bulletin GR 98-5, 9–11, September/October 1998.
8. Physicians Guide to Prevention and Treatment of Osteoporosis. Belle Meade, NJ: Excerpta Medica Inc., 1998.

Suggested Readings

Helms CA. Fundamentals of Skeletal Radiology. Philadelphia: Saunders, 1995.

Kraft GH. Electromyography: doctor's questions answered. Phys Med Rehabil Clin North Am 1990;1:1–16.

5 Musculoskeletal History and Physical Examination

Ralph M. Buschbacher

The complete musculoskeletal examination is far beyond the scope of this chapter. There are, however, some principles common to examining any body part, and this chapter focuses on such common items. Table 5.1 lists some of the issues that are helpful to include in the general musculoskeletal examination. More specific body parts are covered in Chapters 6–13.

History

A detailed history often suggests the most likely diagnosis and in some conditions is more valuable than any other part of the examination. It should include the obvious questions of what the major and secondary complaints are, how they started, what aggravates or alleviates them, and how much they bother the patient in daily activities.

In addition, the patient should always be asked whether the same or similar symptoms have been present at any time in the past. It is surprising how few patients volunteer this information on their own, even if they have experienced an identical condition in the past.

Patients should be asked about the onset of their problem: Was it due to trauma? Did it start all of a sudden or creep up on them gradually? Have they received any treatment to date (either medical or home remedies)? When possible, open-ended questions such as "When did your pain begin?" are preferred over yes or no inquiries. Also, the questions should be asked in a way that a nonmedical person can understand. If a lot of jargon-filled yes or no questions are rattled off by the examiner, patients may simply nod their heads without really understanding the questions.

Past medical or surgical illness, current and past medications, drug use and abuse, and family history are all important areas to be addressed. The patient's age should be noted, as it may make some problems more likely than others. Occupation should be explored. Many work-related hazards predispose work-

TABLE 5.1   Items that may be of importance in the musculoskeletal examination report*

History
    Current symptoms
    Course of the current problem
    Treatment to date, response to such treatment
    What makes symptoms better or worse?
    Sleep history
    Is there radiating/referred pain?
    Do symptoms spread with coughing/sneezing/straining (i.e., Valsalva-type maneuvers)?
    Are there any associated symptoms?
    Results of tests to date
Past medical history
    Peptic ulcer disease
    Renal disease
    Drug allergies
    Previous injuries, especially to the same area
        What treatment was required? How long was recovery?
    Is patient pregnant?
    Medications—for current and other problems
    Past medical and surgical history
Family history
Social history
    Exercise history
    Work (hobby) history
        Current work status
    Smoking history
Review of systems
    Bowel/bladder
    Fever/chills/night sweats/weight loss
    Numbness/tingling/abnormal sensations
Physical examination
    Non-physiologic response/behavior
    Biomechanics/movement patterns
    Joint stability
    Atrophy
    Side-to-side comparisons
    Waddell signs (see Chapter 14)

This list is not comprehensive, but does include items that may be of special interest and are not commonly included.

ers to one musculoskeletal disorder or another. The same holds true for sports activities or hobbies.

Patients commonly complain of "pain" or "numbness" without adequately defining these terms. One person's weakness may be another's joint instability. The examiner must understand exactly what is meant by the patient.

Sleeping patterns are an often overlooked aspect of a patient's history. Sleep disorders may cause or be caused by musculoskeletal pain conditions. Treating the sleep pattern often will help to restore the patient to health. Similarly, changes in mood and social habits may be associated with pain disorders and should be investigated.

A final point about the history is that it should relate to the patient's function. An elderly sedentary man may be found to have a rotator cuff tear, but if it isn't causing him any pain or dysfunction, it really isn't much of a problem. Finding out what the dysfunction is leads the examiner to the musculoskeletal abnormalities underlying the dysfunction. Once identified and treated, this leads to a more satisfactory outcome than if every non-significant physical finding were to be addressed and the patient's overall function ignored. Of course, it must also be recognized that different body parts interact. A painless rotator cuff weakness, for instance, may lead to painful tennis elbow. Until the shoulder weakness is corrected the elbow pain will not improve.

Physical Examination

Inspection

Inspection of patients is done throughout the examination, from the time they arrive at the office until they leave. It yields information about function, mood, and the reaction to the examination. Specific areas to be assessed are signs of muscle atrophy, skin changes, posture, and scars. Most textbooks recommend observing the patient undressing to get an idea of dressing and undressing function; however, in practice this is rarely done. It is, however, good to observe the patient performing common activities such as standing up and walking.

Palpation

Palpation techniques vary according to the body part being examined. In general, the soft tissues and the bones should be assessed. Joints are checked for effusion, muscles are checked for hematoma or disruption, and tendons and ligaments are palpated to detect signs of partial or complete rupture. Palpating the origins and insertions of muscles and ligaments often helps with diagnoses of sprains and overuse.

Strength Testing

Muscle strength testing is commonly graded on a 1 to 5 scale (Table 5.2). Although this system is useful in some conditions and helps to standardize

TABLE 5.2   Muscle strength grading*

	Grade (number)	Grade (name)
No motion	0	Zero
Palpable muscle twitch with no joint motion	1	Trace
Joint movement normal with gravity eliminated	2	Poor
Joint movement normal against gravity with no other resistance	3	Fair
Joint movement against gravity with some resistance	4	Good
Normal strength	5	Normal

*In addition, each individual grade is sometimes split into three sub-grades; for instance, 4⁻, 4, and 4⁺.

strength testing, it has the drawback of not being very functional. Patients often have a poor understanding of what is being asked of them in isolating the various muscles. Additionally, some muscle groups, such as in the back, are hard to isolate from each other. When possible, strength should be compared in the comparable muscles from side to side. Some allowance for slight differences needs to be made because the dominant side is usually stronger. Allowances also need to be made for the general size and physique of the patient and the examiner. When possible, strength should be tested on both sides simultaneously; it is very difficult for patients to give less than optimal effort on one side while simultaneously trying hard on the other.

Substitution movements are used by patients with specific muscle weakness. For instance, patients with weakness in initiating shoulder abduction may be able to hold the arm up once it is there. They may substitute for a weak supraspinatus by swinging the arm up with the trunk or bending to the side. Such substitutions may hide a more profound weakness and should be eliminated in the examination.

Muscles are reproducibly innervated in most people by the same spinal cord levels (within one or two levels). The nerve fibers travel through a characteristic pattern of peripheral nerves to reach their appointed muscles. Therefore, when several muscles are weak, the site of pathology may sometimes be traced to a specific spinal root or peripheral nerve level. Some of the main muscle groups along with their innervation are listed in Table 5.3. A patient who has weakness of foot dorsiflexion as well as hip abduction is likely to have lumbar level 5 (L5) spinal nerve injury, because these actions share a spinal root but not peripheral nerve innervation. A patient with isolated weakness of foot dorsiflexion is more likely to have peripheral nerve damage, possibly of the deep peroneal nerve. The muscle distribution that belongs to a spinal nerve is called a *myotome.*

Neurologic Examination

Because neurologic conditions often lead to musculoskeletal symptoms, a good neurologic examination is usually necessary. It may include testing of

TABLE 5.3   Myotomal and peripheral nerve innervation of the major muscle groups

	Major cranial or spinal nerve level	Peripheral nerve
Upper extremity		
Shoulder muscles		
Elevators	CN11, C_4, C_5	Spinal accessory nerve, posterior branches of spinal nerves
Protractors	CN11, C_5, C_6, C_7	Long thoracic nerve and pectoral nerves
Retractors	CN11, C_5, C_6, C_7, C_8	Dorsal scapular nerve, spinal accessory nerve, and thoracodorsal nerve
Upward rotators	CN11, C_5, C_6	Long thoracic nerve and spinal accessory nerve
Downward rotators	C_6, C_7, C_8	Thoracodorsal nerve and pectoral nerves
Abductors	C_5, C_6	Axillary and suprascapular nerves
Extensors	C_6, C_7, C_8	Thoracodorsal, axillary, and pectoral nerves
Flexors	C_5, C_6	Axillary, musculocutaneous, and pectoral nerves
Internal rotators	C_5, C_6	Pectoral nerves, thoracodorsal and subscapular nerves
External rotators	C_5, C_6	Axillary and suprascapular nerves
Elbow flexors	C_5, C_6	Musculocutaneous nerve
Elbow extensors	C_7	Radial nerve
Wrist extensors	C_6, C_7	Radial nerve
Wrist flexors	C_7, C_8	Median and ulnar nerves
Finger extensors	C_7	Radial nerve
Finger flexors	C_7, C_8	Median and ulnar nerves
Intrinsic hand muscles	T_1	Ulnar and median (thumb) nerves
Trunk and back		
Abdominal muscles	T_7–T_{12}	Segmental innervation
Back muscles	C_2–L_5	Segmental innervation
Lower extremity		
Hip flexors	T_{12}, L_1, L_2	Lumbosacral plexus
Hip extensors	L_5, S_1, S_2	Inferior gluteal nerve
Hip abductors	L_4, L_5, S_1	Superior gluteal nerve
Hip adductors	L_2–L_4	Obturator nerve
Knee flexors	L_5, S_1	Sciatic nerve
Knee extensors	L_2–L_4	Femoral nerve
Foot dorsiflexors	L_4, L_5	Deep peroneal nerve
Foot plantarflexors	S_1	Tibial nerve
Foot inverters	L_4	Deep peroneal and tibial nerve
Foot everters	L_5, S_1	Superficial peroneal nerve

C = cervical level; CN = cranial nerve; L = lumbar level; S = sacral level; T = thoracic level.

light touch and pinprick sensation, temperature sensation, proprioception, balance and coordination, and deep tendon (muscle stretch) reflexes.

Deep tendon reflexes (muscle stretch reflexes) are graded from 1 to 4 as shown in Table 5.4. They are caused by a stretching of the muscle spindle, usually by a reflex hammer. This sends an impulse to the spinal cord, where it immediately stimulates the motor neuron to send a message for the muscle to contract.

Pain is sometimes felt at sites distant to the site of disorder. For instance, irritation of a spinal nerve by a herniated disk may cause pain down the leg and into the foot. When this follows a dermatomal pattern, it is called *radicular pain*.

Other types of distantly felt pain are referred and radiating pain. Referred pain occurs because nerve cells that are close together in the spinal cord may correspond to widely separate parts of the body. When a pain signal comes in from one part, it often "spills over" to the nerves related to the other part, and the person perceives pain to be coming from a wholly unrelated area. For instance, gall bladder pain may be referred to the shoulder and cardiac pain referred to the left arm. This type of pain is usually due to internal organ problems.

Radiating pain occurs when a proximal musculoskeletal disorder causes pain to spread down the limb. For instance, palpation of tender spots in the neck muscles may cause pain or dysesthesia to be felt down the arm into the fingertips. This type of pain is often confused with radicular or neurogenic pain.

Sensory testing is similar to muscle strength testing in that patches of skin are innervated both by a distinct pattern of spinal nerves and by distinct peripheral nerves. The spinal nerve innervation pattern is called a *dermatome* and is depicted in Figure 5.1. The sensory nerve distributions and dermatomes, however, are not really as clear-cut as depicted in this diagram. There is a lot of overlap among the nerves, which makes localization of any problem difficult.

Joint Examination

Joints should be examined for swelling, erythema, excessive warmth, and range of motion. The range of motion should be compared from left to right body sides and also with active and passive movement. It is often measured with devices called goniometers (Figure 5.2), or in the back with an inclinometer. If a patient has restriction of active but not passive movement, it is likely due to muscle weakness. If both are restricted there may be joint contracture or a bony block. The end point of range should always be assessed when testing range of motion.

TABLE 5.4   Deep tendon reflex grades

0	No response
1+	Low normal
2+	Average normal
3+	Brisker than normal, but not necessarily pathologic
4+	Hyperactive, usually with clonus

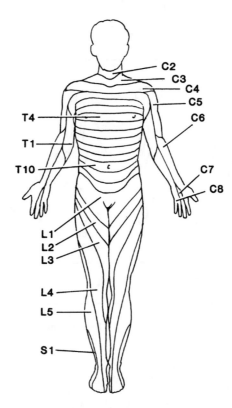

FIGURE 5.1   *Sensory dermatomes.*

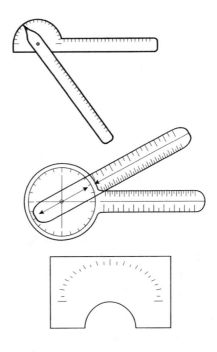

FIGURE 5.2   *Common goniometers.*

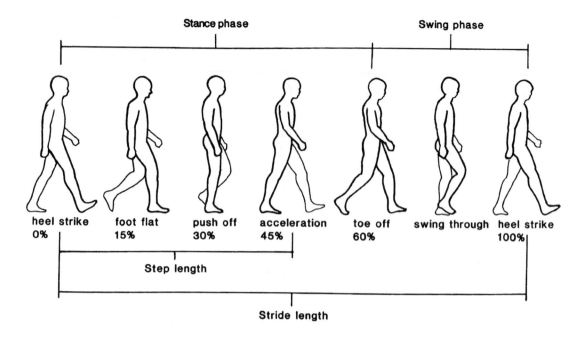

FIGURE 5.3   *The normal gait cycle: Stride length is defined as the distance from one heel strike to the next heel strike on the same foot (the right heel is depicted in this figure). Step length is from heel strike of one foot to heel strike of the other. Ordinarily, the gait cycle is viewed from the perspective of one foot or the other. The cycle consists of 60% stance phase and 40% swing phase. The stance phase is divided into stages by increments of 15% of the total stride as depicted in the figure.*

A hard, rigid end point may be indicative of a bony block. Firm end points are normal, whereas pain on a firm end point may be indicative of a ligamentous sprain. Softer than usual end points are signs of partial ligamentous rupture, and lack of an end point is a sign of a complete ligamentous tear.

Gait

Because gait abnormalities can be manifestations of a large variety of disorders, the normal gait cycle must first be understood. The normal gait pattern is presented in Figure 5.3. As depicted, a full cycle, or stride, goes from heel strike of one foot to the next heel strike of that same foot. Step length is the distance from heel strike of one foot to heel strike of the opposite side. Ordinarily, 60% of the gait cycle is in stance phase, whereas 40% is in swing phase. Approximately 25% of the time both feet are in contact with the ground. The purpose of normal gait is to propel the body's center of mass along a smooth sinusoidal wave to minimize energy consumption. Any deviations from this pattern will increase the energy requirements of ambulation.

Gait must be analyzed by observing the patient from the side, front, and rear (Table 5.5). From the side, the stride length, knee and ankle motions, and foot clearance can be assessed. Common abnormalities seen are a foot drop or back-bending (hyperextension) of the knee, called *genu recurvatum*. The tilt of the pelvis and the ankle are best viewed from the rear. Weakness

TABLE 5.5   Major muscle groups involved in ambulation, the time of the gait cycle they are active in, and the gait abnormalities that occur when they are weak

Muscle groups	Active during	Weakness results in
Hip flexors	Acceleration	Abnormal acceleration and swing (patient compensates by thrusting trunk backward to passively swing the leg)
Hip extensors	Heel strike	Forward lurch of trunk on heel strike (patient compensates by excessive lordosis)
Hip abductors	Stance phase	Trendelenburg gait (see Figure 5.4)
Hip adductors	Heel strike, toe off	Abnormal rotation of leg and pelvis
Knee extensors	Heel strike, acceleration	Knee buckling, especially when walking downhill
Knee flexors	Deceleration, heel strike	Knee snaps out too hard at end of swing, knee buckling at heel strike
Foot dorsiflexors	Swing phase, heel strike	Foot drop, steppage gait, foot slap at heel strike
Foot plantar flexors	Push-off	Short step on unaffected side, poor push-off

of the hip abductors causes the pelvis to drop during stance in what is called an *uncompensated Trendelenburg gait.* In more severe weakness of the abductors, the patient lists to the side of weakness during stance to compensate for excessive pelvic drop in what is called the *compensated Trendelenburg gait* (Figure 5.4). The ankle is assessed for excessive varus or valgus

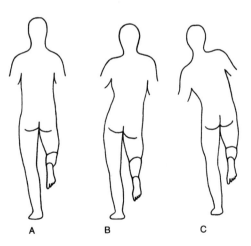

A   B   C

FIGURE 5.4   **A.** *Normal stance allows the opposite hip to drop slightly. This drop is controlled by the hip abductors on the stance side, which keep the pelvis from dropping too much.* **B.** *An uncompensated Trendelenburg gait results when the hip abductors are weak and allow the opposite pelvis to drop.* **C.** *When the hip abductors are even weaker, the person resorts to a compensated Trendelenburg gait. Weight is shifted to the side of the weak abductors to keep the pelvis from dropping excessively.*

position and the foot is checked for excessive pronation. The centers of the heels should normally hit the ground within a side-to-side distance of 5–10 cm (2–4 in.).

Gait should be assessed with shoes both on and off. In addition, shoes should be examined for abnormal wear patterns.

Points of Summary

1. Sleeping patterns are an often overlooked but important part of the history.
2. History taking should concentrate on function.
3. Strength testing is most reliable when comparing the two sides of the body for differences.
4. Radicular pain is due to nerve root irritation and follows a dermatomal pattern.
5. Referred pain is due to "spillover," which occurs when pain from a body organ is transmitted to the spinal cord in the vicinity of other sensory fibers. The body misinterprets the pain signals as coming from another area, such as arm pain during a myocardial infarction.
6. Radiating pain is when stimulation of an area causes pain to be felt distally.

Suggested Readings

Cutter NC, Kevorkian CG. Handbook of Manual Muscle Testing. New York: McGraw-Hill, 1999.

Hawkins RJ. Musculoskeletal Examination. St. Louis: Mosby, 1995.

Hoppenfeld S. Orthopaedic Neurology, a Diagnostic Guide to Neurologic Levels. Philadelphia: Lippincott–Raven, 1997.

MacGee DJ. Orthopedic Physical Assessment (2nd ed). Philadelphia: Saunders, 1992.

II Management of Specific Anatomic Regions

6   Head and Neck

Ralph M. Buschbacher

The neck, perhaps more than any other body structure, reflects who we are and how we feel. When we are happy, we hold our heads high. When sad, we allow our necks to droop. Neck posture is affected by occupation and by habit. When posture is poor, it can set off a series of events leading to pain, continued poor posture, and degeneration. Because of its anatomy, the neck is also particularly vulnerable to trauma.

Anatomy

Bones, Joints, Disks, and Ligaments

There are seven cervical vertebrae (C1–C7) (Figure 6.1). The upper two, called the *atlas* (C1) and the *axis* (C2) (Figure 6.2), differ from the rest in form and function. The atlas holds the head on two concave surfaces. The occipital condyles of the base of the skull rest on these somewhat shallow planes and are held in place to a large extent by ligamentous support.

The atlas and axis articulate through a pivot joint, with the dens of the axis, a finger-like upward projection, providing a point around which the atlas can turn. The atlas and axis are bony rings. The atlas, unlike the rest of the vertebrae, has no vertebral body. The space the body would usually occupy is taken up by the dens. The dens is kept from slipping out of place by the transverse ligament.

The axis attaches to the C3 vertebra by way of an intervertebral disk and two posterior facet joints. There are disks between all the cervical vertebrae at and below this level, but none between the occiput and atlas or the atlas and axis. The C3–C7 vertebrae are all basically similar. Each consists of a body to which a ring, consisting of two laminae and two pedicles, is attached. At the lamino-pedicular junction, bony processes articulate with the corresponding processes above and below to form the facet joints (zygapophyseal joints.) The facet joints are synovial plane joints lined with hyaline cartilage and surrounded by a syn-

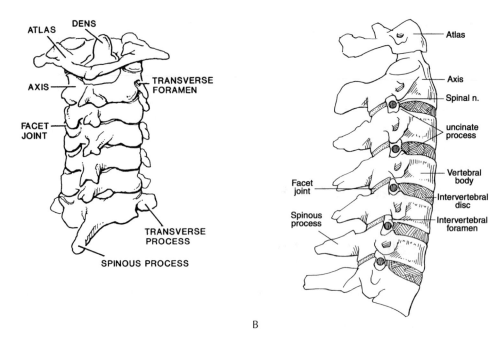

FIGURE 6.1 *The cervical vertebrae viewed from a posterolateral angle* **(A)** *and from a lateral view* **(B)**. *(n. = nerve.)*

ovial membrane and capsule. They face posterosuperiorly at approximately a 45-degree angle and allow a relatively large amount of motion in all directions. The rings of the vertebrae are stacked on top of one another to form the spinal canal, through which the spinal cord and its associated structures pass. The bodies of the cervical vertebrae have an upper and lower vertebral end plate lined by hyaline cartilage. They are curved to allow them to glide on one another.

There are lateral and posterior projections of the rings of the vertebrae called, respectively, the *transverse* and *spinous processes*. These are sites of muscular and ligamentous attachments. The spinous process of C7 (or sometimes T1) is particularly prominent on physical examination and is used as a bony landmark as the "vertebra prominens." The transverse processes contain holes, the transverse foraminae, through which the vertebral arteries and associated autonomic nerves pass.

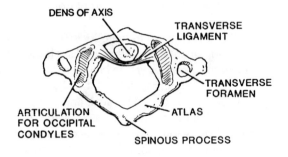

FIGURE 6.2 *The atlas and axis viewed from above.*

The disks between the vertebral bodies are composed of an inner nucleus pulposus and an outer annulus fibrosis. The nucleus is made up of a gelatinous connective tissue with a high water content. It is connected to the vertebrae on its top and bottom at the vertebral end plates, which are lined with cartilage. The nucleus has no direct innervation or blood supply. It receives its nutrition through a regular loading and unloading of weight (or force), which pushes water in and out of the disk by hydraulic pressure. This seems like a tenuous way to receive nutrition, but it works fairly well most of the time. During a day of standing the disk gradually loses water, which leads to a shortening in body height of approximately 3/4 in. per day. The fluid returns and restores height during sleep.

The annulus fibrosis is composed of collagenous fibers that encircle the nucleus in an angular manner. The structure somewhat resembles a radial tire.

There are several ligaments that help hold the vertebral column together (Figure 6.3). The anterior longitudinal ligament runs along the anterior surfaces of the vertebral bodies and disks. The posterior longitudinal ligament runs along the posterior vertebral bodies and disks. This posterior ligament is broader in the neck than in the low back, and thus helps protect the vertebral canal to a greater extent. The ligamentum flavum (yellow ligament), which starts at C2, has a high elastin content. It runs along the posterior part of the spinal canal. Its elasticity allows it to stretch to accommodate neck flexion and to retract without buckling during extension. Between the spinous processes lie thick, strong, interspinous ligaments, which prevent excessive flexion. Running posterior to the spinous processes is a strong supraspinous ligament, the ligamentum nuchae.

On the posterolateral vertebral bodies there are rims of bone, the uncinate processes, which project upwards and downwards. They interact with the corresponding projections above and below them in a pseudoarthrosis (false joint) known as the *uncovertebral joint of Luschka*. This pseudoarthrosis, which is not present at birth, protects the vertebral canal.

Behind the joints of Luschka and in front of the facet joints is a hole, the intervertebral foramen, through which the spinal nerve passes. Both afferent and efferent nerve fibers pass through this tunnel.

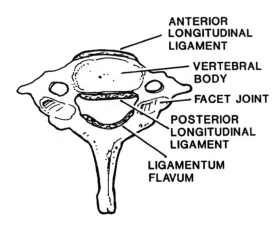

FIGURE 6.3   *The ligaments of the cervical spine from a top view. Note the holes in the transverse processes, which hold the vertebral arteries and associated sympathetic fibers.*

Compared to the lumbar spine, the cervical vertebrae are relatively resistant to disk herniation. This is because cervical disks are intrinsically more wedge-shaped (the lumbar disks assume this shape because of body position). In addition, the posterior longitudinal ligament is broader in the cervical spine, the nucleus is more anteriorly placed within the disk, and the uncovertebral joints protect from herniation. The cervical disks also do not have to support as much weight as do the lumbar disks, and do not have the same pressure increase with lifting, carrying, or straining.

Muscles

The muscles of the neck are numerous and complex, and a complete verbal dissection of them is not important to the focus of this chapter. They are depicted in Figure 6.4.

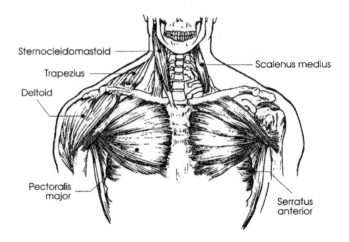

A

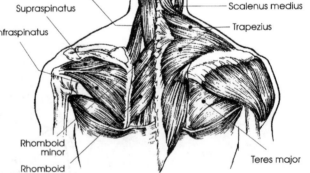

B

FIGURE 6.4   *The muscles of the neck and shoulder girdle. Anterior view (left-superficial, right-deep)* **(A)** *and posterior view (right-superficial, left-deep)* **(B)**.

Nerves

The spinal cord passes through the vertebral canal, giving off segmental spinal nerves (see Figure 6.1). There are eight cervical spinal nerves. The first exits above the atlas. The last exits below C7. They pass out of the vertebral canal through the intervertebral foraminae. After exiting the foraminae, they give off small recurrent branches called the *sinuvertebral nerves*, which innervate some of the structures within the spinal canal. The upper cervical nerves also give rise to the sensory nerves of the scalp, including the greater occipital nerve, which passes from the neck into the scalp a few centimeters lateral to the midline of the base of the skull. The dorsal primary rami innervate the paraspinal muscles (and facet joints), whereas the ventral primary rami innervate the rest of the muscles. Ventral nerve roots C5–T1 form the brachial plexus (Figure 6.5).

Pain-Sensitive Structures

When discussing the spine, it is probably easier to focus on the structures that don't cause pain rather than those that do. The intervertebral disk is commonly believed not to contain pain-sensitive nerve fibers, although there may be pain receptors in the very outer layers of the annulus fibrosis. Also, with tears of the annulus there may be an ingrowth of nerves into the disk. This may be a cause of pain in disk degeneration.

Another structure that does not have pain innervation is the interior of the vertebral body. The exterior, or periosteum, does contain pain innervation; thus, vertebral fractures cause pain.

Finally, the ligamentum flavum and the interspinous ligaments are not believed to be pain sensitive. All other structures, including the anterior and

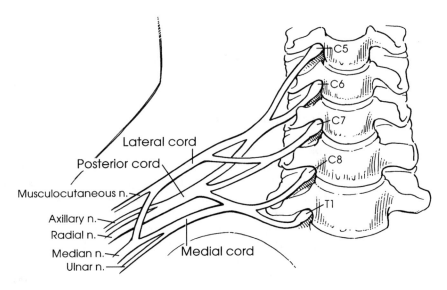

FIGURE 6.5   *The brachial plexus. (n. = nerve.)*

posterior longitudinal ligaments, the facet joints, muscles, dura, dorsal root ganglia, and spinal nerves can be sources of neck pain.[1] In addition, pain can be referred to the neck from distant sites.

Head and Neck Motion

Motion of the head and neck consists of flexion, extension, lateral bending, and rotation. Aside from a few segmental exceptions, the motion at each functional unit (two vertebrae and the disk between them) is small. Overall, however, the motion of the head and neck is quite remarkable.

Approximately 50% of total flexion and extension occurs at the atlantooccipital joint, with the base of the skull essentially rocking on the atlas. The rest of the flexion and extension motion is spread throughout the vertebrae and is preferentially concentrated at the C4–C6 level. Because of the slight concave–convex interface of the vertebral bodies, flexion involves not just a "bending" of the spine but a slight gliding of the upper vertebrae forward on the ones below. Extension involves a reversal of this glide. The facet joints, which face posterosuperiorly at approximately a 45-degree angle, allow flexion and extension to occur. Ordinarily, flexion is limited by the chin hitting the sternum. Extension is limited by the stretch of the anterior longitudinal ligament. During flexion, the anterior disk is compressed while the posterior edge widens. Extension reverses this deformation. Thus, flexion opens up the intervertebral foraminae, whereas extension causes their narrowing. Extreme flexion stretches the spinal nerve roots.

Pure rotation is possible only at the atlantoaxial joint, which contributes approximately 50% of total rotation. The remainder of the rotatory movement is intertwined with lateral bending. It is nearly impossible to laterally bend without also rotating the spine, or to rotate it without bending. When rotating or bending, the disk deforms and the intervertebral foraminae are narrowed on the side being turned or bent toward. The foraminae on the opposite side widen.

Examination and Testing Techniques

History and Physical Examination

A proper history must always be elicited. It should include information about when and how the neck problem started, what exacerbates or relieves it, and how severe it is, as well as any treatments and past medical problems. Of particular importance are a history of any radiating symptoms, bowel or bladder abnormalities, weakness or sensory deficits, aggravation of radiating pain with Valsalva maneuvers (coughing, sneezing, straining, having a bowel movement), and sleep history.

Physical examination starts with the observation of posture, mood, and any abnormal movements. Muscular contour is observed to detect signs of atrophy. The ligaments, joints, and soft tissues of the neck are palpated. The facet joints are felt approximately 1 in. lateral to the midline. Palpation of the muscles often will reveal trigger or tender points.

Range of motion is performed actively and passively in flexion, extension, lateral bending, and rotation. In addition, passive motion of the individual spinal segments can be assessed by the examiner with the patient lying supine, with the head and neck relaxed. Anterior and lateral gliding movements of each vertebra can be performed without exerting much force (Figure 6.6). This examination is pleasant and helps the patient relax.

Neurologic and muscular strength testing must include sensation, reflexes, and motor strength, not only of the neck but also of the head, upper back, and upper extremities (and possibly lower extremities as well.) Obviously, a detailed description of such an examination is beyond the scope of this chapter, but it can be obtained elsewhere.[2,3] It should also be noted that when the neck is injured, the shoulder is often injured too, and vice versa. Neck problems can cause pain to be felt in the shoulder, and vice versa. Therefore, when examining one of these areas, the other should be evaluated as well. What follows are descriptions of a few of the more specialized tests to assess the cervical region.

Compression Test

The compression test is performed by pushing straight down on the sitting patient's head (Figure 6.7). Pain is a positive although somewhat nonspecific finding. It may be due to a narrowing of the intervertebral foraminae, but also could be due to increased pressure on the facet joints. When pain is reproduced in a particular radicular distribution, it may help to localize the level of pathology.

Distraction Test

The distraction test is the opposite of the compression test (Figure 6.8). The examiner pulls up on the head while the patient sits or lies down. Pain relief can be due to a number of causes, including opening up the intervertebral foraminae, unloading the facet joints, or relieving muscle spasm. If pain is reduced, the patient may be a good candidate for traction therapy. Distraction should be sustained for at least 30 seconds to allow the neck time to relax and elongate.

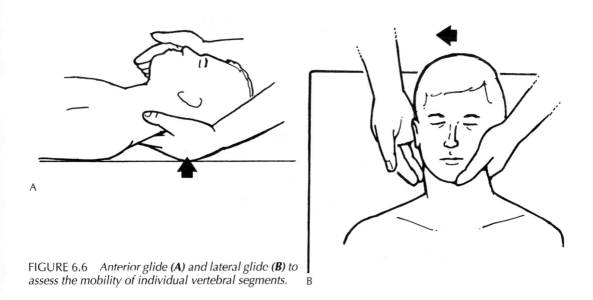

A

B

FIGURE 6.6   *Anterior glide (**A**) and lateral glide (**B**) to assess the mobility of individual vertebral segments.*

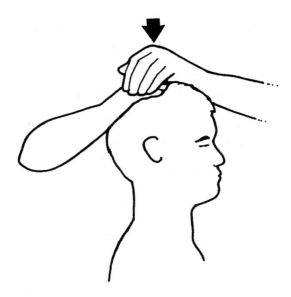

FIGURE 6.7   *Compression test.*

Spurling's Maneuver

Spurling's maneuver, a variation of the compression test (Figure 6.9), is performed by having the patient turn to the side and extend the neck, then applying downward pressure. It may help to localize the site of pathology, as the intervertebral foraminae and facet joints are more compressed on the side the subject turns to. Again, reproduction of radicular symptoms may help localize the level of dysfunction, and such radicular symptoms are required for the test to be labeled positive; local pain alone is a negative result. Spurling's maneuver is a relatively insensitive but very specific test[4]; it is often negative, even in cases of radiculopathy. When positive, however, a radiculopathy is likely to be present. If extension causes problems of dizziness, nystagmus, or vertigo, it may indicate vertebral artery dysfunction. Caution is in order here, as continuing to stress the neck in extension may result in stroke.

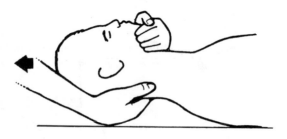

FIGURE 6.8   *Distraction test.*

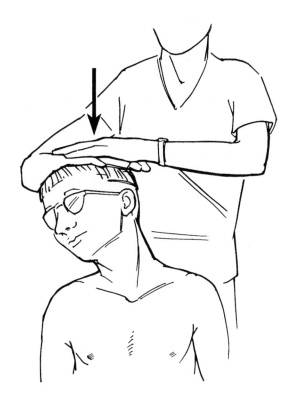

FIGURE 6.9   *Spurling's maneuver.*

Valsalva Maneuver
Increasing venous "back pressure" raises the pressure within the spinal column. This can be done by the Valsalva maneuver, which is basically just holding one's breath and bearing down as if having a bowel movement or lifting a heavy weight. The same increase in pressure is elicited by coughing or sneezing. Pain may be due to intraspinal tumor, but is usually considered a classic sign of a herniated disk.

Valsalva type maneuvers are not without risk. In patients with cardiac disorders they can cause syncope, so they should be performed with care and not where a fall is likely to result in injury.

Adson's Test
Adson's test is performed by palpating the radial pulse and then extending, abducting, and externally rotating the arm. The patient is asked to turn the head towards the arm being examined, then to extend the neck and take a deep breath. Diminution of the pulse is a positive finding and has been considered to be indicative of intermittent arterial compression. The test is often equivocal or positive in asymptomatic individuals and is insensitive to true compression as well.[5] It is of doubtful value.

Trigger or Tender Point Palpation
Palpating the neck muscles, especially the trapezius, sternocleidomastoid, and rhomboids, often causes a reproduction of local pain (tender points) or of pain

radiating into the head or limbs (trigger point). Finding such points is indicative of myofascial pain or fibromyalgia (see Chapter 16).

Shoulder Depression Test

If the examiner manually pushes the head to one side while depressing the shoulder, the spinal nerve roots, mainly levels C5–C7, may be stretched. If radicular pain results, it may indicate nerve root or intervertebral foraminal disease.

Blood Pressure

Although not usually considered a specialized test, blood pressure monitoring in both arms can be useful, possibly helping to diagnose subclavian steal syndrome or other conditions of blood flow impairment to one limb.

Ancillary Diagnostic Testing

In an acute injury in which there is a possibility of spinal fracture or subluxation, x-rays should be obtained, first in neutral, then, if cleared to be safe, in flexion and extension. In subacute injury, chronic injury, or when there is no risk of serious bony disruption, the neck can be x-rayed in anteroposterior views; open mouth (odontoid) views (to visualize the dens); lateral views in neutral, flexion and extension; and oblique views.

The anteroposterior views give a general measure of bony alignment and the structure of the uncovertebral joints. The odontoid view shows whether the dens is fractured, a potentially life-threatening condition that must be ruled out. Lateral views must include all seven cervical vertebrae. These give information about the intervertebral disks, the facet joints, and signs of soft tissue swelling, as well as subluxation or dislocation. Oblique views are used to visualize the intervertebral foraminae.

Other radiologic tests that can be performed include conventional tomography, computed tomography (CT), myelography, and magnetic resonance imaging (MRI). Conventional tomography is used mainly to demonstrate fractures and subluxations. CT testing gives the best general information to assess bones, and detects most fractures, joint disease, and spinal masses. Herniated disks are also well visualized. Myelography gives information about spinal cord or root compression or avulsion. It can be combined with CT to be an even more exact diagnostic tool. MRI is mainly used to visualize soft tissues and is the best test to assess herniated nucleus pulposus and some spinal cord tumors.

Other tests that can be helpful include bone scanning to detect stress fractures, bone tumors, and infection, and fluoroscopy to evaluate movement of the cervical spine.

Laboratory tests help detect connective tissue disease and infection. Electromyography (EMG) is used to detect neuropathy or myopathy.

Diagnosis and Treatment of Specific Disorders

The most important initial decision to be made in assessing the neck is whether neurologic compromise is present. If so, it must be addressed. Other important things to keep in mind are whether the pain is a result of intrinsic neck pathology, an extrinsic problem referring pain to the neck, or a systemic disorder. It is helpful to know if the pain was initiated by trauma and whether it comes from joints or muscles. Referred pain, either to or from the neck, must be differentiated from radicular pain.

This section deals with specific musculoskeletal disorders commonly encountered in a subacute outpatient setting. Medical emergencies such as fractures, dislocations, and spinal cord injury are not covered.

Acute Cervical Sprain/Strain

The prototypical cervical sprain/strain injury occurs in a rear-end auto collision and involves a hyperextension-hyperflexion (whiplash) injury of the neck. Not all cervical injuries, however, are of this type. Other mechanisms of abnormal or extreme neck motion can be caused by trauma in any plane, direct compression from objects falling on the head, or by heavy or awkward lifting.

Any injury that violently hyperflexes or hyperextends the neck will cause some soft tissue damage. When the neck is relaxed, a violent force that pushes the body forward or backward under the head will cause the neck to suddenly move backwards or forwards. The muscles involved in such a quick elongation may be partially torn. They may also be injured if contracted forcefully in a stretch reflex. The vertebral bodies and disks may be compressed as the body moves under the head, and the joints and ligaments may be stretched and possibly subluxated at the extremes of motion. The facet joints are compressed. Because the cervical vertebrae normally glide on each other during flexion and extension, the intervertebral foraminae may be narrowed sufficiently to compromise the spinal nerves, especially in a spine with pre-existing bony spurring. In addition, the sympathetic nervous system may be damaged, either at the foraminae or as the sympathetic fibers pass with the vertebral arteries through the transverse foraminae. The disk is more likely to be damaged if there is a rotatory component to the trauma. Sometimes the disk is torn from the vertebral body, in which case the anterior longitudinal ligament may be torn as well.

The symptoms of whiplash syndrome vary. Headache, neck pain, neck soreness, muscle tightness, decreased range of motion, dizziness, and difficulty swallowing are common problems. Often they start a day or two after injury,[1] which can create the impression that they are due to the anticipation of litigation rather than true injury. Radiation of pain is a common complaint and can sometimes be reproduced on the physical examination. Radicular symptoms (not the same thing as radiation of pain) imply nerve root damage. Other neck structures, such as the trachea, esophagus, or vocal cords, are occasionally damaged.

Hyperextension injury can be more serious in the older individual. The ligamentum flavum loses elasticity with age, and when a hyperextension injury occurs it may "buckle" the ligament and cause acute spinal cord compression.

Whiplash injuries have a worse prognosis if they are associated with advanced age, neurologic signs, muscle spasm (as manifested by an abnormal spinal curvature), neck stiffness, and pre-existing degenerative disease.[6]

Diagnosis

Cervical strain or sprain is diagnosed mainly by history. In the acute stage, the physical examination is often normal. In the subacute stage, there may be signs of muscle splinting, muscle tightness, soreness, and decreased range of motion. Distraction of the neck may relax the neck muscles and relieve pain. In most patients the symptoms resolve in a few weeks. A chronic condition may ensue in more severe injuries or in people who persist in maintaining poor posture and muscle splinting. Rigid muscular splinting of the neck may relieve pain early on, but if maintained, it leads to contracture, chronic isometric muscle contraction, and persistent closing of the intervertebral foraminae.

X-ray findings in cervical strain are usually normal or equivocal, but are important in ruling out other structural injury. There are usually no fractures or obvious dislocations present, but there may be a "reduction of the normal cervical lordosis." This is a nonspecific finding that doesn't aid much in clinical management, although it may indicate the presence of muscle splinting that can lead to later muscle fatigue and pain. Persons with neck injury often have underlying degenerative change with bony spurring and disk-space narrowing. Such x-ray findings are also not of much clinical use. It is possible that the underlying disease predisposed the patient to injury, but often the pain doesn't correspond to the x-ray findings.

In some cases, especially chronic states, the facet joints are irritated.[1] This condition cannot be diagnosed clinically or by imaging study, but only by fluoroscopic injection, which determines whether an anesthetic will block the pain.[7] However, this procedure is usually unnecessary.

Treatment

Acute injury is treated with a few days to a week of relative rest and activity or work restriction, possibly aided with a soft collar, analgesia, and treatment with ice. "Muscle relaxants" may also be useful. As symptoms improve, the soft collar is gradually removed as tolerated, and either heat or ice treatment is used as a modality. After a week or two, range-of-motion exercises are initiated, avoiding early flexion-extension motion to the extremes of range. If symptoms don't resolve within 2–3 weeks, the patient may benefit from a physical therapy referral to work on range of motion, posture, relaxation, and neck isometric strengthening. This can be taught as part of a home exercise program with good results. If resolution is slow, further diagnostic studies, usually just plain film x-rays, are considered. Massage, ischemic compression, ice massage, and trigger/tender point injection may also help. Before the condition becomes chronic, further imaging studies, such as MRI or bone scan, may be indicated. The patient may benefit from transcutaneous electrical nerve stimulation (see Chapter 2), heat or cold, aerobic exercise, adjunctive medications, and possibly a referral to a pain clinic. Subacute or chronic symptoms may develop into a myofascial pain presentation. Chronic cases due to facet joint pain may respond to radiofrequency neurotomy of this joint,[7] but such pain relief may only be temporary.

Myofascial Pain/Overuse Syndrome/Poor Posture

Almost any situation of overuse, poor posture, or unaccustomed work habits can lead to myofascial pain syndrome, which particularly likes to attack the neck and upper back region. Symptoms typically include local or regional muscle pain and stiffness, loss of range of motion, and specific tender spots or trigger points in the muscles. Stress (mental and physical) and previous trauma are important contributors to the problem. "Tension headache" often results from this stress. The causes of myofascial pain are unknown, but may be due to local muscle tears or ischemia.

Diagnosis

A good history gives the most information in diagnosing myofascial pain. New activities, stress, complaints of muscle tightness and soreness, and regional pain complaints are the hallmarks of this disorder, and it is common to see at least some element of myofascial pain in any problems of the neck. The pain often occurs a few days to a week after prolonged work in an exacerbating posture or after trauma. Moderate aerobic activity may relieve it.

Myofascial pain may involve symptoms that are felt distally in the upper extremity, in some cases mimicking a radiculopathy. Most persons with myofascial pain have tenderness in the muscles. Often the muscles contain particularly sensitive, tender spots that are firm and hard, like a local area of "spasm." When palpating such tender spots causes a reproduction of the patient's symptoms and radiation of the pain or paresthesias distally, they are called *trigger points* and are particularly suggestive of myofascial pain as the cause of symptoms. Radiation of pain is required to label a point a trigger point, but in many persons with myofascial pain there are local tender spots that do not cause any such radiation. Tender spots and trigger points are commonly located in the trapezius and rhomboid muscles. The sternocleidomastoid and the scapular attachment of the levator scapula are often affected as well.

Treatment

Treatment is aimed at resolving the symptoms and removing the underlying cause. The problem can be explained to patients as "tight" muscles that have not relaxed after injury as expected. When the muscles relax, the pain will resolve. All aspects of the treatment plan are geared to helping the muscles relax.

Patients usually respond to a short period of relative rest (1–2 weeks), with work or activity restrictions as needed. Nonsteroidal anti-inflammatory medications (NSAIDs), heat or cold therapy, and gentle range-of-motion exercises are useful.

If symptoms do not resolve in 2–3 weeks, relaxation training, ischemic compression (see Chapter 16), ice massage, heat, trigger point/tender spot injection, and a home stretching and aerobic exercise program may be instituted. Medications such as cyclobenzaprine hydrochloride or nortriptyline hydrochloride given at bedtime can help to relax the muscles and improve sleep. Usually a 2–4 week regimen of exercise therapy, medication, and injection is enough to completely resolve the problem. If symptoms persist, one must be particularly careful to address any biomechanical or activity-related perpetuation of the symptoms. When there are tender spots or trigger points of the lateral portion of the pectoralis major, the posterior deltoid, the teres major, or the latissimus dorsi, they usually respond very well to injection, although such injection commonly causes more bruising than in other muscles.

In the long run, treatment aims at building muscle strength, improving posture and flexibility, and reducing stress. In refractory cases, a course of work hardening or conditioning and permanent work or activity restrictions may be needed.

Degenerative Joint Disease/Cervical Spondylosis

Degenerative joint disease occurs in the spine just as it does in many other parts of the body. The cause is unknown but may involve aging, overuse, trauma, or genetic predisposition. It is associated with heavy lifting, smoking, diving (from a board), and possibly with driving or operating vibrating equipment.[8] It preferentially affects the C5–C7 vertebrae. In the spine, the degeneration affects the intervertebral disk and the facet joints.

As the disk ages and is subject to repetitive trauma and motion, the annulus fibrosis develops small tears, which may gradually coalesce and lead to a weakening. The nucleus, which has a somewhat tenuous nutritional supply mechanism (possibly worsened by constant tension and too infrequent loading and unloading of the joint) loses water content, develops fissures, and may project into the coalescent radial annular tears. As this degenerative process progresses, the disk loses height and the annulus bulges outward. The vertebral end plates become sclerotic and grow bony spurs in an attempt to maintain structural strength, and the facet joint surfaces are brought closer together and may shift on each other. This causes synovitis, capsular stretch, and degeneration of these joints. The joints can also degenerate independent of disk disease, primarily by faulty neck motion and repetitive microtrauma, but in most people these processes proceed together. The overall results are the nonspecific degenerative findings commonly seen on x-ray. Sometimes they cause pain and sometimes they do not. The reasons for this are unknown. In the spine, such degenerative change is called *spondylosis*.

When pain occurs, it probably comes to some extent from the disk, the facet joints, the uncovertebral joints, and from the nerves and other spinal column contents that are compressed by the spurs and bulging disk. Symptoms develop insidiously and include morning pain and stiffness.

If the spurring continues, it eventually compresses the contents of the spinal canal. If it encroaches on the spinal canal, it is called *central* (or *spinal*) *stenosis*; if it narrows the intervertebral foraminae, it is called *lateral stenosis*.

Central stenosis can lead to cervical myelopathy, a condition of ischemic compression of the spinal cord. Lateral stenosis can result in radiculopathy.

Diagnosis

The diagnosis of degenerative spine disease is straightforward, because almost everyone older than 50 years of age has some evidence of it. This can be demonstrated on plain x-rays, CT, or MRI. Determining that the degeneration is the cause of pain is more difficult. The patient may complain of an aching pain in the neck or upper back with intermittent exacerbations. Pain is often worse in the morning and is improved with moderate activity. A period of rest after activity may trigger a worsening of symptoms. There may be joint crepitus and decreased range of motion (flexion is relatively spared.) The area over the facet joints may be tender to palpation. Compression testing worsens symptoms, whereas distraction may relieve them. X-rays will reveal diffuse bony spurring and disk space narrowing, sometimes with local areas of worse disease. In most patients these symptoms and signs will stabilize and lessen in time as the spine becomes stiffer (but more stable). In some, however, the bony proliferation produces further problems.

Treatment

Conservative treatment is almost always successful in degenerative disease of the cervical spine. In uncomplicated osteoarthritis of the neck, range-of-motion exercises, NSAIDs, cervical pillows, and modalities such as heat and cold are the mainstays of treatment. Occasionally traction or facet joint injections are required. The patient can expect to have intermittent exacerbations but is unlikely to develop symptoms severe enough to significantly limit function. Exacerbations are minimized by avoiding unaccustomed activity, high impact exercise, or holding the neck in one position (especially extension) for a prolonged period of time. The patient should be taught a long-term moderate stretching and strengthening exercise program as well as a more general aerobic conditioning program. Water aerobics are particularly well tolerated. Bicycling, in which the head is held in an extended posture, is not, although recumbent or exercise bikes may be acceptable.

Radiculopathy and Myelopathy

Radiculopathy is pathology of the nerve root. Such pathology can cause local pain and dermatomal symptoms and myotomal weakness into the arm. Radiculopathy can develop acutely or more insidiously. Although commonly due to a disk herniation, the term is not synonymous with "herniated disk," and can occur in the face of no disk pathology whatsoever. In the person with pre-existing degenerative joint disease, acute radiculopathy often occurs after prolonged abnormal activity such as painting a ceiling or holding the neck in prolonged extension. The activity irritates the spinal nerve root to such an extent that it becomes inflamed. This inflammation (and swelling) in an already narrowed space precipitates symptoms.

Pain is often referred in a dermatomal pattern or to the posterior shoulder. Paresthesias, weakness, and reflex changes may occur, although it is important to realize that radiculopathy is not always painful. Compression of the dorsal root ganglion causes a shooting pain down the arm. Usually the symptoms resolve, but occasionally marked segmental muscle weakness and atrophy develop. There may be more than one nerve root involved.

Acute radiculopathy can also be caused by disk herniation or trauma. In the case of trauma, it is usually clear what caused the injury. Typically, this occurs when a patient is rear-ended in a motor vehicle accident or if an object falls on the patient's head, causing an acute compression of the nerve root, often with no anatomic abnormality noted on imaging study. The nerve suffers acute compression but there is no ongoing damage. Unfortunately, there is often only a limited amount that can be done for such patients except to allow natural healing to take place; they often have poorer outcomes than those with radiculopathies due to herniated disks.

Disk herniation typically occurs in a disk that has had some pre-existing degeneration. It primarily involves the 30 to 55-year age range and cervical levels C5–C6, C6–C7, and C4–C5. When radial annular tears coalesce, the nucleus pulposus may protrude into the spinal canal to compress the spinal cord or spinal nerves. This can happen suddenly or insidiously. It is much less common in the cervical region than in the lumbar spine.

Although the herniated disk may cause local nerve root damage or compression of the spinal cord, it may also just cause pain with no neurologic symptoms.

Trauma or a session of particularly heavy lifting or straining can precipitate the herniation. Sometimes it is difficult to know the exact cause. Herniation can cause radiculopathy either by local compression or, more commonly, by focal chemical irritation to the nerve root. A recently herniated disk releases various mediators of inflammation directly onto the root.[9] This can cause symptoms and nerve damage. As the inflammation resolves, the irritation ceases and the symptoms abate.

Chronic radiculopathy may develop due to progressive narrowing of the intervertebral foramen over time. Abnormal posture or trauma aggravates the symptoms and causes exacerbations.

Cervical myelopathy involves damage to the cervical spinal cord. It can produce far-reaching signs and symptoms. Locally, it may produce pain in the neck from ischemia and spurring, but often such local symptoms are relatively minor. It also may cause lower motor neuron damage at the level of pathology, which usually results in upper extremity dysesthesias, paresthesias, weakness, and depressed reflexes. These changes have an insidious onset. Upper motor neuron damage at the cervical level causes leg weakness, gait disturbance (often slow, wide based, ataxic), and lower extremity spasticity and hyperreflexia. There is also a loss of sensation, and Babinski testing will be positive. Reflexes above the level of the spine pathology, such as the jaw reflex, remain normal. The condition is sometimes mild and may stabilize. In other cases, it progresses rapidly, sometimes even in relatively young patients, and may result in bowel and bladder dysfunction.

Diagnosis

Symptoms of radiculopathy include local pain, radicular pain and paresthesia, dysesthesia, weakness, and reflex changes. These findings may be subtle at times. The symptoms may be worsened or reproduced by Valsalva maneuver, Spurling's maneuver, or compression testing. Distraction with manual traction may relieve symptoms somewhat.

Radiculopathy is best diagnosed by electrodiagnostic study, commonly known as *electromyography*. EMG tells the practitioner whether there is actual nerve damage present. It is a physiologic test that is somewhat operator dependent, but in the right hands it gives a good sensitivity and has an extremely low rate of false-positive results. EMG can help localize which nerve root is damaged, as well as rule out confounding conditions such as carpal tunnel syndrome or brachial plexopathy. If EMG is positive, it is usually worthwhile to obtain an MRI or CT, which can be correlated to the EMG findings to determine the anatomic cause of the nerve root damage. Obtaining the imaging study first would yield a much higher rate of false-positive results because approximately 20% of asymptomatic patients have major cervical MRI abnormalities.[10] This is even higher in older patients. Another advantage to EMG is that it detects nerve root damage in the absence of a herniated disk or other anatomic compression. Such damage is sometimes present after trauma such as a rear-end auto collision.

When diagnosing radiculopathy, oblique x-rays may help by demonstrating foraminal narrowing. Myelogram or CT may be useful to evaluate the extent of bony encroachment. Abduction of the arm may decrease radicular pain in cervical extradural compressive radiculopathy and has been advocated as a diagnostic test for this condition.[11,12]

Diagnosis of cervical myelopathy due to stenosis is made by the clinical picture (lower motor signs at the level of the cervical spine, upper motor neuron signs below this level), electromyography, and measurement of the diameter of the spinal canal through imaging studies. MRI or myelogram may help to delineate the area of cord compression. Affected patients are sometimes developmentally predisposed to the condition by having a narrow spinal canal.

Treatment

In radiculopathy, early treatment involves rest and avoiding aggravating activities such as straining, bending, or lifting. Sometimes a few days of limited bed rest can be helpful. A soft collar can help restrain the patient from aggravating movement and may give some support to the neck. Stool softeners decrease the straining associated with bowel movements. Analgesics, opioids, muscle relaxants, and NSAIDs may be helpful. A brief course of oral steroids can be considered, but epidural steroid injections are very rarely needed and carry with them significant risks due to the proximity of the spinal cord.

After a few days or weeks, gentle range-of-motion exercises (avoiding excessive extension or extension/rotation) can be instituted. Heat or cold can help minimize secondary muscle splinting, and traction can minimize symptoms—both of the radiculopathy, by decompressing the nerve roots; and of muscle pain, by relaxing the cervical musculature.[13] Patients generally do not tolerate much physical therapy in the first weeks of their condition, and should be placed on work or activity restrictions.

More vigorous exercises, including strengthening, stretching, and functional activities, are instituted over a period of 2–8 weeks, as tolerated. Most cases resolve within 3 months, usually even sooner. Surgical decompression generally is not needed, but should be considered in cases of progressive neurologic deficit, significant atrophy, intractable pain, or no signs of improvement within 8–12 weeks. Patients with predominant complaints of neck pain with no neurological deficit or radicular symptoms do not get a better long-term outcome from surgery than from conservative care.[14]

In cases of herniated disk, the herniated portion of the disk is phagocytosed and disappears within approximately 3–6 months. Symptoms may not persist for this long, but in some cases they do. Given such a natural history it is unclear why patients and physicians alike are so eager to surgically remove the disk. Patients (and often employers) must be counseled that this is not simply a "neck strain." If they understand that symptoms often take 2–3 months or even longer to resolve, they will be less impatient with their progress.

Mild, nonprogressive cases of cervical myelopathy can be treated similarly to radiculopathy. Gentle flexion exercises may help to open up the spinal canal. In some cases surgical decompression is necessary, and may be successful if the narrowing is localized to a small area. In diffuse stenosis, surgical results are often poor. Most patients with conservatively treated cervical myelopathy see a stabilization or improvement of their symptoms, but more significant cases benefit from early surgical decompression.[15]

Vertebral Artery Insufficiency

The vertebral arteries pass through the transverse processes of the vertebrae on their way to supply the brain with blood. If bony spurs press on the arteries, they can restrict blood flow to the brain. This is a potentially life-threatening condition and may cause posterior circulation stroke.

Diagnosis

Symptoms of vertebral artery compression include neck pain, headache, light-headedness, dizziness, vertigo, syncope, ataxia, diplopia, dysphagia, dysarthria, and facial dysesthesia. Symptoms are brought on by positions that compress the arteries, usually turning towards the side of the compression, or extension. This condition should be suspected if the patient experiences characteristic symptoms during the physical examination, especially on lateral bending, rotation, and Spurling's maneuver. Plain x-rays may reveal marked spurring, often at the upper cervical and occipital level. Definitive diagnosis is by arteriography.

Treatment

Surgical removal of the offending structures should be considered. Traction and manipulation are absolutely contraindicated. This condition is best managed by a spine surgeon or other physician well versed in its treatment.

Occipital Neuralgia

After trauma, the occipital nerve can become irritated at the junction of the skull and neck, causing pain that radiates from the posterior to the anterior scalp, as well as pain behind the eyes. Headache parallels the sensory distribution of the nerve. Retro-orbital pain is due to a looping of some of the nerve fibers around cranial nerve V; thus it is considered a referred pain.

Diagnosis

Diagnosis is made by the clinical symptoms described above and by reproduction of the symptoms with palpation of the nerve. The nerve may be inflamed and swollen.

Treatment

Occipital neuralgia generally improves with time. Treatment with local anesthetic-steroid injection around the nerve is often successful (which also helps to confirm the diagnosis.) Care must be taken not to inject the nearby vertebral artery. Most affected persons will respond to 1–3 injections. Other treatment options include ice application, ultrasound treatment, electric stim-ulation, and anti-inflammatory medications. Medications useful for treating neuropathic pain, such as tricyclic antidepressants and gabapentin, may also be helpful.

Temporomandibular Joint Dysfunction

This condition causes radiation of pain into the neck and can occur after neck extension injury[16] or have no discernible cause at all.

Diagnosis
The symptoms of temporomandibular dysfunction are pain in the region of the joint, radiation of pain into the neck, a painful "click" on opening the mouth, and painful or restricted range of motion of the jaw. Ultrasound examination of the joint, as well as pressure on the cartilaginous disk of the joint (by manual pressure on the jaw with the joint in neutral), may help make the diagnosis.

Treatment
This condition can be treated with NSAIDs; avoidance of hard, chewy foods; ice treatment; ultrasound treatment; massage of associated tender points; bite plates; or, more definitively, a filing of the teeth to give a better dental occlusion. If symptoms persist despite conservative treatment, a referral should be made to a dentist or other physician specializing in this disorder.

Brachial Plexopathy and Thoracic Outlet Syndrome

Brachial plexopathy and thoracic outlet syndrome are described in Chapter 8.

Connective Tissue Disease

Rheumatoid arthritis, diffuse idiopathic skeletal hyperostosis, ankylosing spondylitis, and other connective tissue diseases may affect the neck. These are primarily rheumatologic disorders and will not be covered in detail in this book; however, a few basic principles will be addressed.

Rheumatoid arthritis (as well as the other rheumatologic diseases) is a systemic condition and must be treated as such. Of special interest in the neck is rheumatoid involvement of the atlantoaxial joint at the dens. As described earlier, this joint is a synovial joint. If it degenerates during the course of connective tissue disease, it can lead to atlantoaxial subluxation.[17] This allows the dens to slip into the spinal cord and brain stem and is potentially fatal. Thus, traction, manipulation, and forceful neck mobilization are contraindicated in these individuals. Risk factors for atlantoaxial instability include steroid use, long duration of disease, older age, and erosive peripheral joint involvement.[15]

Diffuse idiopathic skeletal hyperostosis is a condition characterized by an overproduction of bone, primarily in the spine. It creates a "flowing osteophytosis" on x-ray. It presents in middle age with spinal stiffness and tenderness. Occasionally, patients have trouble swallowing due to osteophytes pushing on the esophagus (as well as the immobile cervical spine). Treatment is general flexibility and conditioning training. Cervical manipulation and traction are again contraindicated.

Ankylosing spondylitis is a disease mainly of young whites, mostly symptomatic in men. It involves calcification and inflammation of spinal tendons and ligaments at their attachments to bone. It typically presents with low back and sacroiliac joint pain and may eventually involve the entire spine. The spine loses mobility and may become fused. Treatment is aimed at maintaining range of motion and avoiding spinal fusion in a stooped posture. Again, traction and manipulation are to be avoided in these patients.

Other Disorders

A number of other disorders must be kept in mind when diagnosing neck pathology. These include fractures, neoplasm, osteomyelitis, meningitis, referred pain (e.g., from myocardial infarction), migraine, conversion disorder, Pancoast tumor, pharyngeal infection, torticollis, malingering, and psychogenic pain. In addition, many shoulder or arm disorders can mimic neck problems. Although the list may seem intimidating at first, a systematic approach and an understanding of anatomy and biomechanics usually leads to a correct diagnosis.

Points of Summary

1. Pain-producing structures in the neck include bones, anterior and posterior longitudinal ligaments, facet joints, dura, nerve roots, and the outer annulus.
2. The intervertebral foraminae narrow with extension and rotation/bending.
3. Herniated disks are less common in the neck than in the lumbar spine. They can cause radiculopathy and usually respond well to conservative care.
4. Not all radiculopathies are caused by herniated disks. Radiculopathy is best diagnosed by electromyography (EMG); magnetic resonance imaging (MRI) will confirm any anatomic cause of compression, but yields a high rate of false-positive results.
5. Injections, ischemic compression, and ice massage are useful in treating myofascial pain.
6. Degeneration of the disk and facet joints may lead to osteoarthritis, radiculopathy, myelopathy, or none of these.
7. X-ray findings in the spine often do not correlate with symptoms.
8. Proper posture and biomechanics are key to preventing chronic neck pain.

References

1. Dreyer SJ, Boden SD. Nonoperative treatment of neck and arm pain. Spine 1998;23:2746–2754.
2. McGee DJ. Orthopedic Physical Assessment (2nd ed). Philadelphia: Saunders, 1992.
3. Hoppenfeld S. Physical Examination of the Spine and Extremities. Norwalk, CT: Appleton-Century-Crofts, 1976.
4. Viikari-Juntura E, Porras M, Laasonen EM. Validity of clinical tests in the diagnosis of root compression in cervical spine disease. Spine 1989;14: 253–257.

5. Glassenberg M. The thoracic outlet syndrome: an assessment of 20 cases with regard to new clinical and electromyographic findings. Angiology 1981;32:180–186.
6. Norris SH, Watt I. The prognosis of neck injuries resulting from rear-end collisions. J Bone Joint Surg 1983;65B:608–611.
7. Bogduk N, Teasell R. Whiplash: evidence for an organic etiology. Arch Neurol 2000;57:590–591.
8. Kelsey JL, Githens PB, Walter SD, et al. An epidemiological study of acute prolapsed cervical intervertebral disc. J Bone Joint Surg 1984;66A:907–914.
9. Saal JS, Franson RC, Dobrow R, et al. High levels of inflammatory phospholipase A2 activity in lumbar disk herniations. Spine 1990;15:676–678.
10. Boden SD, McCowin PR, Davis DO, et al. Abnormal cervical MR scans in asymptomatic individuals: a prospective and blinded investigation. J Bone Joint Surg 1990;72A:1178–1184.
11. Davidson RI, Dunn EJ, Metzmaker JN. The shoulder abduction test in the diagnosis of radicular pain in cervical extradural compressive mononeuropathies. Spine 1981;6:441–446.
12. Fast A, Parikh S, Marin EL. The shoulder abduction relief sign in cervical radiculopathy. Arch Phys Med Rehabil 1989;70:402–403.
13. Swezey RL, Swezey AM, Warner K. Efficacy of home cervical traction therapy. Am J Phys Med Rehabil 1999;78:30–32.
14. Dillin W, Booth R, Cuckler J, et al. Cervical radiculopathy, a review. Spine 1986;11:988–991.
15. Scherping SC, Boden SD, Borenstein DG, Wiesel SW. Neck Pain (3rd ed). New York: Lexis Publishing, 2000.
16. Roydhouse RH. Torquing of neck and jaw due to belt restraint in whiplash-type accidents. Lancet 1985;1:1341.
17. Reiter MF, Boden SD. Inflammatory disorders of the cervical spine. Spine 1998;23:2755–2766.

Suggested Reading

Nachemson AL, Jonsson E (eds). Neck and Back Pain: The Scientific Evidence of Causes, Diagnosis, and Treatment. Philadelphia: Williams & Wilkins, 2000.

Saal JA (ed). Neck and back pain. Physical Medicine and Rehabilitation: State of the Art Reviews 1990:4(2).

Scherping SC, Boden SD, Borenstein DG, Wiesel SW. Neck Pain (3rd ed). New York: Lexis Publishing, 2000.

7   Back

Nathan D. Prahlow, Ralph M. Buschbacher, and Andrea R. Conti

Back pain is encountered commonly in almost any medical setting. It is estimated that as much as 85% of the adult population will suffer from low back pain (LBP) at some time. In the United States, back pain is the most common cause of activity limitation in those younger than 45 years of age, the second most frequent reason for a visit to a physician, and the third most common reason for a surgical procedure.[1]

Anatomy

Vertebral Column

The bony spine is composed of 7 cervical, 12 thoracic, and 5 lumbar vertebrae sitting on the sacrum. The individual spinal segments move little, but motion of the spine as a whole is quite remarkable. During quiet standing the spine is balanced so that virtually no muscular activity is required to maintain its position.

The thoracic and lumbar vertebrae are similar to one another except that the thoracic segments articulate with the ribs. The vertebrae become larger in the caudal direction. Each individual vertebra consists of a body, to which is attached a ring consisting of two pedicles and two laminae (Figure 7.1)

At the laminopedicular junction, bony processes extend to articulate with the corresponding processes above and below them to form the facet joints (zygapophysial joints). The spinal nerves exit the spinal canal through the intervertebral foramina (Figure 7.2).

There are two lateral projections and one posterior projection from the ring of each vertebra. These are called the *transverse* and *spinous* processes, respectively. They are sites of muscular and ligamentous attachment.

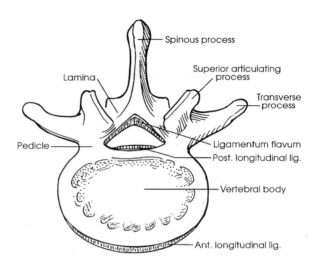

FIGURE 7.1   *Transverse view of a lumbar vertebra. (Ant. = anterior; lig. = ligament; Post. = posterior.)*

The disks between the vertebral bodies are composed of an inner nucleus pulposus and an outer annulus fibrosis (Figure 7.3). The nucleus is made up of a gelatinous connective tissue with a high water content. It is connected to the vertebrae on its top and bottom at the vertebral end plates, which are lined with cartilage. The nucleus has no direct innervation or blood supply. It receives its nutrition through a regular loading and unloading of weight (or force), which pushes water in and pulls it out of the disk by hydraulic pressure. During a day of standing the disk gradually loses water, which leads to a shortening in body height of approximately 3/4 in. per day. The fluid returns and restores height during sleep. This has been demonstrated in vivo by measuring intradiskal pressure; pressure increased 240% after 7 hours in a lying position.[2]

Intradiskal pressure varies with body position and with activity. The pressure is lowest when lying supine (Figure 7.4). Standing and sitting unsupported

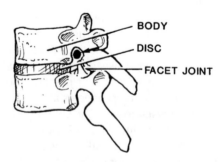

FIGURE 7.2   *Functional unit of the spine: two vertebrae and the intervening disk. The intervertebral foramen houses the spinal nerve (arrow).*

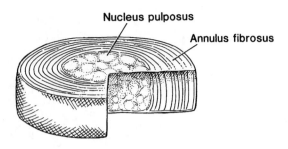

FIGURE 7.3   *The intervertebral disk.*

result in modestly increased pressure, whereas forward leaning and weight lifting increase pressure to a greater degree. "Improper" lifting posture yields a
substantially greater pressure increase than "proper" lifting, with bent legs and
straight trunk.[2]

The annulus fibrosis, which has nociceptive innervation at its periphery, is
composed of collagenous fibers that encircle the nucleus in an angular manner. The structure somewhat resembles a radial tire.

There are several ligaments that help hold the vertebral column together
(Figure 7.5; see Figure 7.1). The anterior longitudinal ligament runs along the

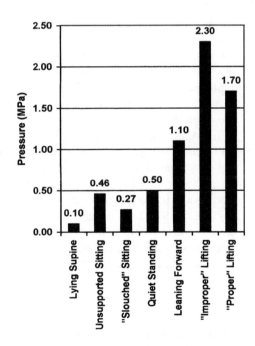

FIGURE 7.4   *Intradiskal pressures in common postures and activities in 70-kg individuals. Lifting weight = 20 kg.*[2]

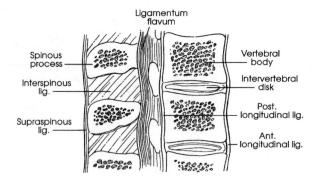

FIGURE 7.5 *A sagittal cutaway view of the vertebral column. (Ant. = anterior; lig. = ligament; Post. = posterior.)*

anterior surfaces of the vertebral bodies and disks. The posterior longitudinal ligament runs along the posterior vertebral bodies and disks, forming the anterior edge of the spinal canal. In the lumbar spine, this ligament is narrower and weaker than in the neck, which is one factor contributing to the higher frequency of disk herniation in the back. The ligamentum flavum (yellow ligament) runs along the posterior wall of the spinal canal. The interspinous ligaments run between the spinous processes, whereas the supraspinous ligament runs dorsal to the spinous processes. Intertransverse ligaments connect the transverse processes.

Muscles of the Back

The muscles of the back are divided into extrinsic muscles and intrinsic muscles (Figure 7.6). For the most part, the extrinsic back muscles contribute to upper extremity motion. They are limb muscles that migrate during embryonic development to cover the back. The intrinsic back muscles maintain posture and control movement of the vertebral column as a whole.

The direction of the fibers of the intrinsic back muscles identifies the different layers. The superficial layer, the splenius muscles of the neck, has fibers that pass superolaterally (from lower spinous process to upper transverse process). The intermediate layer, the erector spinae, runs longitudinally in the groove on each side of the vertebral column. The deeper muscles, the multifidus and rotators, pass superomedially (from lower transverse process to upper spinous process). These deep muscles make up the bulk of the muscles commonly called the *paraspinals*. They control segmental vertebral motion and spinal stabilization during movement.

Nerves

The spinal cord lies in the vertebral canal, giving off pairs of segmental spinal nerves, which exit the spinal canal through the intervertebral foramina. In the thoracic and lumbar spine, the nerves are named and numbered after the vertebral body below which they exit the canal. After passing through the foramina, they give off recurrent branches called the *sinuvertebral nerves* (described by von Luschka in 1850), which innervate some of the structures within the spinal canal.[3]

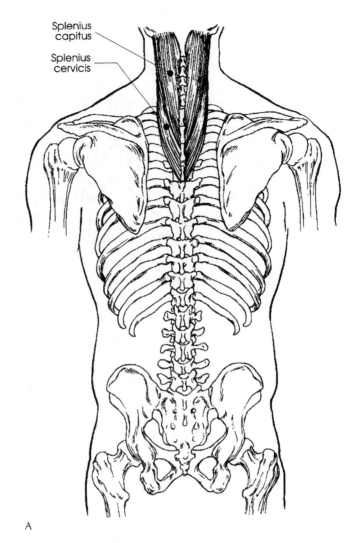

Splenius
capitus

Splenius
cervicis

A

FIGURE 7.6   *The intrinsic back muscles: (A) superficial.*

The spinal cord itself typically ends near the L1–L2 vertebral level. Below this level, the spinal canal contains no cord, just nerve roots traveling caudally to the vertebral levels at which they exit. This collection of nerve roots is called the *cauda equina* (horse's tail).

Pain-Sensitive Structures

The adult intervertebral disk is commonly believed not to contain pain-sensitive nerve fibers, although there are pain receptors in the very outer layers of the annulus fibrosis.[4] The dorsal aspect of the dural sac has been shown to contain no nerve endings, accounting for the relative painlessness of dural punctures.[3] Neither the supraspinous and interspinous ligaments nor the liga-

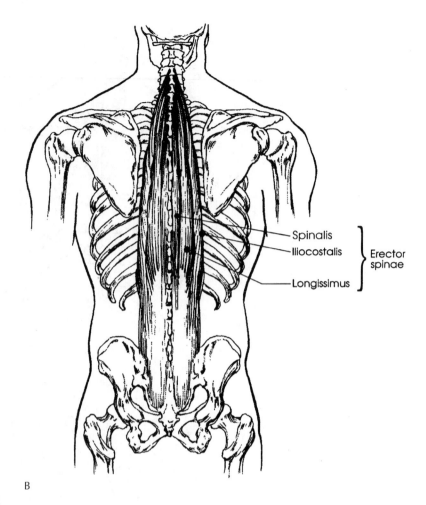

Spinalis
Iliocostalis } Erector spinae
Longissimus

B

FIGURE 7.6   *Continued.* ***B.*** *Intermediate, and* ***(C)*** *deep.*

mentum flavum has pain sensation. Finally, the interior of the vertebral body is not believed to be pain sensitive.[5]

The exterior surface of the vertebral body, the periosteum, does contain pain innervation; thus, vertebral fractures are painful. All other structures, including the anterior and posterior longitudinal ligaments, the facet joints, muscles, dura, epidural blood vessels, and spinal nerves can be sources of spinal pain.[3–5] In addition, pain can be referred to the back from other areas of the body.

Spinal Motion

The thoracic spine has the most limited motion of any area of the vertebral column. The attachment of the ribs and the overlapping of spinous processes limit motion, as does the nearly frontal orientation of the thoracic facet joints. The freest movement allowed is lateral bending. In the lumbar spine, all motions are freer than in the thoracic spine. Because of the oblique orientation of the

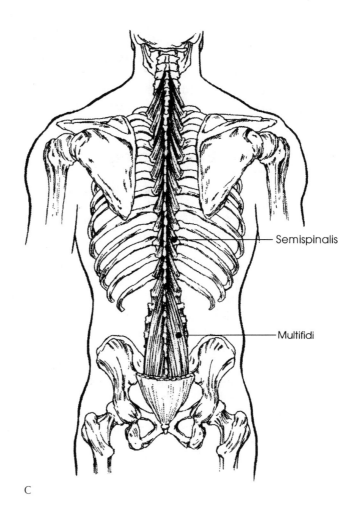

Semispinalis

Multifidi

C

facet joints and the shape of the disks, flexion and extension are the least inhibited.[6]

When bending forward from a standing position, the spine normally flexes to its limit before there is appreciable motion at the hips. As the lumbar spine flexes, the paraspinal muscles contract eccentrically. When full flexion is achieved the back is said to "hang on its ligaments." The paraspinal muscles should relax before the hips flex. Extension involves a reversal of this sequence. This motion pattern reduces the strain on the low back muscles.

In persons with poor back biomechanics, the hips tend to flex sooner in forward bending, and the paraspinal muscles never fully relax and elongate. This causes the muscles to remain isometrically contracted throughout the motion, which can exacerbate back pain.

When the spine rotates, flexes, extends, or bends to the side, the vertebrae should move on one another in a smooth, symmetrical manner. Local areas of asymmetry, hypermobility, or hypomobility are signs of back dysfunction and help identify potential areas of intervention.[7]

The annular fibers of the disk are designed to resist forces in flexion and extension. Because of their overlapping, angled fiber layers, lumbar motion that imposes rotation on a flexed back isolates some of the annular layers and may cause them to tear. Thus, repetitive or strenuous rotation of a flexed back should be avoided. When the back is not flexed, the facet joints prevent the extremes of motion that cause damage.

History and Physical Examination

In evaluating disorders of the back and spine, it is most important to differentiate neurogenic from non-neurogenic causes. The overwhelming majority of LBP patients will have nonspecific myofascial or ligamentous injury; however, herniated disk with radiculopathy, stenosis, or other neurogenic injuries must be ruled out.

The examiner begins with a complete history of the complaint. Specific questions include when and how the problem began. Does the pain radiate from the back into the buttocks or legs? What positions make the pain worse? (Pain that is worse when lying down may be a sign of an intraspinal tumor). Is the pain aggravated by coughing, sneezing, or straining to have a bowel movement (signs of herniated disk)? Patients with significant psychological components to their disorder may report their history either extremely vaguely or in excruciating detail. They may report that "everything hurts" and that no position alleviates the pain, or perhaps relate symptoms of a patently non-physiologic and nonanatomic nature.

Certain "red flags" for potentially serious conditions that come up while taking a history warrant further investigation (Table 7.1). Fracture, tumor, infection, and cauda equina syndrome all must be excluded in any patient with back pain.[8] It is also important to remember that other disorders may cause pain in the back. These include pyelonephritis, renal stones, and dissecting aortic aneurysm.[9]

Observation proceeds with an examination of the general posture and the curves of the spine. Gait should be observed to assess the fluidity of segmental spinal motion. Range of motion of the back in flexion, extension, rotation, and side-bending should be observed and any asymmetries or abnormalities noted. If bending forward (in a patient with a complaint of back and leg pain) causes the patient to bend the knee on the side of the pain, it may be a sign of nerve root compression.[10] A full neurologic examination, including deep tendon (muscle stretch) reflexes, sensation, motor strength, and coordination testing, must be performed. Toe and heel walking are simple screening tests for weakness of dorsiflexion and plantarflexion. Leg length should be measured if there is a suspicion of inequality of length (see Chapter 11).

The back, spine, and buttock must be palpated to detect any abnormalities. Pressing on the spinous processes of individual spinal segments may reveal abnormal areas of hypermobility, hypomobility, stepoff, or pain.

In addition to this general evaluation, a number of specific testing techniques deserve mention. Some of the examination maneuvers listed in Chapter 11 may also be performed, especially those for the sacroiliac joint.

TABLE 7.1   Red flags for potentially serious conditions*

Possible fracture

   Major trauma, such as motor vehicle accident or fall from a height

   Minor trauma or strenuous lifting in older or potentially osteoporotic patient

Possible tumor or infection

   Age older than 50 years or younger than 20 years

   History of cancer

   Constitutional symptoms of recent fever or chills, or unexplained weight loss

   Risk factors for spinal infection, including recent bacterial infection, intravenous drug abuse, or immune suppression (from steroids, transplant, or human immunodeficiency virus)

   Pain worse when supine; severe nighttime pain

Possible cauda equina syndrome

   Saddle anesthesia (perianal/perineal sensory loss)

   Recent onset of bladder dysfunction (retention, frequency, or overflow incontinence)

   Severe or progressive lower extremity neurologic deficit

   Unexplained laxity of the anal sphincter

   Major motor weakness in lower extremities

When suggested by history and physical examination, these findings necessitate prompt investigation.
SOURCE: S Bigos, O Bowyer, G Braen, et al. Acute Low Back Problems in Adults. Clinical Practice Guideline, Quick Reference Guide Number 14. Rockville, MD: U.S. Department of Health and Human Services, Public Health Service, Agency for Health Care Policy and Research, AHCPR Pub. No. 95-0643, December 1994.

Straight Leg Raising

During straight leg raising (SLR), the patient is asked to lie supine while the examiner passively raises the leg. Pain radiating down the leg is a positive finding for nerve root compression. Pain localized only to the low back is atypical, but has been shown surgically to correlate with nerve root compression in one small series.[11]

When performing this test, the spinal nerve roots start to be stretched between 20 and 30 degrees of leg flexion. If the patient complains of pain with less than this amount of flexion, it raises the concern of exaggeration or fabrication (although in some cases it may in fact be legitimate pain).[12] Pain at greater than 70 degrees of flexion is not as helpful, because it may be due to stretching of the hamstrings.

One way to double-check the validity of the test is to perform the SLR while the patient is sitting. This can be incorporated into the muscle strength testing part of the examination without the patient realizing what is actually being tested. A positive supine test is expected to correlate with a positive sitting test; however, this is not always the case. Care must be taken to make sure the patient sits straight. Often a person with true nerve root tension will slouch to lessen the pain.

Another method of validating a supine SLR is to raise the leg to the point where symptoms begin, then gently dorsiflex and plantarflex the ankle or internally and externally rotate the hip. Usually, dorsiflexion of the ankle or internal rotation of the hip increases the radiating pain, whereas the opposite movements may decrease pain.[13]

Sometimes patients complain of pain shooting down the leg when the contralateral leg is raised. This is called the *well-leg SLR (Fajersztajn) test* or *cross-leg pain* and, if positive, is also a sign of nerve root tension or compression.

Femoral Nerve Stretch Test

The femoral nerve stretch test is similar to the SLR test in that it aims to reproduce radiating leg pain. The patient lies prone while the examiner passively flexes the leg at the knee. This preferentially stretches the upper- to mid-lumbar nerve roots, whereas the SLR stretches the lower nerve roots. Pain radiating into the leg, especially the anterior thigh and lower leg, is a positive finding, but must be interpreted with caution, as this test also stretches the quadriceps.

Passive and Active Back Extension Testing

During passive and active back extension testing, the prone patient is asked to prop up on the elbows and allow the back to sag. In conditions of muscle strain this is painless; however, in facet joint disorders, nerve root compression, or other ligamentous or joint conditions, pain may worsen. The patient is then asked to put the arms by the side and lift the chin and chest off the table. This is an active test of the paraspinal muscles, and pain during this maneuver in the absence of pain on passive extension is a sign of muscle strain.

Cat/Camel Exercises

During cat/camel exercises, the patient, while propped on the hands and knees, is told to push the back up towards the ceiling and then let it sag toward the table. This tests whether flexion or extension of the back worsens or lessens symptoms, and may help in deciding which form of exercise (flexion versus extension) should be prescribed.

Rectal Examination

Rectal examination is often performed in patients with back or pelvic pain of insidious onset. It may identify tumors or an enlarged prostate in some cases. It also allows palpation of the undersurface of the piriformis muscle.

Waddell Criteria

Assessment of low back pain can be frustrating and confusing when dealing with a patient suspected of having psychological overlay to his or her physical dysfunction. Waddell et al.[14] have described a simple series of tests to help identify those LBP patients who have significant nonorganic signs (Table 7.2). Objective recognition of these signs can help identify patients who require formal psychosocial evaluation or who are malingerers. However, it is important to realize that these behavioral signs can and do occur concurrently with clear organic findings and that both physical and psychosocial intervention may be warranted.[15]

Ancillary Diagnostic Testing

The majority of cases of LBP of less than 4 weeks' duration do not require imaging studies; a thorough history and physical examination are sufficient. In an acute injury in which there is a possibility of spinal fracture or subluxation, or when red flags suggest an increased risk of neoplasm or infection, radiographs should be obtained.[9] Such radiographs are also valuable in other conditions to evaluate bony alignment and segmental stability, signs of degeneration, and congenital anomalies.

The anteroposterior view gives a general measure of bony alignment. Lateral views reveal additional information about the state of the disks, the facet joint, and the bony alignment. Oblique views are used to visualize the intervertebral foramina and the pars interarticularis (bone between the superior and inferior zygapophysial processes). Flexion and extension or side-bending views help to detect areas of abnormal spinal mobility.

TABLE 7.2   Waddell's nonorganic physical signs*

Nonorganic tenderness

Superficial skin tenderness to light touch over a wide area of lumbar skin not corresponding to a single dermatome, or

Nonanatomic deep tenderness over a wide area not localized to any particular structure are positive findings.

Simulation tests

If axial loading (on the head) or rotation of the whole body (not the lumbar spine) causes low back pain, it is a positive finding.

Distraction testing

If sitting straight leg raise test is negative, whereas supine straight leg raising causes pain it is a positive finding.

Regional pain complaints

If whole regions of the body, such as the entire leg, are affected in a non-physiologic manner, it is a positive finding. This includes sensory or motor deficits.

Overreaction

Excessive grimacing, tremor, collapsing, or complaining during the examination is a positive finding.

*If three or more of the five categories are positive, it is a sign of significant psychologic dysfunction or malingering.
SOURCE: G Waddell, JA McCulloch, E Kummel, et al. Nonorganic physical signs in low-back pain. Spine 1980;5(2):117–125.

Magnetic resonance imaging (MRI) has become an invaluable tool in evaluating the spine and is the best test to assess the disks, the soft tissues, and some spinal cord tumors.

Computed tomography (CT) testing reveals most fractures, joint disease, and spinal masses. Herniated disks are also well visualized.

It should be noted that in asymptomatic adults, up to 25% show degenerative changes on plain films of the spine, and 30% are found to have a major abnormality on MRI. Therefore, correlation between physical and radiographic findings is crucial.[9,16]

MRI reports often describe a "bulging" disk. This is not the same thing as a herniation and is not generally clinically significant; patients should not be made to worry needlessly about these bulges.

Other studies that may prove helpful include electromyography (EMG), myelography, bone scan, and diskography. EMG can diagnose and often localize radiculopathy. It gives information about the actual state of the nerves, as opposed to MRI, which simply shows anatomy, regardless of clinical significance. Myelography gives information about the spinal cord and roots, and is typically combined with CT for better accuracy; however, it is seldom used today. A bone scan may detect stress fractures, bone tumors, and infection. Diskography involves the injection of saline or radiopaque contrast into the disk to see if there is leakage of contrast out of a damaged disk or if the injection reproduces pain.

A practical suggestion for ordering imaging studies comes from Staiger et al.[9] For non-radicular LBP without a history of trauma or warning signs of a potentially serious condition, it is reasonable to wait 4 weeks before ordering anteroposterior and lateral spine films, if pain persists. If occult infection or neoplasm are suggested, a bone scan or MRI, along with a complete blood count and erythrocyte sedimentation rate, should be obtained without delay. For radicular LBP, excluding cauda equina syndrome and rapidly progressing neurologic compromise (both of which require prompt evaluation and management), it is reasonable to wait 4 weeks before proceeding with spine films, EMG, and MRI.

It may be reasonable to perform the EMG first. If it is negative, an MRI is not usually necessary; this avoids the detection of coincidental but clinically insignificant findings. If the EMG is positive, an MRI is warranted to detect the anatomic cause (if any) resulting in nerve damage.

In addition to these imaging studies, connective tissue screening tests, blood counts, blood chemistries, and other laboratory tests may at times be warranted.

Specific Disorders of the Back and Spine

Acute Back Strain or Sprain

Nonspecific strain or sprain is by far the most common condition of the back. It is usually attributed to a single incident, such as lifting a heavy object while twisting, but the underlying cause is usually a lifetime of improper back motion. Structures that may be injured include the paraspinal muscles, the intervertebral ligaments, the iliolumbar ligaments, the facet joint capsules, or even the annular fibers of the intervertebral disks.

Once the injury has occurred, the muscles of the low back splint the damaged area in what is commonly called *muscle guarding* or a *back spasm*. This spasm is typically present supine and standing, and often causes a scoliosis or "listing" to one side. To differentiate spasm from voluntary contraction, the patient is asked to place all his or her weight on one foot and then the other while the examiner gently palpates the paraspinal muscles. The normal response is relaxation of the paraspinal muscles on the weight-bearing side. If relaxation is noted, it usually means true muscle spasm is not present.[13] In time, if the painful muscle splinting and improper posture persist, the patient will develop local soft tissue contracture and chronic or recurrent back pain.

Back strain occurs mostly in the 30- to 60-year age range and appears to have a higher incidence in poorly conditioned persons and in those with poor back extensor muscle endurance, although recent studies have refuted this finding.[17] It is also commonly believed to be more prevalent in persons with poor flexibility, coordination, posture, and muscle strength, although a direct cause-and-effect of these factors has not been proven. It has been associated with heavy lifting, whole body vibration, spinal loading, postural stress, and dynamic trunk motion.[18] Back strain recurs frequently, and one of the best predictors for future back pain is a history of back pain.[19]

Diagnosis

The patient with back strain or sprain usually relays a history of acute back pain associated with lifting or bending. Often the back is injured while performing unaccustomed activity, such as shoveling the first snow of the year or raking leaves. The pain may be minor the day of injury, but the patient may wake up the next day with severe discomfort. Movement is generally restricted in all directions due to pain.

On physical examination the patient may have an antalgic gait, resist quick movements, and resist extremes of range-of-motion and muscle-strength testing due to pain. Neurologic testing is normal, but there may be local muscle tenderness or splinting, especially in the paraspinal muscles. Straight leg raising is negative, and other provocative tests are normal, except for possibly causing local back pain. Radiographic studies, if obtained, are usually normal as well.

Treatment

Acute strains and sprains generally recover within a few days to a week, regardless of treatment. A few days of relative rest, ice (and later, ice or heat), and nonsteroidal anti-inflammatory drugs (NSAIDs), followed by a gradual return to activity, is usually successful. Muscle relaxants are also helpful in the early period, especially when prescribed as a single bedtime dose to help the patient get a restful night's sleep.[20]

The length of time of rest for back injuries is continuously debated. Just a few years ago, it was not unusual for patients to have prescriptions for 2–5 weeks of complete bed rest for any type of back injury. Patients were instructed to arise only for the purposes of toileting and eating. In a randomized clinical trial, Deyo et al.[21] studied two groups of patients with non-neurogenic back pain who were assigned to 2 days or 7 days of bed rest. They found that, although neither group complied well with the recommendation for bed rest, the group with less rest time fared better and returned to work more quickly. Complete bed rest is probably never indicated for back strain, as it leads to a loss of muscle mass and strength.

From a preventive standpoint, randomized controlled trials, for the most part, have been unable to demonstrate any significant prevention of low back pain through the use of lifting instructions, body mechanics instructions, or lumbar supports, although formal back school programs have been shown to be effective.[22,23] Rate of injury, time off work, cost, and rate of repeat injury were not affected—only the subject's knowledge of safe behavior was shown to increase through education.[24]

After back injury, flexibility and strength deficits need to be addressed, and proper sitting and workstation posture should be taught. Less vigorous day-to-day activities are encouraged, using pain as the activity-limiting factor. As a rule, a vigorous strengthening program should be deferred for approximately 6 weeks after injury to allow the damaged tissues to heal properly.

In approximately 90% of patients, symptoms resolve within 4–6 weeks.[8] If no improvement occurs in the first 2–4 weeks after injury, if there is still persistent pain after 4–6 weeks, or if symptoms are resolving more slowly than expected, a more specialized, conservative treatment program may be indicated. Further diagnostic workup should be considered, and it may be necessary to prescribe a more aggressive treatment protocol. For treatment, deep heat, soft tissue mobilization, and muscle relaxation techniques may be added. Occasionally corticosteroid injections help to relieve local muscle pain. The patient should work with a back therapist to correct posture and back biomechanics and start on a progressive stretching and strengthening program. Patients should be reminded that activity is not harmful and that it does not necessarily worsen pain. Exercise can decrease pain, illness behavior, and distress, while simultaneously improving function.

This approach is almost always successful. In persons with a behavioral aspect to their pain, psychological treatment may be added. In cases refractory to treatment, a work conditioning program and possibly permanent work or activity restrictions may be needed.

Disk Herniation and Radiculopathy

When the annulus fibrosis of the disk develops a defect, the inner nucleus pulposus may protrude outward. This can occur with a traumatic event, such as a fall on the buttock, but most often the annular tears develop slowly from a lifetime of repetitive trauma. Then, one day, an acute herniation of the nuclear material occurs due to a minor event, or no event at all.

Disk herniation by itself is painful. But the herniated portion releases inflammatory chemicals that can irritate the nerve root,[25,26] or may directly compress the nerve root. In either of these cases, the herniation leads to radiculopathy. Not all herniated disks cause radiculopathy, and not all radiculopathies are caused by herniated disks.

Radiculopathy can cause pain to radiate into the buttock and leg and may cause sensory, motor strength, or reflex changes in the leg as well. The local disk injury results in pain in the low back. It is often said that the radiating pain must go below the level of the knee to be due to a radiculopathy, but this is not the case.

It is important to use the term *radiculopathy* correctly. It is not synonymous with *herniated disk*, nor with *radiating pain*. It is pathology of the nerve root. It is sometimes called *sciatica*, although technically sciatica could be due to sciatic neuropathy more distal to the nerve root level.

Diagnosis

Radiculopathy is suspected when the patient complains of both back and leg pain arising over the course of a few hours or, in some cases, a few days. Ninety-five percent of lumbar disk herniations occur at the L4–L5 or L5–S1 disks, irritating the L5 and S1 nerve roots, so special attention should be paid to the distribution of these roots.[27] Usually there are sensory, reflex, or motor changes in the extremity, although these may be subtle and difficult to detect due to generalized pain and muscle guarding. The L5 level is the most commonly affected by radiculopathy, and there is no good L5 reflex. Straight leg raising would be expected to be positive, but sometimes is normal. Femoral nerve stretch is sometimes positive.

The patient presents with a resistance to movement of the back and associated painful paraspinal muscle splinting. Coughing, sneezing, or straining to have a bowel movement (or any other maneuver that raises intra-abdominal, and therefore intradiskal, pressure) often exacerbates the leg pain.

Definitive diagnosis of radiculopathy is made with EMG testing and clinical impression, whereas mechanical disk herniation can be demonstrated by CT, MRI, or myelography. MRI is the best of these tests at imaging the disk, but given the number of asymptomatic positives on MRI studies, it is important to correlate MRI and EMG findings, especially when surgery is considered.[16]

Certain individuals develop LBP that fails conservative treatment and becomes chronic and function-limiting. A subset of these patients have pain that is generated by the pain fibers in the annulus fibrosis. This discogenic pain typically is described as LBP that may be exacerbated by sitting, bending, lifting, and axial loading. Radicular signs and symptoms are absent, although there may be some referral of pain into the lower extremity. Imaging studies do not reveal nerve root compression. Diagnosis of discogenic pain may be confirmed by provocative diskography.

Treatment

Almost all herniated disks can be treated conservatively. Treatment is aimed at reducing the intradiskal pressure to prevent a progression of the herniation until the annular tear heals, which usually occurs within 6–8 weeks.

As with acute lumbar strain, careful study shows that for patients with documented nerve root irritation, bed rest is not more effective than relative rest with participation in daily activities.[28] In some cases, bed rest may be prescribed for 5–7 days in cases of acutely herniated disks.[22,29] Activities should be limited to those which do not increase pain or neurologic symptoms. NSAIDs and muscle relaxants may be prescribed, and opioid analgesics are often necessary for adequate pain control. Stool softeners, fluids, and a high-fiber diet make it easier to have bowel movements with less straining. Back flexion is avoided. A trial of gentle extension exercises may help to reduce symptoms; if symptoms worsen, exercises should be discontinued. Traction may be tried in treatment as well. Its benefits are not well documented and it may not be well tolerated, but in some patients it is quite effective.

Although the clinical significance of intradiskal pressure variations is not completely understood, it makes sense that persons with herniated disks would benefit from lower pressures. This may prevent further herniation. Consequently, in the early rehabilitation of patients with herniated nucleus pulposus (HNP), lifting while flexing the trunk and practicing flexion exercises are avoided.

Epidural steroid injection or oral steroids should be considered in treatment, especially when conservative measures fail.[30] Corticosteroids reduce the swelling and inflammation around the nerve root and may hasten recovery.

After the acutely painful period has passed, the patient starts a slowly progressive program of return to activity. Prolonged sitting or driving, excessive back flexion, lifting, bending, and twisting should be avoided for 6–8 weeks.

After this initial treatment time, proper back mechanics are taught, strengthening exercises are begun (starting with isometrics and stabilization exercises), and the patient gradually returns to a normal life. In rare cases, patients have some permanent nerve damage and do not recover completely. These patients may benefit from a trial of aggressive strengthening exercise and possible permanent work/activity restriction.

Most patients can be expected to improve within 6 weeks using the conservative program outlined here.[27] One exception is those with HNP with concomitant lateral stenosis.[31] The presence of such stenosis is not an absolute indication for surgery, but it reduces the success rate for conservative care from approximately 90% to the 65–75% range.[32] If patients have not responded to conservative care by 8 weeks, they should be given the option to proceed to surgery.[33] They should be advised that they have not yet "failed" conservative care, just that they are slow responders. It is still appropriate to continue conservative care, although resolution of symptoms might be faster with surgery. Long-term outcome is probably unchanged, even if surgery is postponed for 3 months.[34]

Other considerations for surgery include persons with central disk herniation with myelopathy (mainly thoracic), persons with intractable pain, and those with progressive neurologic deficits. Patients should always be asked what their worst pain complaint is: back or leg pain. If back pain is the answer, surgery is probably not the cure. Surgery may alleviate leg pain, but it is not as useful for back pain.[35]

Saal and Saal[31] discovered that patients with HNP, leg pain, and radiculopathy—who would usually be considered to have met the criteria for surgery—could be treated just as well with aggressive rehabilitation. They found that a failure of nonoperative treatment was not a sufficient reason to operate, and that the presence of weakness did not adversely affect the outcome of conservative treatment. They also noted that conservatively treated patients fared just as well as those treated with surgery, even within the first year. Furthermore, they found that patients treated with delayed surgery (more than 16 weeks) had good to excellent outcomes as well. They considered progressive neurologic deficit to be an indication for surgery and identified a subgroup of patients with HNP plus spinal stenosis who were less likely to respond to conservative care. Patients with simple extruded disks did well without surgery.

In another study, Saal et al.[33] found that the natural history of extruded disks was one of eventual resorption with no residual perithecal or perineural fibrosis (often cited as reasons to perform surgery early).

Recently, a nonsurgical treatment has become available for patients with chronic, discogenic pain. Known as *intradiskal electrothermal annuloplasty and nuclectomy*, this procedure uses a thermal catheter to denervate the pain-sensitive structures in the surrounding annulus fibrosis. The catheter is placed in the intact nucleus pulposus under fluoroscopic guidance and is heated to 90°C on a specific protocol. The study population was treated conservatively for at least 6 months before undergoing the procedure. Initial results are promising for the successful treatment of chronic, non-radicular low back pain; however, long-term follow-up studies are pending.[36]

Degenerative Joint Disease and Spinal Stenosis

Degenerative joint disease (DJD) (Figure 7.7) occurs in the spine just as it does in many other parts of the body. The cause is unknown but may involve aging, overuse, trauma, or genetic predisposition. In the spine, it is also known as *spondylosis.*

As age increases, progressive degenerative changes occur in the intervertebral disk, the facet joints, and the vertebral body. The water content of the disk decreases, making it more vulnerable to shear and compression. As this occurs, the disk itself thins, leading to decreased space between vertebrae and over-riding of the facet joints. These joints undergo osteoarthritic changes, with formation of bony osteophytes. Osteoporosis and subsequent vertebral body collapse can compound these degenerative changes.[37] Also, certain individuals have congenitally narrow canals, which makes them more susceptible to problems due to these degenerative changes.

The combination of osteophytes and decreased intervertebral space can narrow the intervertebral foramina (lateral stenosis) and the spinal canal

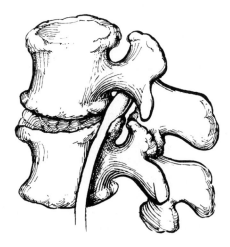

FIGURE 7.7   *Degenerative disease of the spine, involving bony spurring, disk-space narrowing, and foraminal encroachment.*

(central stenosis), resulting in a decrease in physical space surrounding the cauda equina and spinal nerve roots. Bulging disks and redundant folds of the ligamentum flavum further decrease the available space.[38] When these degenerative elements cause sufficient narrowing of the spinal canal or foramina, they can lead to compression of the nerve roots and other contents of the canal.

Diagnosis

The symptoms of DJD include nonspecific complaints of back pain, often exacerbated by extension and relieved by moderate activity. The condition usually has an insidious onset, with increased prevalence associated with advancing age. Patients complain of morning stiffness, decreased back range of motion, and pain on extremes of movement. In advanced cases, radiographs show signs of disk-space narrowing, facet degeneration, and bony spurring.

In central spinal stenosis, the compression of the spinal contents classically causes symptoms of bilateral leg pain, numbness, and weakness, which are brought on or worsened by spine extension. These patients often complain of pain when walking or standing that is relieved only by sitting, lying down, or lumbar flexion.[39] The pain is not due to the exercise itself, as affected people can walk pushing a cart or in a stooped posture without developing the leg pain. This is known as *pseudoclaudication*, which is often confused with *intermittent claudication*, a condition of poor arterial blood supply to the legs. Intermittent claudication causes ischemic leg pain with exercise regardless of the position of the spine. The pain is relieved by rest in any position.

The characteristic history of symptoms of central spinal stenosis helps in making the diagnosis. Patients often have signs of multilevel radiculopathy, with mild reflex, sensory, or motor changes as well. Imaging studies, such as CT or MRI, reveal the spinal narrowing, whereas EMG can help detect the nerve damage. Isolated lateral stenosis can cause the symptoms of radiculopathy described earlier. EMG may be positive, but imaging studies will reveal bony narrowing, rather than disk herniation (sometimes both are seen together).

Treatment

Because DJD is not reversible, patients often have a series of recurring flare-ups of their back pain. These exacerbations become less frequent and less severe with aging as the spine stabilizes. Treatment is aimed at alleviating pain and maintaining mobility.

Acute exacerbations of DJD are treated with rest, heat, and NSAIDs. This is followed by a maintenance program of gentle strengthening, flexibility, and aerobic exercises. Water aerobics are particularly well tolerated.

For patients with central spinal stenosis, flexion exercises often keep symptoms of pseudoclaudication tolerable. They often do better with bicycling than with walking, because bicycling is done with a flexed back.[38] Various modalities have been used, although none has proven to be particularly helpful. Patients may benefit from using NSAIDs, a cane or walker, and soft shoe inserts. A rigid plastic brace designed to decrease lumbar lordosis may be beneficial, although the need for custom fitting, the cost, and the discomfort decrease its utility.[39] Epidural steroid injections are of questionable value for the treatment of spinal stenosis,[38] although some advocate a trial of one or two doses.[39] If symptoms are limiting enough, surgical decompression of the spinal canal is necessary.[38]

Sacroiliac Dysfunction

See Chapter 11.

Spondylolysis and Spondylolisthesis

A defect in the pars interarticularis is known as *spondylolysis. Spondylolisthesis* is a forward slippage of one vertebra relative to the vertebra it sits on (backward slippage is called *retrolisthesis*). It can be due to a traumatic event, degeneration of the facet joints, or a defect of the pars interarticularis of the arch of the vertebrae (also known as *isthmic spondylolisthesis*).[40]

Spondylolysis can present as a stress fracture or a true fracture with bony separation.[41] It is not present at birth, but cases have been reported in infants from 6 weeks to 10 months in age.[40] Fredrickson et al.[42] followed 500 first-grade children over 25 years. They reported a prevalence of 4.4% at age 6, rising to 6.0% by adulthood. Spondylolysis occurs twice as often in men as in women, but the most severe cases are usually seen in women.[40] Spondylolysis in children is not generally associated with pain or with spondylolisthesis. Most people with spondylolysis are asymptomatic and never seek medical attention; however, among adolescents referred for evaluation of back pain, the prevalence of spondylolysis ranges from 13% to 47%.[41,43]

The cause of spondylolysis is unclear. Factors that may play a role include congenital predisposition (associated to some degree with spina bifida occulta), bony degeneration, trauma, growth, posture, repetitive stress, and athletic training (specifically, activities that require repetitive hyperextension and rotation, such as gymnastics, soccer, wrestling, and football).[40,41] It occurs most commonly at the L5–S1 junction and less frequently at L4–L5.

Patients with spondylolisthesis are typically asymptomatic. Those who develop pain complain of dull, chronic, midline lumbosacral pain that is located along the beltline. They commonly have tight hamstrings and may have symptoms of sciatica. Pain is exacerbated by spinal extension.[41] Spondylolisthesis predisposes to developing disk disease above the level of the defect; in some cases, this may be the actual source of the symptoms.

Diagnosis
In the adolescent athlete complaining of LBP, inspection and palpation of the spine may reveal a stepoff from one vertebral spinous process to the next, suggesting spondylolisthesis. If pain is produced by extension or by extension with rotation, this should raise suspicion of spondylolysis.

Lumbosacral spine films including oblique views are obtained when either spondylolysis or spondylolisthesis is suspected. The characteristic finding for spondylolysis is the broken neck of the "Scottie Dog"—the fractured pars interarticularis—seen on the oblique view. If radiographs are normal but spondylolysis is still suspected, a bone scan or single-photon emission CT scan may be helpful in demonstrating stress fractures. CT and MRI are less helpful.[41] The severity of spondylolisthesis is classified according the degree of anterior slippage or translation of the superior vertebral body on the inferior one on lateral spine films, as originally described by Meyerding in 1933.[44] Grade 1 is a slippage of less than 25% of the diameter of the vertebral body; grade 2 is less than 50%; grade 3 is less than 75%; and grade 4 is more than 75%.

Treatment

For symptomatic spondylolysis, pain relief, healing of the lesion, and prevention of further injury are the goals. Rest from competitive sports may be indicated for athletes, and physical therapy may be helpful for lumbar stabilization, abdominal strengthening, and hip flexor and hamstring stretching.[41]

Grade 1 and 2 spondylolistheses often cause no symptoms and require no treatment. Children with grade 1 slippage should be advised to avoid any future occupation with heavy labor, and those with grade 2 displacement should be warned against participation in contact sports or sports involving lumbar hyperextension, such as football or gymnastics. Radiographic observation should continue every 4–6 months until age 10, every 6 months until age 15, and every year thereafter until growth stops.[40] Progression of a slip is unlikely after adolescence.[42]

Symptomatic slippages up to 50% may be treated nonoperatively with antilordotic bracing (often for several years), abdominal flexion strengthening exercise, stretching programs, activity modifications, and radiographic follow-up as above. Surgical evaluation is indicated for any grade 3 or 4 slippage in a growing child, for persistent pain despite conservative treatment in grade 1 or 2 slippages, and in any grade slippage with progressive neurologic deficits or severe pain.[40]

Osteoporotic Vertebral Compression Fractures

Osteoporosis is a common disease associated with considerable morbidity and mortality. In the spine, vertebral fractures secondary to osteoporosis number approximately 700,000 each year.[45] Patients typically have multiple fractures over the years, as the vertebral bodies "crumble" away. Each fracture is painful for 4–6 weeks, until it heals. However, the vertebral body does not regain the height lost due to the fracture, so a kyphosis gradually develops.

Diagnosis

Diagnosis is typically made using a dual-energy x-ray absorptiometry scan, with results compared to age-corrected standards. A result from 1.0 to 2.4 standard deviations below normal bone mass indicates significant bone loss and osteopenia; a result below 2.5 standard deviations indicates frank osteoporosis.[46]

Treatment

Acute osteoporotic fractures of the spine are treated with pain medicine as needed over the 4–6 weeks that the fracture takes to heal. Other issues that must be addressed during this time include deep venous thrombosis prevention (if the patient is nonambulatory) and avoidance of nicotine or corticosteroids (which may slow fracture healing), and adequate caloric intake.[47]

Recently, two minimally invasive procedures for management of acute vertebral fractures have been developed. Known as *vertebroplasty* and *kyphoplasty*, they involve the injection of a bone cement into the fractured vertebral body. Neither controlled trials nor long-term follow-up studies have been completed.[47]

Prevention and treatment of osteoporosis focuses on building and maintaining healthy bones. Adequate calcium intake during childhood (700 mg per day) and adolescence (1,300 mg per day) is essential to build peak bone mass, which is achieved at age 25. Maintenance of that bone mass requires 800 mg per day for adults, but varies with pregnancy (1,500 mg per day), lactation (2,000 mg per day), and during recovery from a major fracture (1,500 mg per day). Post-menopausal women require 1,500 mg per day. In addition to calcium intake, a woman's hormonal status and exercise level are crucial for achieving and maintaining bone mass.[46]

Medications such as estrogen for menopausal women, calcitonin, bisphosphonates, and oral calcium all play a role in prevention and treatment.[48] It is important to remember that women who are post-menopausal due to oophorectomy require pharmacologic treatment earlier in life.[46] An investigational study involving parathyroid hormone has shown promising results, with a decrease in the risk of fractures and an increase in bone density.[49]

In addition to medication, exercise (walking or jogging three times a week for 50–60 minutes) has been shown to increase bone mineral density in post-menopausal women. Resistance training can increase bone mass, but only when it is strength-oriented, rather than endurance-oriented. Gains that can be made with exercise are, unfortunately, lost quickly if activity is halted. It is important to remember that these individuals often have other medical problems; careful screening is necessary before prescribing any exercise program.[50]

Chronic Back Pain/Failed Back Syndrome

It is no surprise that chronic back pain and failed back syndrome are often considered to be synonymous, as a "failed back" is generally considered to be one that has not responded to surgery. Indeed, it is hard to find a patient with chronic back pain who has not had back surgery; many have had several operations. This is not to say that surgery causes all chronic back pain, just that it is not a particularly good treatment for it.

Chronic back pain is the end result of back dysfunction in some individuals, who never recover normal function, flexibility, and strength after acute back strain, disk herniation, or surgery. They generally wind up with inflexible spines, excessive muscle splinting, and poor back biomechanics. These patients often become obsessed with their pain, allowing it to dominate their private and working lives. Several factors have been identified as having an impact on the transition from acute to chronic pain, as well as on return to work. These include financial issues, length of time off work, and job satisfaction.[51,52]

Once a person has developed chronic back pain, it is difficult to treat. Therefore it is important to make sure that acute back patients are not allowed to slip into a passive role in which they "protect" their backs from activity or exercise; rely on narcotic analgesia, injections, or indefinite physical therapy; and make back pain the focus of their existence.

When chronic pain has developed, it must be treated with a multidisciplinary approach to restore mobility and strength, teach relaxation, regain a sense of proportion, and help the patient to regain control over life.

Pain clinics, work hardening, and functional restoration programs may be useful in these patients. Further discussion of chronic pain is found in Chapter 21.

Facet Joint Pain

There appears to be a subset of LBP patients who have primary facet joint pathology. Although there has been much debate about the existence of a "facet syndrome," it is generally accepted that the facet joints are a source of LBP. However, with prevalence data ranging from 6% to 94%, there remains controversy as to the best way to diagnose the problem.[53]

History and physical examination alone are not sufficient to diagnose facet problems. Diagnostic injection of the facet joint under fluoroscopic guidance is required. However, the difficulty then becomes selecting appropriate patients to refer for diagnostic injection. Revel et al.[54] find that patients may be selected for facet joint injection if they have LBP that is not exacerbated by coughing, by forward flexion, by hyperextension, by extension with rotation, or when rising from forward flexion, and in whom pain is well-relieved in the recumbent position. If these criteria are met, then 92% of the patients who will respond to injection are selected, whereas 80% who would not respond are excluded.

One difficulty with single diagnostic blocks is their high false-positive rate. Schwarzer et al.[53] suggest that techniques using controls with either extra-articular injection of saline or a series of two local anesthetic blocks may be more reliable for diagnosis of facet joint pain.

Once the diagnosis of facet joint pain has been confirmed, it is treated more permanently with radiofrequency denervation of the facet joint. This is also done under fluoroscopic guidance. Results have been promising for this technique, with significant alleviation of pain and functional disability shown for 12 months.[55]

Other Causes of Back Pain

Numerous other conditions may cause or be associated with back and spinal pain. They include scoliosis, Scheuermann's disease, and spina bifida. In addition, myofascial pain, fibromyalgia, tumors, disk infections, and referred pain syndromes may cause back pain.

Points of Summary

1. Acute low back sprain or strain should not be treated with bed rest.
2. Imaging studies for most episodes of low back pain are not needed, unless pain persists for more than 4 weeks.
3. Potentially serious conditions such as cancer, infection, fracture, and cauda equina syndrome must be investigated promptly if history or physical examination raises suspicion.
4. Almost all herniated disks, even when they are associated with weakness and neurologic deficits, can be treated conservatively.

5. The subset of patients with herniated disks and lateral stenosis may respond more slowly to conservative care.
6. Degenerative disease of the spine causes the insidious onset of low back pain, decreased and painful range of motion, and morning stiffness.
7. Spondylolysis is a defect in the pars interarticularis. Spondylolisthesis is a forward slippage of one vertebra on the one below it.
8. Prevention of osteoporosis begins by building peak bone mass and continues throughout life with maintenance of healthy bone.
9. The Waddell criteria can be useful in objectively measuring nonorganic examination findings.
10. EMG is useful in diagnosing nerve damage, but cannot determine the anatomic cause of that damage; MRI depicts anatomy, but cannot determine whether there is nerve damage.
11. MRI has a high rate of "coincidental" findings.
12. Symptoms of pseudoclaudication are relieved by bending forward, whereas those of intermittent claudication are relieved by rest.

References

1. Andersson GBJ. Epidemiological features of chronic low-back pain. Lancet 1999;354:581–585.
2. Wilke HJ, Neef P, Caimi M, et al. New in vivo measurements of pressures in the intervertebral disk in daily life. Spine 1999;24(8):755–762.
3. Bogduk N. The innervation of the lumbar spine. Spine 1983;8(3):286–293.
4. Cavanaugh JM, Ozaktay AC, Yamashita T, et al. Mechanisms of low back pain: a neurophysiologic and neuroanatomic study. Clin Orthop 1997;335:166–180.
5. Jackson HC, Winkelmann RK, Bickel WH. Nerve endings in the human lumbar spinal column and related structures. J Bone Joint Surg Am 1966;48A(7):1272–1281.
6. Jenkins DB. Hollinshead's Functional Anatomy of the Limbs and Back (7th ed). Philadelphia: Saunders, 1998.
7. Mayer TG, Robinson R, Pegues P, et al. Lumbar segmental rigidity: Can its identification with facet injections and stretching exercises be useful? Arch Phys Med Rehabil 2000;81:1143–1150.
8. Bigos S, Bowyer O, Braen G, et al. Acute Low Back Problems in Adults. Clinical Practice Guideline, Quick Reference Guide Number 14. Rockville, MD: U.S. Department of Health and Human Services, Public Health Service, Agency for Health Care Policy and Research, AHCPR Pub. No. 95-0643, December 1994.
9. Staiger TO, Paauw DS, Deyo RA, et al. Imaging studies for acute low back pain. Postgrad Med 1999;105(4):161–172.
10. Rask M. Knee flexion test and sciatica. Clin Orthop 1978;134:221.
11. Kosteljanetz M, Bang F, Schmidt-Olsen S. The clinical significance of straight-leg raising (Lasègue's sign) in the diagnosis of prolapsed lumbar disc. Spine 1988;13(4):393–395.
12. Breig A, Troup JDG. Biomechanical considerations in the straight-leg-raising test. Spine 1979;4(3):242–250.

13. Cocchiarella L, Andersson GBJ (eds). Guides to the evaluation of permanent impairment (5th ed). Chicago: AMA Press, 2000.
14. Waddell G, McCulloch JA, Kummel E, et al. Nonorganic physical signs in low-back pain. Spine 1980;5(2):117–125.
15. Main CJ, Waddell G. Behavioral responses to examination. Spine 1998;23(21):2367–2371.
16. Boden SD, Davis DO, Dina TS, et al. Abnormal magnetic-resonance scans of the lumbar spine in asymptomatic subjects. J Bone Joint Surg Am 1990;72A(3):403–408.
17. Malanga GA, Nadler SF. Nonoperative treatment of low back pain. Mayo Clin Proc 1999;74(11):1135–1148.
18. Frank JW, Kerr MS, Brooker A, et al. Disability resulting from occupational low back pain. Spine 1996;21(24):2908–2917.
19. Smedley J, Inskip H, Cooper C, et al. Natural history of low back pain. Spine 1998;23(22):2422–2426.
20. Cherkin DC, Wheeler KJ, Barlow W, et al. Medication use for low back pain in primary care. Spine 1998;23(5):607–614.
21. Deyo RA, Diehl AK, Rosenthal M. How many days of bed rest for acute low back pain? N Engl J Med 1986;315(17):1064–1070.
22. van Tulder MW, Koes BW, Bouter LM. Conservative treatment of acute and chronic nonspecific low back pain. Spine 1997;22(18):2128–2156.
23. van Poppel MNM, Koes BW, van der Ploeg T. Lumbar supports and education for the prevention of low back pain in industry. JAMA 1998; 279(22):1789–1794.
24. Daltroy LH, Iversen MD, Larson MG, et al. A controlled trial of an educational program to prevent low back injuries. N Engl J Med 1997;337(5): 322–328.
25. Rosomoff HL. Do herniated disks produce pain? Clin J Pain 1985;1(2): 91–93.
26. Goupille P, Jayson MIV, Valat J, et al. The role of inflammation in disk herniation-associated radiculopathy. Semin Arthritis Rheum 1998; 28(1):60–71.
27. Della-Giustina DA. Emergency department evaluation and treatment of back pain. Emerg Med Clin North Am 1999;17(4):877–893.
28. Vroomen PC, de Krom MC, Wilmink JT. Lack of effectiveness of bed rest for sciatica. N Engl J Med 1999;340(6):418–423.
29. Deyo RA, Loeser JD, Bigos SJ. Herniated lumbar intervertebral disk. Ann Intern Med 1990;112(8):598–603.
30. Rivest C, Natz JN, Ferrante M, et al. Effects of epidural steroid injection on pain due to lumbar spinal stenosis or herniated disks: a prospective study. Arthritis Res 1998;11(4):291–297.
31. Saal JA, Saal JS. Nonoperative treatment of herniated lumbar intervertebral disk with radiculopathy: an outcome study. Spine 1989;14(4): 431–437.
32. Saal JA. Intervertebral disk herniation: advances in nonoperative treatment. Phys Med Rehabil Clin N Am 1990;4(2):175–190.
33. Saal JA, Saal JS, Herzog RJ. The natural history of lumbar intervertebral disk extrusions treated nonoperatively. Spine 1990;15(7):683–686.
34. Shvartzman L, Weingarten E, Sherry H, et al. Cost-effectiveness analysis of extended conservative therapy versus surgical intervention in the

management of herniated lumbar intervertebral disc. Spine 1992;17(2): 176–182.

35. Postacchini F. Management of herniation of the lumbar disc. J Bone Joint Surg Br 1999;81B(4):567–576.
36. Saal JS, Saal JA. Management of chronic discogenic low back pain with a thermal intradiskal catheter. Spine 2000;25(3):382–388.
37. Mazanec DJ. Evaluating back pain in older patients. Cleve Clin J Med 1999;66(2):89–99.
38. Spivak JM. Degenerative lumbar spinal stenosis. J Bone Joint Surg Am 1998;80A(7):1053–1066.
39. Nagler W, Hausen HS. Conservative management of lumbar spinal stenosis. Postgrad Med 1998;103(4):69–88.
40. Lonstein JE. Spondylolisthesis in children. Spine 1999;24(24):2640–2648.
41. Garry JP, McShane J. Lumbar spondylolysis in adolescent athletes. J Fam Pract 1998;47(2):145–149.
42. Fredrickson BE, Baker D, McHolick WJ, et al. The natural history of spondylolysis and spondylolisthesis. J Bone Joint Surg Am 1984;66A(5): 699–707.
43. Micheli LJ, Wood R. Back pain in young athletes. Arch Pediatr Adolesc Med 1995;149:15–18.
44. Meyerding HW. Diagnosis and roentgenologic evidence in spondylolisthesis. Radiology 1933;20(1):108–120.
45. Ledford D, Apter A, Brenner AM, et al. Osteoporosis in the corticosteroid-treated patient with asthma. J Allergy Clin Immunol 1998;102(3): 353–362.
46. Lane JM, Russell L, Khan SN. Osteoporosis. Clin Orthop 2000;372:139–150.
47. Klibanski A, Adams-Campbell L, Bassford T, et al. Osteoporosis prevention, diagnosis, and therapy. JAMA 2001;285(6):785–795.
48. Deal CL. Osteoporosis: prevention, diagnosis, and management. Am J Med 1997;102(1A)(suppl):35S–39S.
49. Neer RM, Arnaud CD, Zanchetta JR, et al. Effect of parathyroid hormone (1-34) on fractures and bone mineral density in postmenopausal women with osteoporosis. New Engl J Med 2001;344(19):1434–1441.
50. Sharkey NA, Williams NI, Guerin JB. The role of exercise in the prevention and treatment of osteoporosis and osteoarthritis. Rheumatology 2000;35(1):209–221.
51. Hunter SJ, Shaha S, Flint D, et al. Predicting return to work. Spine 1998;23(21):2319–2328.
52. Williams RA, Pruitt SD, Doctor JN, et al. The contribution of job satisfaction to the transition from acute to chronic low back pain. Arch Phys Med Rehabil 1998;79:366–374.
53. Schwarzer AC, Aprill CN, Derby R, et al. Clinical features of patients with pain stemming from the lumbar zygapophysial joints. Spine 1994;19(4): 1132–1137.
54. Revel M, Poiraudeau S, Auleley GR, et al. Capacity of the clinical picture to characterize low back pain relieved by facet joint anesthesia. Spine 1998;23(18):1972–1977.
55. van Kleef M, Barendse GAM, Kessels A, et al. Randomized trial of radiofrequency lumbar facet denervation for chronic low back pain. Spine 1999;24(18):1937–1942.

Suggested Readings

Bigos S, Bowyer O, Braen G, et al. Acute Low Back Problems in Adults. Clinical Practice Guideline, Quick Reference Guide Number 14. Rockville, MD: U.S. Department of Health and Human Services, Public Health Service, Agency for Health Care Policy and Research, AHCPR Pub. No. 95-0643, December 1994.

Della-Giustina DA. Emergency department evaluation and treatment of back pain. Emerg Med Clin North Am 1999;17(4):877–893.

Klibanski A, Adams-Campbell L, Bassford T, et al. Osteoporosis prevention, diagnosis, and therapy. JAMA 2001;285(6):785–795.

Lonstein JE. Spondylolisthesis in children. Spine 1999;24(24):2640–2648.

Spivak, JM. Degenerative lumbar spinal stenosis. J Bone Joint Surg Am 1998;80A(7):1053–1066.

van Tulder MW, Koes BW, Bouter LM. Conservative treatment of acute and chronic nonspecific low back pain. Spine 1997;22(18):2128–2156.

8 Shoulder Girdle and Arm

Ralph M. Buschbacher

The shoulder is the most mobile connecting structure in the body. It moves in several planes, with motion occurring at many joints and involving several bones. In a larger sense, it can be thought of as the "shoulder girdle," of which the shoulder proper is just a small part.

Shoulder and Arm Anatomy

Bones of the Shoulder

The bones of the shoulder are depicted in Figure 8.1.

Scapula
The triangular scapula is split into two sections by the "spine of the scapula." The upper section is the supraspinatus fossa and the lower is the infraspinatus fossa. The inner surface of the scapula is known as the subscapular fossa. All three fossae are sites of muscle attachment. The lateral projection of the spine ends at the acromion or "tip of the shoulder." The lateral angle of the scapula widens into an articulating surface, the glenoid fossa. Projecting anteriorly from the scapula is the coracoid process.

Clavicle
The S-shaped clavicle is convex anteriorly in its medial section and concave laterally. It provides the only bony attachment of the shoulder and arm to the axial skeleton.

Humerus
The humerus is a long bone and has an articulating head superiorly, which lies in the glenoid fossa. Anteriorly, the humerus has a prominence known as the *lesser tubercle* (tuberosity), which is separated from the lateral greater tubercle by the intertubercular groove.

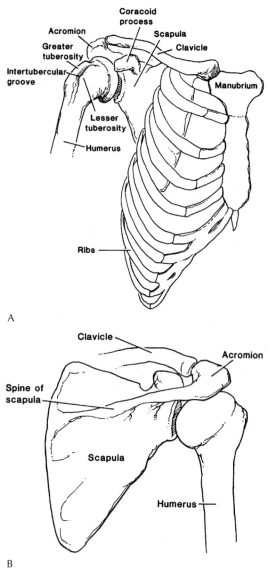

FIGURE 8.1 *A. The anterior bones of the shoulder girdle. B. Posterior bones.*

Joints of the Shoulder

Glenohumeral Joint

The glenohumeral joint is the articulation between the humerus and the scapula. The glenoid fossa has an upward tilt. This tilt helps hold the humerus in place without active muscle contraction. The glenoid fossa is surrounded by a rim called the *glenoid labrum*, which was once described as a discrete piece of fibrocartilage, but which is now believed to be a fold of the joint capsule.[1] The labrum increases the depth of the joint and the surface of articulation, both of which improve the stability of the joint.

To maintain mobility, the glenohumeral joint capsule is relatively loose in all directions. It does, however, have some areas that are reinforced for stability. Superiorly it is reinforced by the coracohumeral ligament, and anteriorly it has three thickened areas known as the *superior, middle,* and *inferior gleno-humeral ligaments.*

Acromioclavicular Joint

The acromioclavicular (AC) joint is a plane joint that is strengthened by the superior and inferior AC ligaments. More important, the clavicle is kept in place in relation to the acromion by the coracoclavicular ligaments (conoid and trapezoid) (Figure 8.2).

Scapulothoracic Joint

The scapulothoracic joint is a gliding joint between the scapula and the thoracic wall. It is lubricated by a bursa at its inferomedial pole.

Other Joints

Other joints involved to a lesser extent in shoulder motion are the sternoclavicular, costovertebral, sternocostal, and vertebral joints.

Muscles of the Shoulder

The muscles of the shoulder (Figure 8.3) can be divided into intrinsic and extrinsic muscles (Table 8.1). The intrinsic muscles arise on and insert into the shoulder girdle. Four of the intrinsic muscles, the supraspinatus, infraspinatus, subscapularis, and teres minor, are collectively known as the *rotator cuff.* They surround the glenohumeral joint. In addition to performing specific actions, the rotator cuff, as a group, serves two main purposes:

Depression of the humeral head to prevent upward migration of the humerus.

Centering of the humeral head in the glenoid fossa during motion.

In addition, the supraspinatus is important in the initiation of abduction. The rotator cuff tendons contain areas of relative avascularity.[2] This predisposes them, especially the supraspinatus, to injury. This area becomes hyperemic in the recumbent position, which explains the common finding of night pain when this area is injured.

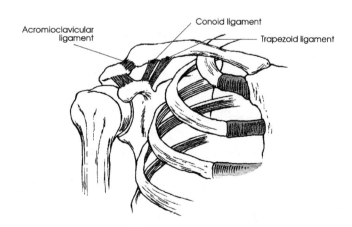

FIGURE 8.2 *The supporting ligaments of the acromioclavicular joint.*

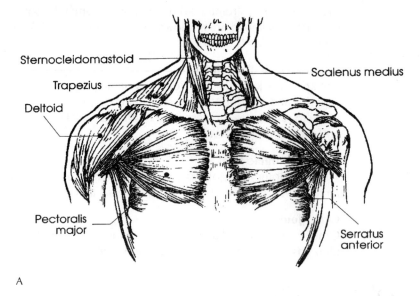

A

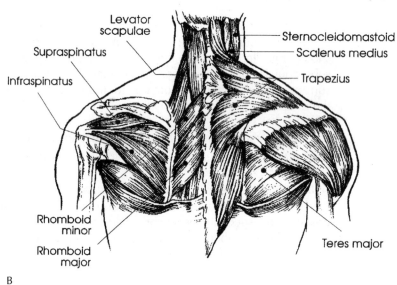

B

FIGURE 8.3   *The shoulder girdle muscles: (**A**) anterior view (left-superficial, right-deep); (**B**) posterior view (right-superficial, left-deep).*

Other Important Structures of the Shoulder

Coracoacromial Arch

The coracoacromial arch is formed by the acromion, the coracoid process, the coracoacromial ligament, and the scapula below (Figure 8.4). It contains the supraspinatus, subacromial (subdeltoid) bursa, the tendon of the long head of the biceps, and the coracohumeral ligament. It protects the enclosed structures as well as the humeral head below, but because it has a fixed volume, it is subject to problems that increase the pressure within the arch. Any condition that causes inflammation, edema, or bleeding can result in such a pressure increase.

TABLE 8.1   Muscles of the shoulder

Intrinsic shoulder muscles
   Supraspinatus ⎫
   Infraspinatus ⎪
   Teres minor   ⎬   Rotator cuff
   Subscapularis ⎪
   Teres major ⎭
   Deltoid
   Coracobrachialis
Extrinsic shoulder muscles
   Pectoralis major
   Pectoralis minor
   Sternocleidomastoid
   Trapezius
   Levator scapulae
   Latissimus dorsi
   Rhomboid major
   Rhomboid minor
   Serratus anterior
   Biceps
   Triceps

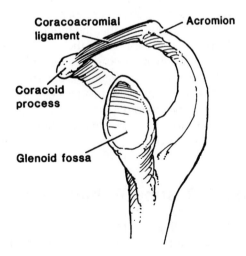

FIGURE 8.4   *The coracoacromial arch, lateral view.*

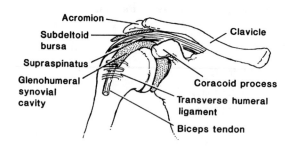

FIGURE 8.5 *The glenohumeral synovial cavity and subdeltoid (subacromial) bursa in an anterior shoulder view.*

Brachial Plexus

The brachial plexus (see Chapter 6) is a group of interconnecting nerves that emerges from the neck. It passes between the clavicle and first rib to reach the axilla, where it forms the great nerves of the arm.

Bursae

The subacromial (subdeltoid) bursa (Figure 8.5) lies between the rotator cuff and the coracoacromial arch and deltoid muscle. It does not normally communicate with the glenohumeral joint cavity. The scapulothoracic bursa lies between the inferomedial angle of the scapula and the chest wall.

Glenohumeral and Scapulothoracic Motion

Ordinarily, scapulothoracic motion complements glenohumeral motion in what is described as the *scapulohumeral rhythm.* During abduction, the scapula rotates 1 degree for every 2 degrees of glenohumeral motion (Figure 8.6). When assessing shoulder motion, the exact ratio of motion is unimportant. What is important is that the motion is smooth and symmetric on both sides. Scapular movement keeps the deltoid operating near its maximal power length, and therefore is sorely missed when defective. The humerus can be fully abducted only when it is externally rotated.

At rest, the humeral head is kept from drifting downward by the upward angle of the glenoid fossa and by the coracohumeral ligament, which is taut in this position. In conditions of motor weakness in which the scapula is allowed to rotate downward, the shoulder may subluxate.

Examination and Testing Techniques

When dealing with the shoulder, it is important to assess the neck as well. Many shoulder and neck problems are interrelated and may have similar symptoms.

History

Before proceeding with a physical examination and diagnostic tests, a good history of the nature of the shoulder complaint is indicated. Included in the history should be a description of when and where the dysfunction or pain

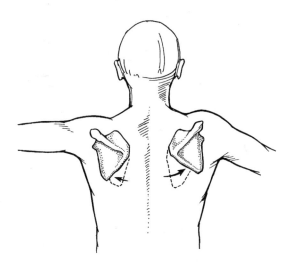

FIGURE 8.6   *The scapulohumeral rhythm. On the left (normal), the scapulothoracic joint moves 1 degree for each 2 degrees of glenohumeral abduction. On the right, the person with adhesive capsulitis or other limitation of glenohumeral motion moves the arm primarily at the scapulothoracic joint.*

began, what activity caused it and exacerbates it, and any past history of injury or surgery to the area. This often leads the examiner to the most productive line of inquiry and testing. Discussing functional limitations such as dressing, eating, and hair combing may be useful. A general review of systems is also helpful because abdominal, cardiac, or other diseases may cause pain to be referred to the shoulder.

Physical Examination

As always, the physical examination must include the following: inspection, palpation, passive range of motion (ROM), active ROM, strength, and stability testing.

Inspection may reveal signs of muscular atrophy, such as a prominent scapular spine. Atrophy may result from cervical nerve root compression, brachial plexus or peripheral nerve damage, or muscular tears or inactivity. If the biceps tendon is ruptured, the muscle retracts and creates a distal lateral enlargement of the biceps. Visualization should be from the front and back to see all the muscles of the shoulder girdle and to check the general alignment of the scapulae.

Anterior dislocation is accompanied by prominence of the humeral head anteriorly, with a depression in back. Posterior dislocation causes a posterior bulge and the coracoid becomes prominent anteriorly. Inferior subluxation, seen after cerebrovascular accident or brachial plexus or axillary nerve injury, causes a stepoff between the acromion and the humeral head.

Palpation of the shoulder structures may reveal tenderness at the site of injury. Tenderness at the intertubercular groove is common in noninjured people, and bicipital tendonitis should not be over-diagnosed by this isolated finding. The supraspinatus insertion can be palpated anterolateral to the acromion, especially with the arm extended a bit. The AC joint can easily be palpated, as it is so superficial. It has also been reported that full-thickness rotator cuff tears can be detected by transdeltoid palpation with excellent results.[3]

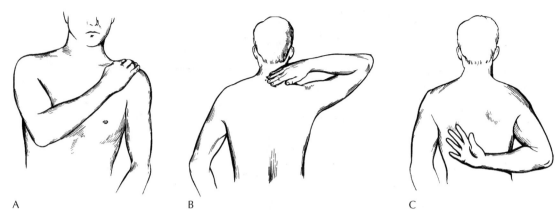

A   B   C

FIGURE 8.7   *The Apley scratch test. The patient is asked to touch the opposite shoulder blade in three ways: from across the opposite shoulder (**A**), from behind the neck (**B**), and from behind the lower back (**C**). This tests all the major planes of range of motion.*

Active ROM may be assessed in the seated, not standing, position to avoid trunk and leg contribution to ROM. Passive ROM is tested in the seated and supine positions.

An easy functional way to assess ROM is the Apley scratch test (Figure 8.7). The patient is asked to touch to opposite scapula across the opposite shoulder, behind the neck, and from behind the lower back. Active ROM testing reveals areas of inflexibility, specific muscle weakness, and painful arcs. Active abduction and external rotation are decreased in rotator cuff disease. In cuff problems the patient tends to shrug the shoulder when asked to abduct the arm.

Discrepancies between active and passive ROM are noted. If both active and passive motion are limited, there is likely to be a joint contracture, adhesive capsulitis, fixed dislocation, or bony abnormality. When passive motion is greater than active, a rotator cuff tear is suspected.

ROM of the scapulothoracic joint is observed, along with that of the glenohumeral joint. The scapulohumeral rhythm is evaluated using the nonaffected side as a control. Excessive scapulothoracic motion is a sign of glenohumeral stiffness and is commonly seen in rotator cuff tears, adhesive capsulitis, and in degenerative joint disease (see Figure 8.6).

To test anterior stability of the shoulder, the patient is seated or asked to lie supine at the edge of the table. The arm is held over the edge of the table in a position of abduction and external rotation. The examiner tries to move the humeral head anteriorly by exerting pressure on the proximal humerus (Figure 8.8). Pain on this maneuver is a sign of anterior subluxation; apprehension is indicative of a prior dislocation and is called a *positive apprehension test*. Pushing the humeral head back into place relieves the pain and apprehension.

Pushing the proximal humerus posteriorly tests for posterior subluxation (Figure 8.9). This is less likely to cause pain or apprehension, and the degree of posterior movement may be subtle. With the arm flexed and internally rotated, the examiner pushes the patient's elbow with one hand while feeling for movement behind the shoulder with the other. This may reveal posterior movement

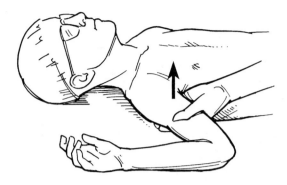

FIGURE 8.8   *Test for anterior shoulder stability. The examiner pushes the proximal upper arm anteriorly.*

of the humerus. A posterior translation of the humeral head of up to 50% of its diameter has been described as being normal.[4]

Inferior stability is assessed by applying inferior traction to the relaxed arm. If this causes a stepoff to appear between the humeral head and the acromion, it is called a *positive sulcus sign* and indicates inferior instability. This can be done with the patient seated or supine (Figure 8.10). In the seated position, the examiner can place one hand on the shoulder to feel for inferior movement. The patient's forearm is relaxed on the lap, and the examiner's other hand applies inferior traction by pushing down on the proximal forearm.

Strength testing at the shoulder must systematically isolate the various muscle groups. The deltoid is tested in its anterior, middle, and posterior portions. Internal rotation, external rotation, and abduction can be tested with the patient seated with the arms by the sides and the elbows flexed. It is very diffi-

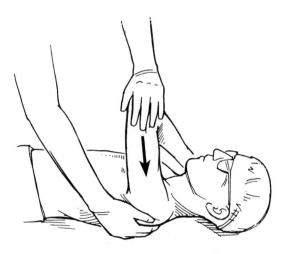

FIGURE 8.9   *Test for posterior stability. The examiner pushes back on the internally rotated and flexed upper arm while palpating behind the shoulder with the other hand.*

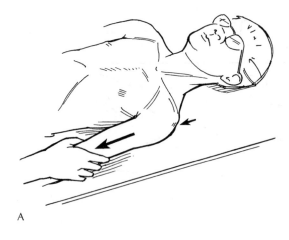

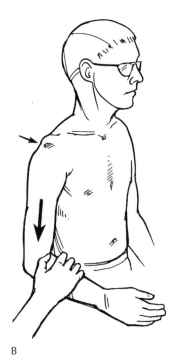

FIGURE 8.10 *Inferior stability testing in the supine (**A**) and seated (**B**) positions, with a positive sulcus sign (small arrows).*

cult to give good effort on only one side, so it is helpful for the examiner to test both sides simultaneously. Patients are able to overcome the examiner's resistance in internal rotation, but the examiner can detect any asymmetry of strength. Examiners must take care not to apply so much resistance that they injure their own shoulders in the process. Weakness in external rotation is seen relatively often even in the absence of pain with this maneuver. This is in contradistinction to supraspinatus strength testing, in which true weakness is often difficult to distinguish from pain inhibition. Such unilateral external rotation weakness is often a subtle sign of a cuff tear.

Serratus anterior weakness is accompanied by winging of the medial scapula when pushing against a wall (Figure 8.11). Trapezius weakness may cause a similar winging (but with more lateral displacement of the scapula) with the same maneuver, and leads to a weak shoulder shrug. The scapular retractors are tested by pushing posteriorly with the arm behind the lower back (palm facing to the rear).

After assessing the basics as described above, a number of more specialized tests and observations may be indicated.

Impingement Testing for Supraspinatus Pathology

In the Neer test, the arm is internally rotated and then flexed to its limit (Figure 8.12). Pain in the shoulder is a positive finding. The Hawkins test is performed by flexing the arm to 90 degrees and then internally rotating it to its limit (Figure 8.13). Impingement again is painful. Patients should be asked where they feel pain, because these tests sometimes aggravate myofascial pain in the upper back, and this is obviously not a positive finding. In both of these maneuvers pain is relieved after injection of local anesthetic into the subacromial space. This "impingement injection test" rules out other causes

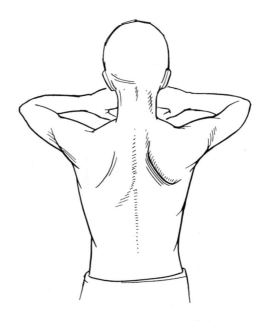

FIGURE 8.11   *Serratus anterior weakness causes a medial "winging" of the scapula when the patient pushes against a wall with the elbows pointed outward.*

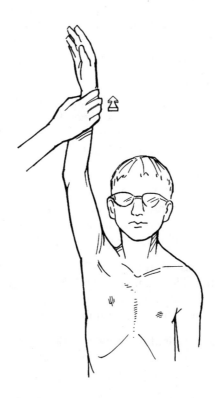

FIGURE 8.12   *The Neer impingement test.*

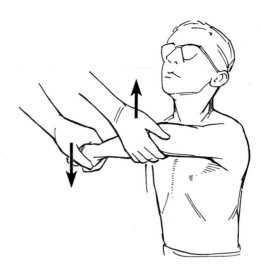

FIGURE 8.13   *The Hawkins impingement test.*

of shoulder pain, such as AC pain and adhesive capsulitis, which are not relieved by the injection. Also, pain relief allows more accurate muscle and ROM testing.

Drop Arm Test
The drop arm test is used to evaluate a possible rotator cuff tear, specifically in the supraspinatus muscle. The patient sits or stands while the examiner abducts the arm. The patient is asked to hold the arm in place and to lower it slowly. Severe pain or inability to lower the arm slowly is a positive finding.

The Painful Arc
In impingement or partial cuff tear, the supraspinatus tendon forms a mass or swelling that passes under the coracoacromial arch in the arc of 70–120 degrees of abduction. Therefore, pain in the arc of 70–120 degrees of abduction is suggestive of an inflamed or swollen supraspinatus tendon.

Speed's Test
In Speed's test (Figure 8.14), the patient's forearm is placed in extension and supination with the arm held a bit to the side. The patient is asked to flex the shoulder (not the elbow) against resistance. Pain at the biceps tendon is a positive finding for bicipital tendonitis.[5]

Yergason's Test
The elbow is flexed to 90 degrees and the forearm is pronated (Figure 8.15). The examiner resists combined flexion and supination of the forearm. Again, pain at the biceps tendon is significant for bicipital tendonitis.[6]

Supraspinatus Strength Testing
The supraspinatus can be relatively isolated and tested by holding the arm abducted to 90 degrees, flexed to 30 degrees, and internally rotated so the

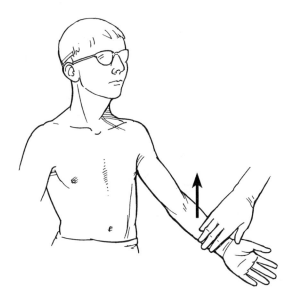

FIGURE 8.14 *Speed's test for bicipital tendonitis. The patient flexes the arm at the shoulder, not the elbow.*

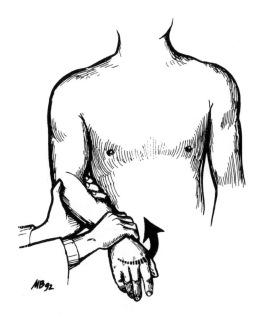

FIGURE 8.15 *Yergason's test for bicipital tendonitis. The arm is held at the side with the elbow flexed to 90 degrees and the forearm pronated. The examiner resists while the patient attempts to supinate the forearm. Pain at the intertubercular groove at the shoulder is a positive finding.*

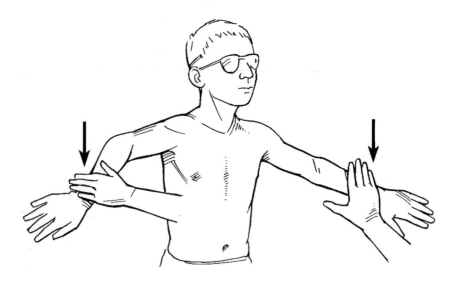

FIGURE 8.16   *Supraspinatus testing: The arm is abducted 90 degrees and flexed forward 30 degrees, with the thumbs pointing down. This lines the humerus up in the plane of the scapula and isolates the supraspinatus to testing.*

thumbs point down (Figure 8.16). Pain or weakness to downward pressure in this position is indicative of supraspinatus pathology.

Horizontal Adduction

The AC joint can be compressed by horizontal adduction (Figure 8.17). Pain on this maneuver is a sign of AC sprain or degeneration. The examiner should

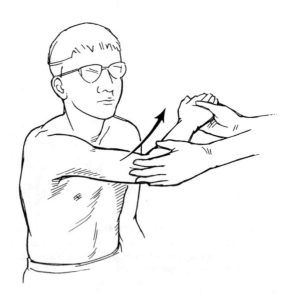

FIGURE 8.17   *Horizontal adduction causes compression of the acromioclavicular joint.*

ask the patient where the pain is felt, as this maneuver can also stretch the posterior structures of the shoulder. Only pain felt directly at the joint is a positive finding. The patient can also place the hand on the opposite shoulder while the examiner pushes down on the elbow and the patient resists this motion. This can also cause a reproduction of AC pain.

Ancillary Diagnostic Testing

There are numerous ancillary diagnostic procedures that may be performed about the shoulder. They include x-rays, magnetic resonance imaging (MRI), diagnostic ultrasound, computed tomography (CT), electromyography (EMG), arthroscopy, and arthrography. Arthrography is especially good at detecting full-thickness rotator cuff tears. MRI is best at detecting any soft tissue abnormality, such as partial or complete rotator cuff tears, tendonitis, or labral tears. CT or CT arthrogram is useful in assessing the internal anatomy of the glenohumeral joint, especially the labrum. Ultrasound can detect some cuff tears as well as cysts. EMG is useful in detecting radiculopathy, plexopathy, or neuropathy. Bone scan can detect stress fractures, osteomyelitis, degenerative processes, reflex sympathetic dystrophy, and tumors.

It is difficult to know when an x-ray is needed. There are no hard and fast rules, but Table 8.2 gives some general guidelines as to when an x-ray evaluation might be appropriate. Three basic x-ray views should be obtained: an anteroposterior view, an axillary lateral view, and a scapular lateral or Y view. The anteroposterior view gives a good depiction of the glenohumeral joint. The axillary view helps to detect dislocations, and the Y view, so named because it is angled toward the Y shape of the body of the scapula, spine of the scapula, and coracoid process (similar to the view depicted in Figure 8.4), gives information about the rotator cuff and coracoacromial arch, including the shape of the acromion.[2] In addition, anteroposterior views can be obtained with the arm in internal and external rotation.

TABLE 8.2   Guidelines on when to order x-ray studies

When there is severe, unremitting, or prolonged pain

When there is joint swelling

When range of motion is decreased (active or passive)

After any dislocation to rule out associated fracture

When the shoulder is unstable

If there is evidence of a mechanical block or articular "grinding"

When the joint is incongruent to examination

After a clavicular or acromial "contusion" to rule out fracture or acromioclavicular separation

In adolescents or preadolescents with a diagnosis of "ligamentous" sprain, to rule out growth plate injury (ligaments may be stronger than growth plate)

Diagnosis and Treatment of Specific Disorders

When approaching problems of the shoulder, a number of questions should be kept in mind. First, is the problem truly coming from the shoulder? Neck pathology can often be experienced as shoulder pain, so the neck should always be examined in addition to the shoulder. Second, is the problem nerve-related? Radiculopathy, mononeuropathy, plexopathy, and thoracic outlet syndrome are all treated quite differently than a musculoskeletal disorder. Third, is an inflammatory or infectious condition causing the symptoms? Again, the treatment is very different if this is the case. Finally, is there a bony or other anatomic block limiting motion? Certain exercises and treatments are contra-indicated if so. It should also be remembered that other conditions, such as cholecystitis and myocardial infarction, can cause pain to be referred to the shoulder. What follows are more detailed discussions of some of the more common shoulder conditions.

Impingement Syndrome

Impingement syndrome is a condition of pain, inflammation, and edema of the structures within the coracoacromial arch. It occurs mostly at the supraspinatus muscle. It is due to repetitive microtrauma, usually from overhand arm motions, and is exacerbated by motions that increase the encroachment of the humeral head into the coracoacromial arch, most notably internal rotation and raising the arm. Certain activities and occupations predispose to the development of impingement, including sports such as swimming and overhead throwing or racquet sports, and jobs that require frequent or prolonged overhead activity, such as painting. When degenerative arthritis causes bony spurs to encroach on the already tight space in the arch, it may also lead to tendon injury. Some people may also have an acromial or coracoid shape that predisposes to impingement.[2]

Impingement may progress to rotator cuff tear. True impingement of the supraspinatus is almost always intertwined with the other conditions of rotator cuff tendonitis, subdeltoid (subacromial) bursitis, and bicipital tendonitis, although isolated overuse of the biceps may occur in some repetitive underhand motions.

As described previously, the supraspinatus tendon is chronically ischemic. Repetitive use of the hands at or above shoulder height increases the load on the shoulders and worsens the ischemia. Degeneration occurs slowly with age and repetitive movement, making the cuff muscles weaker. As they weaken, the deltoid overpowers the cuff and pulls the humerus into the coracoacromial arch, thereby compressing the supraspinatus and damaging it further.

Sometimes calcific deposits form within the rotator cuff tendons. This is also a part of the continuum of overuse injury and is found most commonly in the middle-aged. Presentation is identical to impingement. Although calcific deposits are found in some patients with shoulder pain, they are not always the cause of the pain. It is important to remember that such deposits are formed as the body reacts to impingement and damage; they are not the primary cause of the damage.

TABLE 8.3 Stages of impingement

Stage 1	Edema, hemorrhage, and fibrosis
Stage 2	Tendonitis
Stage 3	Full-thickness rotator cuff tears

There are three stages of impingement (Table 8.3).[2] If left untreated, they progress to include bony changes such as acromial and greater tuberosity sclerosis, and cyst and spur formation. A large cuff tear may eventually lead to a "cuff tear arthropathy," with an upward migration of the humeral head into the acromion.

Diagnosis

Pain in impingement is localized to the anterolateral shoulder, and is often described as a deep ache. Impingement signs may be positive, and abduction in the arc between 70 and 120 degrees may be painful. There may be tenderness at the distal supraspinatus insertion onto the humerus, which is felt anterolateral to the acromion with the arm extended slightly. The drop arm test should not be positive, but may be equivocal due to pain inhibition causing the patient to resist holding the arm up. There may be signs of rotator cuff muscular atrophy.

In the early stage of impingement, pain occurs only after strenuous activity. Later it may occur with almost any movement, and if not treated can progress to nearly constant pain, especially night pain. When the biceps tendon is involved, it is tender to palpation and Yergason's and Speed's tests are positive. Isolated tenderness over the biceps tendon is common in normal individuals and care must be taken not to over-diagnose this condition. Comparing the biceps tenderness from side to side may help detect unilateral pathology.

X-ray findings of impingement are usually minimal. In advanced cases, bony spurring may be detected, but in general this is purely a soft tissue disorder. Under-penetrating x-rays are best at detecting calcific deposits. MRI will usually show at least some degree of chronic tendonitis.

Treatment

In the early stages of impingement, before rotator cuff tear has occurred, the main goals of treatment are to reduce pain and inflammation. This decreases pressure on the tendons and gives the contents of the coracoacromial arch more "room to breathe," which may help to break the cycle of irritation. Relative rest, with no overhead activity, is indicated. Nonsteroidal anti-inflammatory drugs (NSAIDs) and ice are used in this stage.

After the patient begins to have at least some pain relief, an exercise program is started, with below-shoulder internal/external rotation strengthening. Exercises are performed with the arm by the side. As tolerated, gentle ROM exercises are added, especially in external rotation. Pulley stretches, internal rotation, and abduction are avoided.

If there is not a relatively rapid improvement in symptoms, MRI may help to rule out other pathology, such as a cuff tear. Steroid injections into the subdeltoid bursa are considered. They are not a definitive treatment by themselves, but may decrease swelling within the coracoacromial arch, allowing the patient to participate more fully in exercise. As symptoms improve, more aggressive stretching and strengthening exercises are added. Stretching should still emphasize external rotation. The goal of the strengthening exercises is to improve the function of the humeral head depressors. Thus, the rotator cuff muscles and the latissimus dorsi are targeted. Strengthening and flexibility in the direction of external rotation is stressed because a position of internal rotation tends to worsen the impingement. Corner push-ups (stretching into a corner with one hand on each wall) are valuable. If the flexibility program does not bring a return of full ROM, mobilization by a therapist may be indicated.

The rotator cuff muscles can be strengthened with a few specific exercises. Internal and external rotation are practiced with the arm by the side to strengthen the subscapularis and the infraspinatus/teres minor, respectively. This can be done with weights while lying on the side or with elastic bands tied to a doorknob or other support. The supraspinatus is strengthened by holding the arm abducted 90 degrees and flexed forward 30 degrees with the thumb pointing down (same position as for supraspinatus strength testing). The arm is slowly lowered and then brought back up. The patient should be instructed not to raise it above horizontal level. At first, no weights are used; 1- to 5-lb weights can be added later (preferably strapped to the wrists rather than held), but heavy weights are avoided because they aggravate the condition. Ten to twenty repetitions done once or twice per day are adequate.

If conservative treatment fails to improve the symptoms, surgery may be considered. This might consist of a coracoacromial arch decompression or resection of the AC joint. A long period of conservative treatment for uncomplicated impingement is indicated before surgery is considered. In the athlete this can be up to 9 months, as surgical repair rarely allows people to return to an elite level of play.[7]

More advanced stages of impingement (stages II and III) are also initially treated conservatively, as described for the earlier stages. Partial or small rotator cuff tears may respond to this treatment as well, but if no improvement occurs, surgery may be necessary.

In addition to the above guidelines, bicipital tendonitis or chronic bursitis may respond to ultrasound deep heat treatment. Calcific tendonitis may respond to puncture of the tendon with a needle to allow the contents to spill into the bursa and, from there, be resorbed. This relieves intratendinous pressure and reduces swelling.

After recovery (or for prophylaxis), patients should be counseled to avoid activities or work that tend to aggravate impingement. This might include overhead weight lifting (such as the military press), prolonged overhead activity, swimming, overhand racquet sports, or throwing sports. If patients wish to participate in such sports, they may benefit from working with a coach to make sure they are using proper technique.

Rotator Cuff Tears

A tear of the rotator cuff may, of course, be caused in a healthy shoulder by a macrotraumatic injury, such as a glenohumeral dislocation. More commonly, however, this injury is superimposed on chronic pathology. Overuse, age, tendonitis, and inflammation all take their toll on the rotator cuff. The weakened cuff tendon is more easily torn when a traumatic event comes along, and because it is weak, it is less able to avoid such a traumatic event.

Rotator cuff tears may occur in young athletes who are active in sports that stress repetitive motion, or in middle-aged athletes who have been sedentary for a long time. Typically, these middle-aged athletes decide to "get in shape," overdo it, and end up tearing the cuff in their enthusiasm. Training principles such as "no pain, no gain" and "work through the pain" only worsen the condition of the shoulder. Older patients are more likely to have degenerative change in the shoulder. This predisposes them to injury from a macrotraumatic event that would not harm a younger, healthier shoulder.

Rotator cuff tears occur in the tendons of the cuff muscles, most often in the supraspinatus. The tear can be partial or full thickness.

Diagnosis

Acute cuff tears are associated with the acute onset of pain and tenderness about the greater tuberosity, usually after some traumatic event. A classic cause is when a person slips and tries to break the fall, stretching the shoulder. There may be weakness in the initiation of abduction and a positive drop arm test. Supraspinatus strength testing elicits pain and weakness, and impingement testing may be positive. Depending on which tendons are torn, there may be weakness in external rotation, as well as in other motions. Palpation through the deltoid process may reveal a full-thickness tear.[3] On x-ray there may be superior migration of the humeral head. MRI confirms the tear.

Chronic tears are the most common rotator cuff tears, especially in older individuals. They can be due to an old macrotraumatic injury, but more likely are due to chronic degenerative disease of the tendons. There is often a gradual onset of symptoms, including night pain and weakness. Overhead arm activities cause discomfort and fatigue. The drop arm test is often positive, and there is usually weakness in external rotation. Atrophy of the shoulder muscles, especially the supraspinatus and deltoid, is common. Supraspinatus strength testing is painful, and there is a positive impingement sign. X-rays are nonspecific but may show degenerative bony changes and upward migration of the humeral head. The diagnosis should be confirmed with MRI.

Treatment

Conservative care of rotator cuff tears is similar to that for impingement. After controlling pain and inflammation, flexibility is restored. Then isometrics are started, with progression to isotonic exercises as tolerated. The rotator cuff muscles are strengthened in internal and external rotation with the arm held by the side to reduce impingement. Judicious use of intrabursal steroid injection is considered.

If an acute rotator cuff tear is suspected, the patient may be followed conservatively with rest for the first 1–2 weeks. If strength returns and pain resolves, a program of rehabilitation may be initiated. If there is no improvement, an MRI should be obtained. If this reveals a cuff tear, surgery should probably be performed. Surgical outcome for traumatic tears is best if the repair is done soon after injury.[2]

In chronic or degenerative cuff tears, planning the best treatment can be difficult. Massive tears are usually surgically repaired. Partial tears may initially be treated with rest, ice, and NSAIDs. Subsequently, when the pain and inflammation have subsided, a rehabilitation course is instituted. If symptoms recur, the patient may need surgery. The treatment of smaller complete tears depends on the activity level of the patient. An active, motivated individual will probably benefit from surgery, although a 3-month trial of conservative treatment may be tried first. Some patients—those who are unlikely to use the shoulder vigorously in the future, those who pose a great surgical risk, or those who are likely to develop postoperative complications of immobility—may be treated conservatively. After surgery for a massive tear, the patient is immobilized for 6 weeks in an abduction brace to facilitate healing, after which a rehabilitation program of stretching, then strengthening, is started as tolerated. The total rehabilitation after cuff tear repair takes 9–12 months.

Instability

Glenohumeral instability is the most prevalent shoulder problem in young athletes. Although anterior instability is most common, instability can also be present in other directions: posterior, inferior, anterosuperior, and multidirectional. Instability can be due to traumatic injury's disrupting the integrity of the shoulder joint, or there may be laxity of the connective tissues leading to the instability and possibly predisposing to a traumatic injury. In some cases seizures can lead to dislocation (posterior). In others, persons may volitionally dislocate their own shoulders.

Instability may be limited to subluxation, in which the humeral head slips over the glenoid rim but spontaneously relocates. It can also result in frank dislocation in which the humeral head lodges outside the glenoid rim. Instability can result from macrotrauma, repetitive microtrauma, or congenital or neuromuscular abnormalities of the joint.

Anterior dislocation or subluxation occurs when the arm is forcibly abducted, externally rotated, and elevated or extended (Figure 8.18). The anterior labrum is often torn in the process, and the rotator cuff and axillary nerve may be damaged. Posterior dislocations or subluxations may occur from a fall on the outstretched arm or in car accidents (see Figure 8.18). They may also occur during seizures in which the stronger internal rotators overpower the external rotators. Once a shoulder has dislocated or subluxated it is likely to do so again in the future, especially in younger patients. Because the vast majority of patients with instability have it in the anterior direction, the rest of this discussion focuses on this direction, unless otherwise noted.

When obtaining shoulder x-rays, two findings are often made that are associated with prior shoulder dislocation: the Bankart lesion and the Hill-Sachs lesion. The Bankart lesion is an avulsion of the labrum from its attachment at the anterior glenoid rim. A Hill-Sachs lesion is a compression fracture of the posterior humeral head, where it impacts the anterior glenoid fossa in an anterior dislocation. In some cases, a large Hill-Sachs defect can cause the shoulder to lock into a dislocated position, making it difficult to relocate.

Diagnosis

Stability testing reveals abnormal laxity in the affected directions, and apprehension testing is positive. In acute dislocations, the patient may be unable to move the arm out of the locked position.

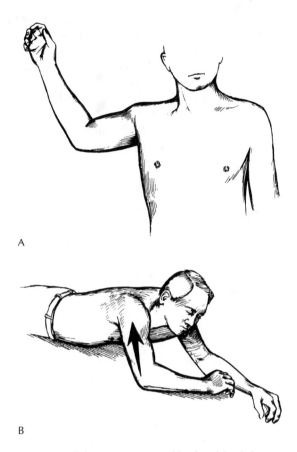

A

B

FIGURE 8.18 **A.** *Anterior dislocation is caused by forcible abduction and external rotation;* **(B)** *posterior dislocation may be caused by a fall on the internally rotated adducted arm.*

X-rays, including the axillary view, confirm diagnosis. They should be obtained to rule out any associated fractures, even after a dislocation has been reduced.

Treatment

Dislocations must, of course, be reduced, and for a discussion of such reduction, the reader is referred elsewhere.[7] After reduction of the dislocation, the patient may be immobilized in a sling for 4–6 weeks. A shorter period of 7–10 days—or no immobilization at all—may be indicated in persons with recurrent dislocation and in older patients, who are less likely to have a recurrence and who are more susceptible to problems of immobility.[7] Recurrent dislocation or subluxation can also be immobilized for a shorter period.

The shoulder is treated early on with ice. Isometric exercises of the distal arm can be performed to prevent disuse atrophy of the rest of the limb. Later, heat and gentle ROM exercises are instituted with the arm below shoulder level. External rotation is limited to 10 degrees less than the good arm.

Because this is a condition of joint laxity, the stretching program is relatively nonaggressive. A strengthening program is begun as tolerated, first with the arm below shoulder level (stressing the internal rotators), then with the addition of other motions, isotonics, isokinetics, and diagonal strength exercises. In all the strengthening exercises, the extremes of ROM are avoided. If symptoms persist, an MRI can be obtained to rule out concomitant rotator cuff tear.

If the patient does not improve with conservative treatment within 3 months, surgery can be considered. The surgery usually involves a capsular shift procedure to tighten the anterior shoulder, with a labral repair if indicated. Postoperatively, the shoulder is immobilized for 6 weeks, and then the whole rehabilitative process is started over again. Stretching of the anterior shoulder is restricted.[7]

Recurrence of shoulder dislocations is high, up to 94% in athletes under age 20.[8] A rehabilitation program may decrease this rate of recurrence to as low as 25%.[9]

Anterior subluxation does not require prolonged sling immobilization. It is treated similarly to a dislocation. Posterior dislocation or subluxation is also treated similarly, although in this condition the anterior shoulder muscles are stretched more, whereas the posterior muscles are strengthened more.

Adhesive Capsulitis

Adhesive capsulitis is a painful condition of decreased ROM of the glenohumeral joint. The cause is unknown, but it often follows an injury or a period of immobilization of the shoulder or arm. There appear to be capsular adhesions within the glenohumeral joint, which restrict ROM. Adhesive capsulitis occurs more commonly in women, in older persons, and in diabetics.[10] The condition is usually described as self-limited, with restoration of normal to near-normal function within 1–2 years. However, during this time span there is much morbidity and loss of function. Muscles atrophy and the patient's lifestyle changes. Clearly, early aggressive treatment is indicated.

Diagnosis

Almost any other injury can lead to the development of adhesive capsulitis; thus, this condition should always be looked for even when the shoulder has other obvious disorders. The hallmark of adhesive capsulitis is that both passive and active ROM are restricted, especially in abduction and external rotation. Pain is evident—often at rest, but especially when attempting ROM exercise. The patient moves the shoulder mainly at the scapulothoracic joint (see Figure 8.6), a sign that the glenohumeral joint is stiff. Local anesthetic injection into the glenohumeral joint relieves the pain but does not change joint mobility.

Treatment

At the first signs of adhesive capsulitis, aggressive pain control and mobilization are indicated. NSAIDs may be prescribed. Frequent ROM exercises, just short of producing pain, are indicated. Treatment may start with a home stretching program—such as "walking" the fingers up the wall, sliding the arm up the wall, or corner stretching—but if improvement does not begin within the first week or so, therapist-assisted exercises are warranted. Moist heat, slow gentle stretching, ultrasound treatment, and joint glide mobilizations are all helpful and should be performed once or twice daily. Pulley exercises may be used, but only with caution. The long lever arm of the pulley may actually injure the shoulder and cause impingement. Treatment with intra-articular steroid injection is controversial, but in the author's experience provides significant benefit. In cases refractory to even aggressive physical management, manipulation under anesthesia is an option.

Adhesive capsulitis may occur after any surgery or period of joint immobilization; thus it is clear that the shoulder should always be mobilized as soon as is feasible. Prevention is important, especially in the elderly or debilitated, and is done with twice-daily shoulder ROM exercises.

Acromioclavicular Problems

The AC joint is usually injured by trauma, such as landing on the acromion, or "tip of the shoulder." This can cause a variety of ligament sprains. Mild sprains to the AC ligaments usually cause no displacement of the joint. More significant sprains involve the coracoclavicular ligaments and may cause displacement of the acromion downward in relation to the clavicle. Other injuries can result in posterior or inferior displacement of the clavicle.

Diagnosis

Diagnosis is usually relatively straightforward, with a history of trauma and pain and tenderness localized to the joint. If there is a stepoff of the joint, this can be seen or felt by palpation, using the opposite side as a control. In moderate or severe sprains, there is pain and limitation of motion in adduction and abduction of the shoulder. Horizontal adduction increases the pain. X-ray taken with weight strapped (not held, to avoid contraction of the deltoid) to the wrist may show an increase in the stepoff.

Treatment

Treatment is usually with rest. A mild case can be padded, and, if due to sports injury, the patient may return to play. More significant injuries respond to rest, ice, ultrasound, NSAIDs, and a short period of wearing a sling (Kinney-Howard sling). In some cases the pain persists, especially in activities such as bench pressing or overhead throwing and racquet sports. These cases benefit from more prolonged activity modification. Sometimes an anesthetic/corticosteroid injection into the joint helps. This also helps confirm the AC joint as the pain generator. In refractory cases causing significant functional limitation, the distal clavicle and joint can be resected, usually with good result.

For most AC sprains, surgery is not necessary. There may be a permanent stepoff at the joint that does not respond to wearing a sling. This can be corrected for cosmetic reasons, but function will not be changed.

Degenerative Joint Disease

Arthritis of the glenohumeral and AC joints may occur, especially in patients with prior injury to these joints. This is known as *degenerative joint disease*. It also occurs in aging, overuse, and in rheumatic conditions. The AC joint can also be affected in those who lift heavy weights; such persons are predisposed to developing an osteolysis of the distal clavicle.

Diagnosis

Joint crepitus, decreased ROM, diffuse pain, and pain with motion are seen in these disorders. Mild activity often lessens the symptoms. X-rays confirm the diagnosis with signs of bony degeneration, spurring (which may be felt also), and sclerosis. If the AC joint is involved, horizontal adduction increases the pain. These patients may have a tender joint, with palpable degenerative changes.

Treatment

For glenohumeral joint arthritis, proper joint mechanics and energy conservation techniques are helpful. NSAIDs and occasional steroid injections are often used. Rarely, joint replacement is indicated.

For AC arthritis, treatment is similar to that for a sprain, with rest, ice, NSAIDs, injections, and, in refractory cases, surgery. The shoulder is surprisingly functional, even after such surgery.

Costochondritis

Costochondritis causes anterior chest pain that, in some cases, mimics cardiac pain. It is seen more commonly in women and is a frequent cause of emergency room visits in young women. It involves pain and tenderness at the rib articulations with the costal cartilage at the sternum, especially at ribs 2–5. It presents similarly to Tietze's syndrome, which is a painful swelling at the costal cartilages. Both conditions are generally self-limiting but may cause pain for a few days to a few weeks.

Diagnosis

Costochondritis is diagnosed by palpation, which reproduces the patient's pain complaints. Cardiac pathology, connective tissue disease, psychogenic aspects, and other internal disorders may need to be ruled out.

Treatment

Reassurance, ice massage, NSAIDs, and rest are prescribed in the acute stage. Local steroid injection may help relieve pain and inflammation in chronic cases.

Neurovascular Compromise/Thoracic Outlet Syndrome

A number of causes of neurovascular compression can result in shoulder and neck pain. Compression of the brachial plexus between the anterior and middle scalene muscles (scalenus anticus syndrome); compression between the clavicle and the first rib (costoclavicular syndrome); an abnormal shape of the first rib; and a cervical rib, among others, have been described. They tend to affect the ulnar distribution predominately, although the median nerve may also be affected. They occur only rarely and are probably over-diagnosed.

These problems occur more commonly in young to middle-aged women, and a poor posture with rounded forward slumping shoulders may be implicated. They sometimes occur after trauma.[7]

Diagnosis

Neurovascular compression causes a burning pain and numbness in the shoulder or the medial arm and forearm. Blood flow studies with a Doppler device or an arteriogram, as well as nerve conduction studies, may be helpful in making the diagnosis, depending on whether the nerves or blood vessels are primarily affected. Overhead activity may worsen or reproduce the symptoms. Night pain is common. There may be weakness of the intrinsic hand muscles. X-rays may reveal a cervical rib or traumatic clavicular anomaly. EMG, in some cases, shows slowing of nerve conduction across the thoracic outlet (although because of technical factors this is not as reliable as detecting some other problems) and rules out similarly presenting conditions such as radiculopathy, carpal tunnel syndrome, and ulnar neuropathy.[2]

Treatment

The shoulder elevators and retractors are strengthened and the anterior chest and neck structures are stretched. Overhead activity is discouraged. Most patients respond well to these interventions. Surgery may occasionally be necessary, although it is probably performed more often than it should be.

Stingers/Brachial Plexopathy

Brachial plexopathy is classically caused by a motorcycle accident or other fall in which the shoulder is depressed and the head is pushed in the other direction. Another cause is birth trauma (although in utero damage is probably even more common). What these injuries have in common is that they stretch the nerves of the brachial plexus, especially the upper plexus. A mild injury can cause a burning pain to radiate down the arm. This is a common football injury and is referred to as a *burner* or *stinger.* The arm may feel weak and useless. Symptoms last from a few seconds to a few minutes.

More severe injury can cause axonal damage to the nerves, resulting in enduring pain and dysesthesia, and possibly even atrophy of the muscles, usually of the shoulder.

Diagnosis is by the history of such an injury, as well as the physical examination. EMG can help detect more significant injury in which there is nerve damage present, and can help rule out a radiculopathy. Milder injury generally is associated with a normal EMG. If EMG is positive, it may be helpful to obtain an MRI of the plexus area to make sure that there is no hematoma or other anatomic abnormality causing ongoing damage to the nerve, which could potentially be treated. When plexopathy occurs without a known cause, tumor compression should be suspected. Persons who have previously received radiation therapy to the area can also have a delayed (for years) plexopathy.

There is generally no treatment for plexopathy unless an underlying anatomic cause can be identified. Aggravating high-risk activity should be avoided, possibly indefinitely. In many cases the nerve recovers fully, although in more significant injury this can take months. Bracing may possibly be helpful to better position a severely affected, nonfuctional arm, but unfortunately often achieves disappointing results.

Neuropathies

There are a number of isolated neuropathies that can occur around the shoulder.[11] The physician should be aware of them, as they can complicate the recovery course. EMG should be obtained if any nerve damage is suspected.

Axillary neuropathy can occur after anterior shoulder dislocation. It is relatively common, although not often clinically significant. The patient may experience weakness and atrophy of the deltoid and sensory loss at the lateral shoulder or upper arm (axillary patch).[12]

Suprascapular neuropathy can occur at the suprascapular notch of the scapula, often due to overuse or a cyst compressing the nerve. This results in weakness and atrophy of the supraspinatus and infraspinatus. Traction injury at the spinoglenoid notch, where the nerve passes around the spine of the scapula, can occur in throwing athletes. This causes weakness and atrophy of the infraspinatus only.

The long thoracic nerve can be damaged by a load being placed onto the shoulder, a "rucksack" or "backpacker's" palsy. This leads to weakness of the serratus anterior and medial winging of the scapula.

Spinal accessory nerve damage can be caused by traction injury or, more commonly, by surgical dissection. This causes significant shoulder dysfunction, as the upper trapezius is the only muscle that directly elevates the lateral tip of the shoulder. Dysfunction of this action leads to downward rotation of the scapula, which reduces the upward tilt of the glenoid fossa and causes inferior shoulder subluxation.

Parsonage-Turner syndrome is a condition of acute pain in the shoulder followed by a reduction in pain, but weakness and atrophy of the muscles innervated by one or more of the nerves of the brachial plexus. It often follows an infection or immunization. The cause is not known. Treatment is symptomatic and aims at reducing long-term dysfunction due to disuse and contractures.

Neuropathies of most other nerves of the arm can also occur, but they are rare.

Points of Summary

1. The rotator cuff muscles depress the head of the humerus and help prevent impingement.
2. The supraspinatus muscle is predisposed to overuse syndromes.
3. Impingement of the supraspinatus is usually combined with subdeltoid bursitis and bicipital tendonitis.
4. Scapulohumeral rhythm describes motion of the scapula of 1degree for every 2 degrees of glenohumeral abduction.
5. The shoulder is uniquely susceptible to problems of immobility.
6. In anterior instability, the internal rotators are strengthened.
7. In posterior instability, the external rotators are strengthened.
8. Thoracic outlet syndrome is over-diagnosed.
9. Arthrography detects complete rotator cuff tears; magnetic resonance imaging detects both complete and partial tears.

10. Adhesive capsulitis should be treated with early aggressive range-of-motion exercise.

References

1. Mosley HF, Övergaard B. The anterior capsular mechanism in recurrent anterior dislocation of the shoulder: morphological and clinical studies with special reference to the glenoid labrum and the glenohumeral ligaments. J Bone Joint Surg 1962;44(B):913–927.
2. Klimkiewicz JJ, Shaffer BS, Wiesel SW. Elbow and Shoulder Pain (2nd ed). New York: Lexis Publishing, 2000.
3. Wolf EM, Agrawal V. Transdeltoid palpation (the rent test) in the diagnosis of rotator cuff tears. J Shoulder Elbow Surg 2001;10:470–473.
4. Jobe FW, Bradley JP. The diagnosis and nonoperative treatment of shoulder injuries in athletes. Clin Sports Med 1989;8(3):419–437.
5. Clarnette RG, Miniaci A. Clinical exam of the shoulder. Med Sci Sports Exer 1998;30:S1–S6.
6. Yergason, RM. Supination sign. J Bone Joint Surg 1937;13(B):160.
7. Nicholas JA, Hershman EB, Posner MA (eds). The Upper Extremity in Sports Medicine. St. Louis, MO: Mosby, 1995.
8. Rowe CR, Sakellarides HT. Factors related to recurrences of anterior dislocations of the shoulder. Clin Orthop 1961;20:40–47.
9. Aronen JG, Regan K. Decreasing the incidence of recurrence of first time anterior shoulder dislocations with rehabilitation. Am J Sports Med 1984;12(4):283–291.
10. Hannafin JA, Chiaia TA. Adhesive capsulitis: a treatment approach. Clin Orthop 2000;372:95–109.
11. Leffer RD. Nerve lesions about the shoulder. Orthop Clin North Am 2000;31:331–345.
12. Perlmutter GS, Apruzzese W. Axillary nerve injuries in contact sports. Sports Med 1998;26:351–361.

Suggested Readings

Conservative management of shoulder injuries. Orthop Clin North Am 2000;31.

Klimkiewicz JJ, Shaffer BS, Wiesel SW. Elbow and Shoulder Pain (2nd ed). New York: Lexis Publishing, 2000.

Nicholas JA, Hershman EB, Posner MA (eds). The Upper Extremity in Sports Medicine. St. Louis, MO: Mosby, 1995.

9   Elbow and Forearm

Robert P. Wilder and William J. Barrish

Disorders of the elbow and forearm are commonly encountered in clinical practice. Evaluation of these injuries is dependent on an understanding of anatomy, the mechanism of injury, history, and presentation. Establishment of a correct pathoanatomic diagnosis is the basis for implementing rehabilitative and, if necessary, surgical management.

Anatomy of the Elbow and Forearm

The elbow consists of three articulations: the humeroulnar, humeroradial, and proximal radioulnar joints. The humeroulnar and humeroradial joints are hinge joints that act together in flexion and extension. The proximal radioulnar joint is a pivot joint that allows pronation and supination. Stability and support are provided by ligamentous and muscular structures.

Osseous Structures

The bones of the elbow and forearm are depicted in Figure 9.1.

Humerus
The long bone of the arm, the humerus, flares medially and laterally at its distal end, terminating in rounded medial and lateral epicondyles. The epicondyles serve as origins for the flexor and extensor forearm musculature. The distal end of the humerus bears two articulating surfaces: the capitellum, which articulates laterally with the head of the radius, and the trochlea, which articulates medially with the ulna.

Ulna
The ulna is the medial bone of the forearm. At its proximal and posterior aspect is the olecranon, a large process that articulates posteriorly with the olecranon fossa of the humerus. When the elbow is flexed, the coronoid process of the ulna fits in the coronoid fossa of the humerus. The fossa is located anteriorly and proximal to the trochlea.

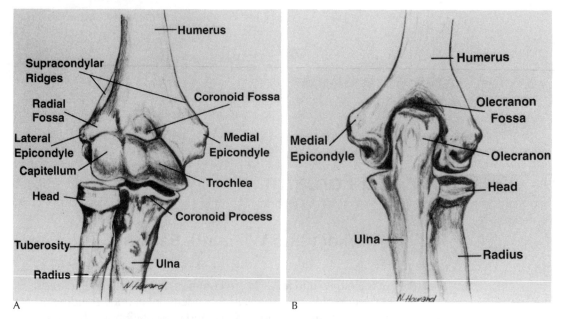

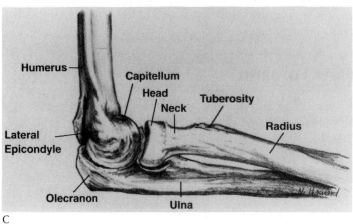

FIGURE 9.1 *Osseous structures of the elbow:* (**A**) *anterior view,* (**B**) *posterior view,* (**C**) *lateral view.*

Radius

The radius is the lateral bone of the forearm. At its proximal aspect, the radial head is expanded and flattened to articulate with the capitellum.

Ligamentous Structures

The ligaments of the elbow are depicted in Figure 9.2.

Lateral Collateral Ligament

The lateral (radial) collateral ligament extends from the lateral epicondyle to the annular ligament. It provides lateral support to the elbow complex.

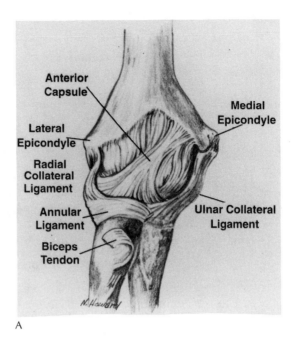

A

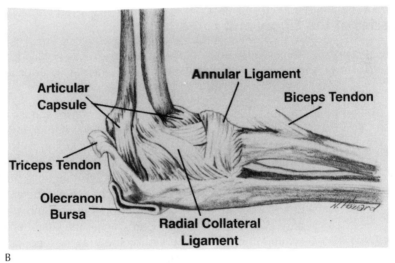

B

FIGURE 9.2   *Ligamentous structures of the elbow: (A) anterior view, (B) lateral view.*

Medial Collateral Ligament

The medial (ulnar) collateral ligament extends from the medial epicondyle to the ulna. It provides medial support to the elbow complex. It is divided into three bundles: anterior, posterior, and transverse, with the anterior bundle providing the greatest degree of stability.

Annular Ligament

The annular ligament cups the radial head and neck, holding them in place in the radioulnar articulation.

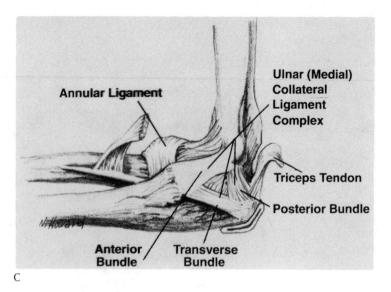

FIGURE 9.2   *Continued.* **C.** *Medial view.*

Muscles of the Elbow and Forearm

The muscles of the elbow and forearm can be divided into four groups based on their anatomic location: lateral, medial, anterior, and posterior (Figure 9.3).

Lateral
The muscles of the posterolateral or extensor surface of the elbow can be divided into two groups. The superficial group includes the brachioradialis, extensor carpi radialis longus, extensor carpi radialis brevis, extensor digitorum, extensor digiti minimi, and extensor carpi ulnaris. The deep group includes the supinator, abductor pollicis longus, extensor pollicis brevis, extensor pollicis longus, and extensor indicis. The extensor carpi radialis brevis, extensor digitorum, extensor digiti minimi, and extensor carpi ulnaris arise from a common aponeurosis near the lateral epicondyle. This is of clinical importance in lateral tennis elbow, as the tendons of these muscles may be involved in overuse injury.

Medial
The flexor muscles of the forearm can be divided into three groups. The superficial group includes the pronator teres, palmaris longus, flexor carpi radialis, and flexor carpi ulnaris. These four muscles arise from a common aponeurosis near the medial epicondyle. Chronic overuse of this group can result in medial tennis elbow (golfer's elbow). The intermediate mass is made up of one muscle, the flexor digitorum superficialis. The deep group includes the flexor digitorum profundus, the flexor pollicis longus, and the pronator quadratus.

Anterior
The anterior muscles, the biceps brachii and brachialis, arise from the shoulder and upper arm. The biceps is a flexor and supinator of the forearm. Its two

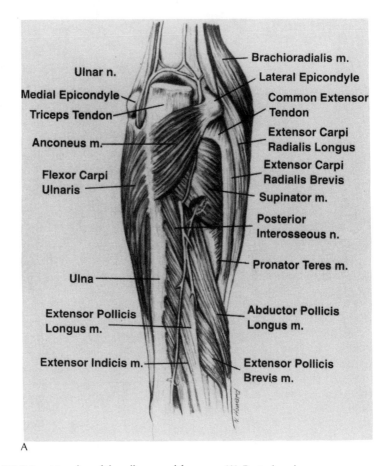

FIGURE 9.3   *Muscles of the elbow and forearm: (A) Posterior view.*

heads unite in the biceps tendon, which inserts on the radial tuberosity, the proximal radius, and the forearm fascia. The brachialis arises from the anterior humerus and inserts on the ulnar tuberosity just distal to the coronoid process. The brachialis functions as a flexor of the forearm.

Posterior
Posteriorly, the three heads of the triceps provide extension to the elbow and insert on the proximal olecranon. The anconeous is attached to the lateral epicondyle, the lateral side of the olecranon, and the adjacent part of the ulna. It provides extension to the elbow and stabilizes against flexion and pronation-supination.

Neurovascular Structures

Brachial Artery
The brachial artery can be palpated just medial to the biceps tendon at the level of, and just proximal to, the antecubital fossa.

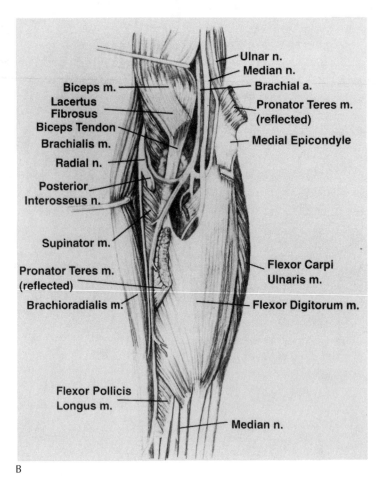

Figure labels:
- Ulnar n.
- Median n.
- Biceps m.
- Brachial a.
- Lacertus Fibrosus
- Pronator Teres m. (reflected)
- Biceps Tendon
- Brachialis m.
- Medial Epicondyle
- Radial n.
- Posterior Interosseus n.
- Supinator m.
- Flexor Carpi Ulnaris m.
- Pronator Teres m. (reflected)
- Brachioradialis m.
- Flexor Digitorum m.
- Flexor Pollicis Longus m.
- Median n.

B

FIGURE 9.3 *Continued. B. Anterior view.*

Median Nerve

At the elbow, the median nerve lies medial to the brachial artery. It passes between the two heads of the pronator teres to enter the volar forearm.

Ulnar Nerve

The ulnar nerve runs in a sulcus between the medial epicondyle and the olecranon process. It passes between the heads of the flexor carpi ulnaris to enter the medial forearm.

Examination and Testing Techniques

History

As with all musculoskeletal injury, evaluation of the elbow begins with a thorough history. A complete history of the injury and symptoms helps focus the physical examination and ancillary testing by developing an anatomically based differential diagnosis.

The location of symptoms can often direct further examination to the medial, lateral, anterior, or posterior structures of the elbow. Subjective complaints, including aching, sharp pain, numbness, tingling, or weakness, can help differentiate between various musculoskeletal injuries and nerve entrapment syndromes.

Rapid versus insidious onset of symptoms helps differentiate between an acute injury and chronic overuse injury. With acute traumatic injuries, a single occurrence often can be identified as the inciting event. Conversely, overuse injuries present with gradual development of symptoms, usually related to repetitive loads being placed on an anatomic structure. Repetitive motions associated with certain athletic activities have an associated predisposition to the development of elbow injuries.

Alleviating and aggravating factors are important to note. Also, the presence of symptoms at rest or exclusively during provocative activity provides information regarding the severity of symptoms. History of locking or catching may indicate bony or intra-articular pathology. Previous interventions, including self-treatment, should be investigated.

Past history of injury should be reviewed, including previous treatments and response. A review of an athlete's training program, with emphasis on recent changes in intensity, duration, or frequency, should also be reviewed. Discussing an athlete's short-term and long-term goals with respect to his or her sport is helpful for the development and implementation of an appropriate treatment plan. Evaluation of equipment and techniques can reveal extrinsic factors that may predispose to injury.

Physical Examination

Physical examination includes inspection, range-of-motion testing, palpation, provocative testing, and neuromuscular testing.[1] Asymmetry in size or positioning between the extremities should be noted. A brief screening examination, including the shoulder, cervical spine, and wrist, is done to evaluate for any primary pathology in these joints that may be causing referred or radiating pain in the elbow or forearm. The arms should be examined in the anatomic position, noting the carrying angle, the angle formed between the arm and forearm (Figure 9.4). Normal carrying angles measure up to 5 degrees of valgus in males and 10–15 degrees in females. An excessive carrying angle, known as cubitus valgus, may be congenital or due to traumatic causes such as fracture or epiphyseal damage. Cubitus varus, a less than normal carrying angle, may result from a supracondylar fracture of the humerus. Posterior elbow swelling should be noted, as it may be a sign of olecranon bursitis or fracture.

Range of motion should include both active and passive testing. Passive limitation warrants further investigation to determine the source of mechanical blockade. Normal values for forearm range of motion are as follows: extension (0 degrees), flexion (150 degrees), pronation (70 degrees), and supination (90 degrees).[2] Coronal plane stability should be assessed with valgus and varus testing in 10–15 degrees of flexion as well as in full extension. Elbow flexion of 10–15 degrees allows for unlocking of the olecranon from its fossa, thus revealing more subtle instability. Anterior-posterior stress should be applied to test for sagittal plane instability. Palpation with the elbow held at 90 degrees identifies areas of tenderness. When examining the elbow, it is helpful to con-

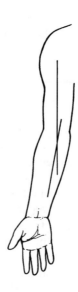

FIGURE 9.4   *The carrying angle is the angle formed between the arm and the forearm. Normal carrying angles measure up to 5 degrees of valgus in men and 10–15 degrees valgus in women.*

centrate on specific areas, such as the lateral, medial, anterior, and posterior regions. What follows is a brief description of some of the techniques of examining those regions.

Lateral

The lateral epicondyle, supracondylar line of the humerus, tendon origins, and radial head should be palpated. Rotation of the radial head is noted with pronation and supination. The lateral collateral ligament and annular ligament (located deep to the extensor aponeurosis) are not directly palpable, although the area should be examined for tenderness.

The extensor forearm muscle group is often subject to overuse injury, and palpable tenderness over the extensor carpi radialis brevis is common in this condition. Pain is intensified with active (resisted) wrist and finger extension and passive wrist flexion, especially with the elbow extended. In more severe cases symptoms are elicited with the elbow flexed as well. Strong gripping motions also reproduce symptoms of lateral overuse.

The tennis elbow (lateral epicondylitis) test (Figure 9.5) is performed with the patient's elbow stabilized by the examiner's thumb, which rests on the patient's lateral epicondyle. The patient is then asked to make a fist, pronate the forearm, and radially deviate and extend the wrist while the examiner resists the motion. A positive sign is indicated by a sudden, severe pain in the area of the lateral epicondyle of the humerus.[3]

Medial

The medial epicondyle, medial supracondylar line of the humerus, and ulnar border should be palpated. Overuse of the flexor mass results in pain and palpable tenderness at the medial epicondyle (and for approximately 1–3 cm distal to the epicondyle). Pain is intensified with provocative testing such as

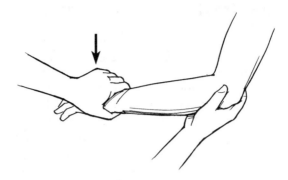

FIGURE 9.5   *The lateral tennis elbow test. The examiner's thumb rests on the lateral epicondyle. The patient is asked to make a fist and then pronate the forearm while radially deviating and extending the wrist. The examiner resists this motion. Pain at the lateral epicondyle is a positive finding.*

active (resisted) wrist flexion and passive wrist and finger extension, especially with the elbow extended (and in advanced cases, with the elbow bent as well).

The ulnar nerve is located in the retrocondylar groove, the sulcus between the medial epicondyle and the olecranon. Tinel's sign (tapping the area of the nerve in the ulnar groove, which results in a tingling sensation down the arm in the ulnar nerve distribution) may be present in patients with nerve entrapment, but is often positive in normal subjects as well. Laxity or pain at the underside of the medial epicondyle that is exacerbated by valgus stress testing (force applied laterally to stress the medial structures) suggests a sprain or tear of the medial collateral ligament.

The golfer's elbow (medial epicondylitis) test is performed with the examiner palpating the patient's medial epicondyle, followed by passive supination and wrist extension. A positive sign is indicated by pain over the medial epicondyle of the humerus.[3]

Ancillary Diagnostic Testing

X-ray testing should include anteroposterior and lateral views. This helps identify bony pathology, including loose bodies, calcification, myositis ossificans, joint-space narrowing, or osteophytes. Special views, such as an oblique view to examine the radial head or an axial projection to examine the olecranon fossa, are obtained as deemed necessary. Arthrography and magnetic resonance imaging (MRI) can identify loose bodies, ligament ruptures, chondral defects, and articular cartilage damage. Triple-phase bone scans are sensitive for stress fractures, infections, and tumors. Ultrasound may be a useful imaging modality for detection of tendon and other soft tissue injury. Computed tomography scans are useful in the evaluation of complex bony anatomy.[4] Arthroscopy is the final diagnostic approach for intra-articular inspection, joint debridement, and removal of loose bodies, as indicated. Electromyography (EMG) can help detect areas of nerve compression.

Diagnosis and Treatment of Specific Disorders

Injuries to the elbow can be divided into those resulting from overuse and those resulting from single-event trauma. Overuse injuries are caused by repetitive loads, which result in chronic pathologic changes in the tissue involved. Several factors have been identified that contribute to such injury (Table 9.1). Intrinsic factors are unique to the individual and include forearm muscle problems such as weakness, imbalance, or inflexibility, as well as instability of the elbow complex and previous injury. Extrinsic factors are related to training errors and include improper conditioning, techniques, and equipment. Rehabilitative management includes correction of such inadequacies, in addition to promoting healing of the injured tissues.

When dealing with problems of the elbow, it is important to keep in mind a few general principles. First, although early rest to the area may be beneficial, this does not mean immobilization, but rather the elimination of specific activities that cause pain (abuse). For example, if lateral tennis elbow symptoms occur only with the tennis backhand stroke, the player is not instructed to avoid playing tennis, but rather to avoid using the backhand. General body conditioning should also be maintained with other exercise, such as running, if necessary.

Cortisone injections are used sparingly, as intratendinous injections can result in tendon atrophy or dissolution. Injections are generally reserved for those cases in which pain interferes with the rehabilitative progress.

Rehabilitative exercises are generally begun with a stretching program. Initially, exercises are performed with the elbow bent; later exercises involve a more straightened elbow. Daily isometric exercises without weights are started within the pain-free arcs of motion. Full-range exercises and weights are gradually added as tolerated. Exercises are performed first with the elbow bent, and then, when tolerated, with the elbow extended. Exercises can be performed throughout the day, avoiding any position that is particularly painful and following a rule of fives: 5 repetitions, 5 seconds per repetition, and 5 times per day.

Sport- or activity-specific exercise is added in a progressive, controlled fashion. Proper biomechanical technique is mandatory, and the help of a technique coach or ergonomics expert may be helpful. Assessment of technique should include attention to biomechanics, equipment, and activity-specific activities, which, when faulty, may cause concentrated force loads that lead to overuse injuries. Lateral tennis elbow seems to be closely related to a faulty

TABLE 9.1   Overuse injury risk factors

Intrinsic factors	Extrinsic factors
Malalignment	Training errors
Muscular imbalance	Equipment
Inflexibility	Environment
Muscular weakness	Technique
Instability	Sports-imposed deficiencies

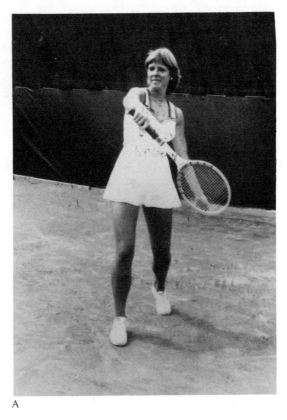

A

FIGURE 9.6   *A. Faulty backhand stroke. Poor lower body mechanics increase forceful stress on small forearm wrist extensors.*

backhand (Figure 9.6) (possibly due to weakness of shoulder external rotation) or delayed forehand with a late wrist snap. Medial tennis elbow appears to be related to overhead serves as well as a late forehand. Control of the intensity and duration of activity is of utmost importance; athletes must follow the training principle of gradual progression. Proper equipment is important to avoid overuse injury.

Return to sports or work activity may commence when the patient has attained full range of motion and 80–90% of strength compared with the uninjured side. Sports activity should initially be limited to every other day, then increased as tolerated. Rehabilitative exercises should continue on return to the sports activity for up to 6 weeks. They may then be decreased as tolerated. Some degree of maintenance rehabilitative exercise assists in decreasing the likelihood of re-injury.

As overuse injuries comprise the majority of elbow disorders seen in a rehabilitative practice, the remainder of this discussion focuses on such injuries. In addition to overuse and traumatic injuries, compartment syndrome can result in elbow and forearm pain as well and is included in this discussion. Overuse injuries are conveniently classified according to their anatomic location (i.e., lateral, medial, anterior, or posterior).

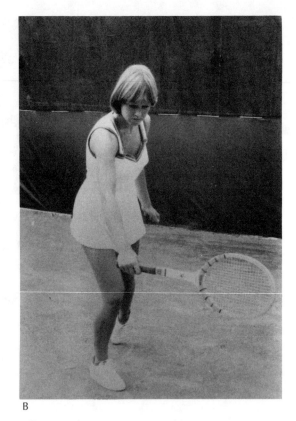

B

FIGURE 9.6 *Continued.* **B.** *Correct backhand stroke. Proper lower body mechanics with forward weight transfer and shoulder circumduction enhance the quality of tennis play and decrease the potential for forearm muscle-tendon overload. (Courtesy of Medical Sports, Inc., Arlington, VA.)*

Lateral Overuse Injuries

Lateral Tennis Elbow (Lateral Epicondylitis)

Lateral tennis elbow results from chronic overuse activity that causes pathologic changes in the forearm extensor tendons. The actual tissue changes have been termed *angiofibroblastic tendonosis.* Histologically, the changes appear as an invasion of young vascular and fibroblastic tissue in a characteristic pattern, with collagen formation in an unorganized fashion. The extensor carpi radialis brevis tendon is the structure most commonly involved. The extensor communis and, rarely, the extensor carpi ulnaris, may be involved as well. It should be noted that this condition presents primarily as a degenerative rather than an inflammatory process (inflammatory cells are rarely present in histologic specimens). Furthermore, changes occur within the tendon itself, not specifically at the epicondyle. Therefore, the term *epicondylitis* is really a misnomer. Most commonly seen in racquet sports and in occupations requiring repetitive extensor forearm use, lateral tennis elbow has been related to poor sport and occupational mechanics (e.g., lifting with the palm down), conditioning, and equipment use. In tennis, weakness of the external rotators of the shoulder cause the player to compensate with wrist extension, which leads to the classic tennis elbow.

Diagnosis

Patients with lateral tennis elbow present with localized tenderness medial and distal to the lateral epicondyle.[5] Pain and tenderness extend distally along the muscle mass of the extensor carpi radialis brevis. Symptoms are exacerbated with provocative stress testing such as active (resisted) wrist and finger extension with the elbow extended (and in advanced cases, with the elbow flexed). Passive wrist flexion can also increase symptoms, especially with the elbow extended. Radiographs are often normal, but may show calcific deposits in the extensor aponeurosis.

Treatment

When treating a patient for lateral tennis elbow, it is important to address weaknesses and biomechanical abnormalities in other parts of the upper extremity, which may be related to this condition.

Early on, relief of pain and any inflammation that is present is achieved through relative rest, ice, and nonsteroidal anti-inflammatory drugs (NSAIDs). Ice can be applied multiple times throughout the day. Other helpful modalities may include ultrasound, electrical stimulation, and other sources of heat.

Rehabilitative exercises are begun with isometric strengthening of the elbow flexors, wrist extensors, and pronators and supinators. This initially is done only within the arcs of pain-free motion, but later is expanded to include full range of motion. Isotonic weight and resistance training is added as tolerated, initially with the elbow flexed and later with the elbow extended. For more competitive athletes, arm cycling and isokinetic exercises may be useful as well. Stretching is often not tolerated early in the treatment course, but as 80% of normal strength is achieved, a stretching program can be initiated. The stretches included in this program are performed in flexion and extension; again at first with the elbow flexed, and later with the elbow extended. Ice application both before and after stretching can be beneficial.

When the patient is starting to feel better and is ready to return to full activity, a gradual progression of return to either sport or job is indicated. Proper technique should be taught, and aggravating activities avoided. As a rule, patients should not lift objects with the palm down, especially heavy objects on a repetitive basis. They should avoid prolonged or strong gripping activities, which cause a contraction of the wrist extensors. They may need to be taught not to grip a briefcase or suitcase overly tightly, but to let the fingers carry the load. Too early a return to activity often causes a recurrence, which can be difficult to treat.

Surgical management, which includes resection of the pathologic tissue while leaving all normal tendon origins in place, is considered only if the patient fails to respond to an adequate rehabilitation program (generally lasting a minimum of 3–4 months).[6,7]

COUNTERFORCE BRACING Counterforce bracing is commonly used by patients even before they seek medical attention. Such bracing is believed to constrain the extensor muscle groups while maintaining muscle balance (Figure 9.7).

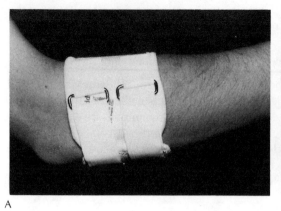
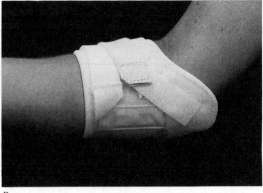

A   B

FIGURE 9.7   *Elbow counterforce braces. Counterforce bracing constrains key muscle groups while main-taining muscle balance, thus controlling intrinsic overload of the elbow tendon. **A.** Lateral tennis elbow coun-terforce brace. **B.** Medial tennis elbow counterforce brace. The medial brace extends over the medial epicondyle, providing additional support to the pronator teres and flexor carpi radialis.*

Elbow counterforce bracing has been shown to decrease EMG muscle activity and elbow angular acceleration, and may therefore be of value in treating tennis elbow.[8]

CORTICOSTEROID INJECTION   Corticosteroid injections into the lateral epicondylar region or into the most painful area of muscle/tendon involvement may in some cases be necessary, but is usually reserved for those persons who cannot participate in a proper rehabilitation program because of severe pain. Because most cases of tennis elbow are not truly inflammatory, it is unclear exactly what the mechanism of action of the steroid is. Some believe that it accelerates the degenerative process and causes a tearing of some of the damaged tissues, in effect mimicking a surgical resection of these tissues. In any case, such injections often provide dramatic relief. If no further treatment is instituted, this relief is likely only temporary.

Posterior Interosseous Nerve Entrapment
The posterior interosseous syndrome is an entrapment neuropathy. It involves damage to the posterior interosseous branch of the radial nerve at the fibrous arch of the supinator muscle or, more distally, within the muscle itself.

Diagnosis
In posterior interosseous nerve compression, lateral elbow pain radiates into the distal forearm and is aggravated by pronation and supination. Tenderness is noted 3–4 cm distal to the lateral epicondyle where the nerve crosses the radial head and penetrates the supinator muscle. Tinel's sign may be present and there may be weakness of the wrist and finger extensors. Numbness is not normally present, as this is a motor nerve at this level. Confirmation of the condition can be obtained with EMG. This neuropathy is sometimes seen in conjunction with lateral epicondylitis, and before patients undergo surgery for the epicondylitis it is sometimes helpful to obtain an EMG to see whether a nerve release should be incorporated into the surgery.

Treatment

Treatment of posterior interosseous nerve entrapment emphasizes rest, NSAIDs, and flexibility and endurance training. Surgical decompression may become necessary in refractory cases.[9]

Radiocapitellar Chondromalacia

Radiocapitellar chondromalacia occurs when repetitive valgus forces, such as those encountered in throwing sports, cause lateral elbow joint compression, possibly leading to damage to the radial head and humeral capitellum.

Diagnosis

Pain in radiocapitellar chondromalacia is localized to the radiocapitellar joint and is exacerbated by activity. Crepitus or "catching" may be present. An axial load applied with passive supination and pronation often provokes pain and can be helpful in differentiating radiocapitellar chondromalacia from lateral tennis elbow. X-ray studies demonstrate a loss of radiocapitellar joint space, osteophytes, and sometimes, loose bodies.

Treatment

Mild cases of radiocapitellar chondromalacia respond to NSAIDs and rehabilitation. Exercises are similar to those described for lateral tennis elbow; however, special caution to perform exercises only within pain-free arcs is necessary to ensure joint safety. Surgical débridement is often necessary, especially in more severe cases.

Posterolateral Synovitis

A potential and not uncommon companion to lateral tennis elbow is synovitis and (probable) chondromalacia of the posterolateral joint in and around the lateral olecranon gutter. This most likely represents an impingement phenomenon of the inflamed synovium.

Diagnosis

In posterolateral synovitis, pain and tenderness are localized to the lateral olecranon gutter to the level of radial head. Joint crepitus may be present, but motion is rarely restricted. Posterolateral synovitis is most often associated with lateral tennis elbow, but may present independently or in association with other elbow maladies.

Treatment

Conservative treatment for posterolateral synovitis emphasizes anti-inflammatory measures (i.e., NSAIDs, ice, relative rest). Rehabilitative exercises are similar to those described for lateral tennis elbow; however, exercises are initiated with the elbow straight. In general, exercises performed with the elbow bent are poorly tolerated by patients with posterolateral synovitis. Recalcitrant cases require surgical débridement.

Osteochondritis Dissecans Capitellum

Lateral compressive forces on the elbow joint can lead to focal avascular necrosis of the capitellum. This is known as osteochondritis dissecans.

Diagnosis

In osteochondritis dissecans, pain at the radiocapitellar joint is increased with pronation and supination. Patients often lack full active and passive elbow extension. X-ray films may reveal a flattening or focal distortion of the capitellum and perhaps even loose bodies. Tomograms or MRI can confirm the diagnosis.

Treatment
Osteochondritis dissecans of the capitellum often responds to rest (3–4 months of nonabusive activity) and rehabilitative effort. Exercises are directed toward minimizing strength loss during the rest period. Specific exercises are similar to those described for lateral tennis elbow, with added emphasis on biceps and triceps strength. Surgery is required if loose bodies are present. Preliminary evidence suggests that electrical bone stimulation may stimulate vascular supply and healing, and thus it is recommended by the authors.

Medial Overuse Injuries

Medial Tennis Elbow (Medial Epicondylitis)
Medial tennis elbow, or golfer's elbow, results from chronic overuse of the flexor forearm musculature.[5] Primary injury occurs in the pronator teres and flexor carpi radialis and, to a lesser degree, in the palmaris longus, flexor carpi ulnaris, and (rarely) the flexor digitorum sublimis.

Diagnosis
In medial tennis elbow, localized tenderness at the tip of the epicondyle extends distally for approximately 1–3 cm along the pronator teres and flexor carpi radialis. Pain is exacerbated by active (resisted) wrist flexion or pronation with the elbow in extension (and in advanced cases, with the elbow flexed). Passive wrist and finger extension also exacerbates the pain, more significantly with the elbow in extension and supination.

Treatment
Rehabilitative management for medial tennis elbow is essentially the same as for lateral tennis elbow, except that the opposite side and direction are emphasized. Wrist flexor isometric exercises are also useful. Injections are rarely necessary, but if performed, great care should be taken because of the proximity of the ulnar nerve. This condition also should not be mistaken for an ulnar neuropathy, which can occur in the same vicinity. Surgical management is considered only after failure of adequate rehabilitative efforts.

Ulnar Nerve Compression or Subluxation
Nirschl has divided the medial epicondylar groove into three zones[10]:

Zone I: Proximal to the medial epicondyle

Zone II: The level of the medial epicondyle (retrocondylar groove)

Zone III: Distal to the medial epicondyle (cubital tunnel)

Repetitive overuse can result in compression of the ulnar nerve in zone II by a tight flexor carpi ulnaris muscle. Nerve irritation can also be caused in zones II and III by a subluxating ulnar nerve (a nerve that slips around the epicondyle during elbow flexion); in zone II by elbow synovitis; in zone I or II by cubitus valgus deformity; or in zone I by the medial inter-muscular septum.

The ulnar nerve can also be damaged by direct trauma, and in some cases, remote trauma to the elbow can cause an ulnar neuropathy. This can occur even years after the injury and is termed *tardy ulnar palsy*.

Diagnosis

In ulnar neuropathy at the elbow there may be pain, numbness, and weakness in the ulnar nerve distribution. Intrinsic hand muscle wasting or hypothenar atrophy may be noted in long-standing cases. A positive Tinel's sign may be elicited over the ulnar nerve within the epicondylar groove, but there is a high rate of false-positive test results. Subluxation of the nerve can sometimes be palpated when the patient's elbow is flexed past 90 degrees, and confronta-tional strength testing is often positive (see Chapter 10). Confirmation of the disorder is made electromyographically. EMG also helps rule out other, simi-larly presenting conditions such as thoracic outlet syndrome, ulnar neuropathy at the wrist, and radiculopathy.

Treatment

Conservative management of an ulnar entrapment neuropathy includes the use of NSAIDs, protection with an elbow pad and night splint, avoidance of extreme repetitive flexion (especially in cases of a subluxating nerve), and exercise emphasizing elbow flexibility and forearm strength and endurance. Patients should be told not to sleep with their hands under their pillows, prop the chin in the hand, or lean on the elbows for prolonged periods of time. Chronic subluxation, failure to respond to conservative management after 3–4 months, or progressive motor or sensory deficits call for surgical decompres-sion of the nerve. In some cases an anterior transposition of the ulnar nerve is indicated. Surgical transposition may be suboptimal, however, if blood supply to the nerve is compromised.

Medial Collateral Ligament Sprain

Medial collateral ligament (MCL) sprain can result from repetitive valgus stress and is common in racquet and throwing sports, especially in baseball pitchers.[5]

Diagnosis

In MCL sprains, elbow pain of insidious onset is increased by valgus stress testing at 30 degrees of elbow flexion. MCL sprain must be differentiated from complete ligamentous rupture, which is more often associated with acute trauma. Instability on examination and abnormal calcification on plain x-rays suggest the presence of ligament rupture. This diagnosis can be con-firmed by MRI.[11]

Treatment

Most cases of MCL sprain respond to rehabilitative management. Emphasis is placed on isometric exercises of the forearm flexors and pronators to enhance their role as secondary stabilizers of the medial joint. Chronic cases, especially if accompanied by heterotopic ossification (abnormal bone deposition), bone spurring, or loose bodies, may require surgical repair (usually with an autoge-nous tendon graft).

Medial Epicondyle Apophysitis (Little League Elbow)

Repetitive valgus stress in an adolescent whose growth plates have not yet fused can result in an avulsion of the medial epicondyle. This is an *apophysitis*. A single traumatic event can also result in a complete avulsion of the epicondyle. This is associated with rupture of the medial capsule.

Diagnosis

In apophysitis, pain and tenderness are localized to the medial epicondyle. The symptoms are intensified by throwing. A widening of the apophyseal line or even complete apophyseal separation are seen on x-ray.

Treatment

Lesions involving less than 0.5–1.0 cm of apophyseal separation are initially treated with rest for 2–3 weeks. This is followed by a rehabilitative effort that is similar to the one described for medial tennis elbow; however, resistance exercises are avoided until isotonic exercises (without weight) can be performed without pain (generally 2–3 weeks). Throwing is avoided for 6–12 weeks. Separation greater than 0.5–1.0 cm, failure to respond to conservative measurement, or sudden traumatic avulsion are indications for surgery.

Anterior Overuse Injuries

Biceps Tendonitis

Biceps tendonitis is an overuse injury resulting from repetitive elbow flexion and forearm supination.

Diagnosis

In biceps tendonitis, localized pain of the biceps tendon in the anterior elbow is exacerbated by resisted flexion and supination.

Treatment

Rehabilitation for biceps tendonitis emphasizes rest, NSAIDs, and later, restoration of strength and flexibility of the flexor mechanism. The biceps rarely rupture at the elbow, and such an injury is generally attributable to a traumatic event. If it occurs, immediate surgical repair is indicated.

Pronator Teres Syndrome

The pronator teres syndrome is an entrapment neuropathy of the median nerve distal to the antecubital fossa. In most cases, the median nerve pierces the two heads of the pronator teres before passing under the muscle. Muscle hypertrophy, trauma, or entrapment by an anomalous fibrous band may injure the nerve at this point.[11]

Diagnosis

In this condition, pain at the pronator teres is exacerbated by resisted pronation. Weakness and sensory changes can be seen in the median nerve distribution, and Tinel's sign may be present. Diagnosis is confirmed electromyographically and rules out other conditions such as carpal tunnel syndrome or radiculopathy.

Treatment

Rehabilitation emphasizes removal of the aggravating activity, rest, NSAIDs, ice, and restoration of proper flexibility and strength of the wrist flexors and forearm pronators. Rehabilitation is most beneficial in those cases in which compression is related to medial elbow tendonosis. Gentle massage along the fibers may aid in breaking up adhesions. Surgical release may be necessary in recalcitrant cases (i.e., those cases related to muscle hypertrophy or entrapment by a fibrous band).

Anterior Capsule Strain

Repetitive hyperextension activity results in small tears of the anterior joint capsule. Associated brachialis muscle tears with myositis may also occur. Anterior elbow pain may also occur after a single traumatic hyperextension event.

Diagnosis

Anterior elbow pain is worsened with passive extension or with hyperextension stress testing of the elbow. Radiographs are advisable to rule out myositis ossifications of the brachialis muscle.

Treatment

Rehabilitation of anterior capsule strain emphasizes active range-of-motion exercise to avoid the formation of a flexion contracture. A gradual strengthening program for the biceps and brachialis accompanies the flexibility program.

Posterior Overuse Injuries

Triceps Tendonitis

Triceps tendon overload injury results from repetitive extension of the elbow.

Diagnosis

In triceps tendonitis, posterior elbow pain is worsened by resisted extension. X-ray evaluation is indicated to rule out olecranon apophysitis in adolescents and an avulsion fracture in adults.

Treatment

Initial management includes rest, NSAIDs, and ice. Rehabilitative exercises emphasize flexibility and strength of the extensor mechanism.

A violent triceps contraction may result in tendon rupture or olecranon avulsion fracture. These conditions are associated with severe pain and often a palpable defect at the triceps insertion. Surgical reattachment is followed by a short period of immobilization, then the gradual addition of range-of-motion and strengthening exercises.

Olecranon Bursitis

Inflammation of the olecranon bursa may be caused by repetitive or single-event trauma. This can occur with prolonged pressure on the bursa, as when leaning on the elbow (so-called *student's elbow*).

Diagnosis

Repetitive irritation, contusion, or direct trauma to the olecranon bursa results in swelling of the posterior elbow. Pain or associated redness may be signs of an associated intrabursal infection. X-ray studies are indicated to rule out loose fragments, prominent exostosis, or chip fractures.

Treatment

Treatment of bursitis involves ice, NSAIDs, and the use of elbow pads. In refractory cases, the bursal fluid should be aspirated. This should also be done in cases in which infection is suspected. Recurrent swelling may necessitate surgical referral for bursectomy.

Olecranon Impingement Syndrome

Repetitive impingement of the olecranon in the olecranon fossa may occur with valgus stress in throwing sports. Stress to both articular surfaces of the joint may result in the formation of loose bodies, chondromalacia, and synovitis.[5]

Diagnosis

In olecranon impingement, posterior elbow pain may be associated with catching, clicking, and crepitus, which are worsened by elbow extension. Full extension may be limited by mechanical blockade. X-ray findings confirm loose bodies, olecranon osteophytes, and commonly associated anterior elbow changes.

Treatment

Mild cases of olecranon impingement respond to rehabilitative management to re-establish normal motion, strength, and endurance; however, continued pain, loose bodies, and mechanical blockade are indications for surgery.[5]

Olecranon Stress Fracture or Apophysitis

Repetitive overload may result in olecranon stress fracture or separation of the olecranon apophysis.

Diagnosis

In these conditions, pain over the olecranon is exacerbated by resisted elbow extension. Swelling may be present, and the bone may be tender to percussion. X-ray studies may confirm the diagnosis; however, a bone scan is sometimes necessary to detect early stress fractures.

Treatment

Treatment involves relaxed immobilization for 4–6 weeks with a 90-degree elbow immobilizer. Daily range-of-motion exercises are performed. Rehabilitation commences after 4–6 weeks if x-ray evaluation and clinical examination show evidence of healing. Separation of the olecranon apophysis is an indication for surgical referral for possible open reduction and internal fixation.

Compartment Syndrome

Increased pressure within the volar and dorsal compartments of the forearm can compromise circulation to the tissues in these spaces. This results from trauma, bleeding, or muscle hypertrophy. Chronic exertional compartment syndrome is a condition in which excessive, intermittent pressure during activity decreases blood flow to the compartment. Intense pain, weakness, and sensory symptoms can result. Compartment pressure may be measured with a catheter. Pressures exceeding 35–40 mm Hg mandate surgical decompression.

Points of Summary

1. Injury to the elbow and forearm can most easily be classified as *overuse* or *traumatic*.
2. Overuse injuries are the result of repetitive microtrauma that, over time, results in inflammation and cellular degradation.
3. In lateral tennis elbow, the tendon most commonly involved is the extensor carpi radialis brevis. This is followed in frequency by the extensor communis and extensor carpi radialis and, to a lesser degree, the extensor carpi ulnaris.
4. In medial tennis elbow, the most commonly involved tendons are those of the pronator teres and flexor carpi radialis. The palmaris longus, flexor carpi ulnaris, and flexor sublimis may also be affected.
5. Provocative testing for lateral tennis elbow consists of active (resisted) wrist and finger extension with the elbow in extension. Testing for medial tennis elbow consists of active (resisted) wrist flexion or pronation with the elbow in extension. Advanced cases elicit pain when tested with the elbow in flexion.
6. The goal of rehabilitative exercise is to restore injured tissue to a normal or near-normal state; fitness exercise is directed toward training normal tissue to a supranormal state.
7. All rehabilitative programs should include assessment of intrinsic and extrinsic risk factors in addition to injury-specific management.
8. Surgical management of tennis elbow (conducted after failure of an adequate trial of rehabilitation) is directed toward removal of degenerated tissue, thus providing an optimum environment for more normal healing.

References

1. Coleman WW, Strauch RJ. Physical examination of the elbow. Orthop Clin North Am 1999;30(1):15–20.
2. Mehloff T, Bennett J. Elbow Injuries. In M Mellion, W Walsh, G Shelton (eds), The Team Physician's Handbook. Philadelphia: Hanley & Belfus, 1990.
3. Magee DJ. Orthopedic Physical Assessment (2nd ed). Philadelphia: Saunders, 1992;143–168.
4. Potter HG. Imaging of posttraumatic and soft tissue dysfunction in the elbow. Clin Orthop 2000;58(suppl 14)(370):9–18.
5. Field LD, Savoie FH. Common elbow injuries in sport. Sports Med 1998;26(3):193–205.
6. Nirschl R, Pettrone F. Tennis elbow: the surgical treatment of lateral epicondylitis. J Bone Joint Surg 1979;61A:832–839.

7. Sevier TL, Wilson JK. Treating lateral epicondylitis. Sports Med 1999; 28(5):375–380.
8. Groppel J, Nirschl R. A mechanical and electromyographical analysis of the effects of various joint counterforce braces on the tennis player. Am J Sports Med 1986;14:195–200.
9. Rosenbaum R. Disputed radial tunnel syndrome. Muscle Nerve 1999; 22(7):960–967.
10. Nirschl R. Soft-tissue injuries about the elbow. Clin Sports Med 1985;5: 637–652.
11. Chumbley EM, O'Connor FG, Nirschl RP. Evaluation of overuse elbow injuries. Am Fam Physician 2000;61:691–700.

Suggested Readings

Coleman WW, Strauch RJ. Physical examination of the elbow. Orthop Clin North Am 1999;30(1):15–20.

Field LD, Savoie FH. Common elbow injuries in sport. Sports Med 1998; 26(3):193–205.

Sevier TL, Wilson JK. Treating lateral epicondylitis. Sports Med 1999; 28(5):375–380.

10   Wrist and Hand

Michael J. Stonnington

The wrist and hand are complex, interrelated structures that optimally combine flexibility, power, dexterity, proprioception, and fine sensibility. Impairment of the wrist or hand can result in significant challenges when it comes to daily living, as well as vocational and recreational function.

Wrist and Hand Anatomy

Bones, Joints, and Ligaments

The wrist consists of a radiocarpal and an ulnocarpal joint (Figure 10.1). There are eight carpal bones, which articulate with the radius proximally and the metacarpals distally (Figure 10.2). The radiocarpal joint is an ellipsoid joint that includes the distal radius and the scaphoid, lunate, and triquetrum. The main stabilizing ligaments of the radiocarpal joint are the volar radiocarpal ligaments. The ulnocarpal joint is mainly composed of the triangular fibrocartilage complex (TFCC). The TFCC, a complex of ligaments and fibrocartilage, originates from the ulnar radius, inserts at the ulnar styloid, and articulates with the carpal bones.

The hand has 5 metacarpals and 14 phalanges. The first carpometacarpal joint is a sellar joint (saddle-shaped), which provides most of the mobility of the thumb. The metacarpophalangeal (MCP) joints of digits 2 through 5 are condylar joints. The MCP joints and interphalangeal (IP) joints are stabilized by a joint capsule, collateral ligaments, a volar (palmar) plate, and the intrinsic muscles. Interestingly, the collateral ligaments of the MCP joint are in a relaxed position when the digits are extended but are taut when the MCP joint is flexed (Figure 10.3). This is important when positioning the hand during immobilization, as debilitating contractures may occur if the joints are splinted in extension.

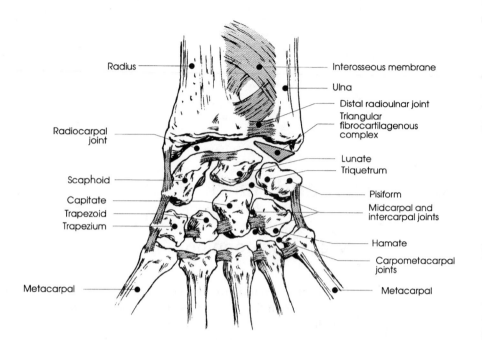

FIGURE 10.1   *The joints of the wrist and hand.*

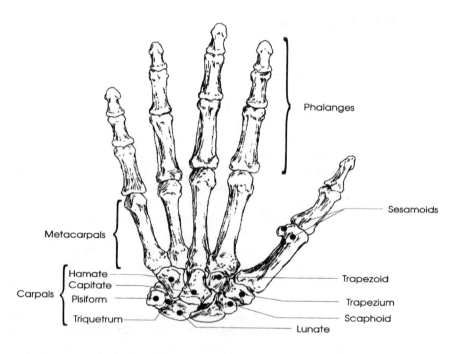

FIGURE 10.2   *The bones of the wrist and hand.*

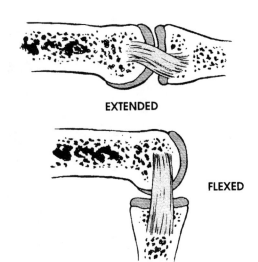

EXTENDED

FLEXED

FIGURE 10.3   *The metacarpophalangeal collateral ligaments. When the finger is extended, these ligaments are lax and allow motion in abduction and adduction. When the finger is flexed, the ligaments are taut.*

Muscles

The muscles of the wrist and hand can be divided into intrinsic and extrinsic muscles. The extrinsic muscles arise from the elbow or forearm, and their tendons insert onto the hand and wrist. The flexor digitorum superficialis (FDS) splits at the proximal interphalangeal (PIP) joint to allow the tendon of the flexor digitorum profundus (FDP) to pass distally to the distal phalanx (Figure 10.4). The FDS flexes the PIP (and MCP) joint, whereas the FDP flexes the distal interphalangeal (DIP) joint (and indirectly, the PIP and MCP joints as well). The extensor tendons have a complex arrangement on the fingers, which is called the *dorsal extensor apparatus.* Because there is only one extensor tendon for each finger, the tendons extend the MCP, PIP, and DIP joints.

The lumbricals and interossei are intrinsic muscles of the hand. The lumbricals originate from the FDP tendons and insert onto the extensor apparatus. They flex the MCP joints and extend the PIP and DIP joints. The interossei originate from the metacarpals and insert onto the phalanges and extensor apparatus. They produce abduction, adduction, and flexion of the MCP joints. The other intrinsic muscles of the hand make up the thenar and hypothenar eminences of the base of the thumb and fifth digit respectively.

Nerves

The radial, ulnar, and median nerves course into the hand. The radial nerve is a sensory nerve in the hand (i.e., radial sensory nerve). It supplies sensation to a large portion of the dorsum of the hand. The median and ulnar nerves

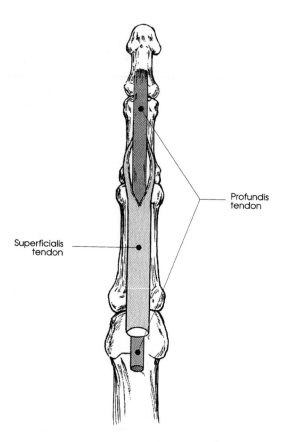

FIGURE 10.4 *The flexor tendons of the fingers. The flexor digitorum superficialis splits to allow the flexor digitorum profundus to pass underneath to the distal phalanx.*

Profundis tendon

Superficialis tendon

supply sensation to the remainder of the hand (Figure 10.5). The median nerve also innervates most of the thenar muscles (abductor pollicis brevis, opponens pollicis, half of the flexor pollicis) and two lumbricals, whereas the ulnar nerve innervates the rest of the intrinsic muscles of the hand. It should be noted that this innervation pattern does not always hold true: There are many persons with anomalous patterns.

Carpal Tunnel and Guyon's Canal

The carpal tunnel is an enclosed space formed by the carpal bones and the transverse carpal ligament (flexor retinaculum) (Figure 10.6). The transverse carpal ligament, which is the roof of the tunnel, attaches medially to the pisiform and hamate and laterally to the scaphoid and trapezium. The carpal tunnel contains nine tendons (eight finger flexors and a thumb flexor) and the median nerve. The transverse carpal ligament also forms the floor of Guyon's canal, which is covered by the volar carpal ligament. Guyon's canal contains the ulnar nerve and artery.

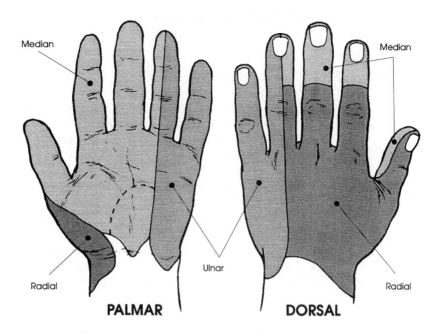

FIGURE 10.5   *The sensory innervation pattern of the hand.*

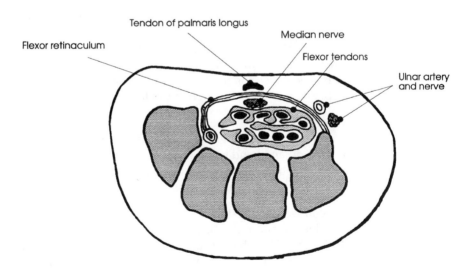

FIGURE 10.6   *The contents of the carpal tunnel: median nerve and flexor tendons of the digits.*

Examination and Testing Techniques

History and Physical Examination

Evaluation should start with a complete history. Hand dominance can be useful in evaluating disability or an overuse injury. A review of systems may lead to a diagnosis of a connective tissue disease such as rheumatoid arthritis, which often presents with hand complaints. With an injury, the mechanism of injury should be sought.

The physical examination should include observations for atrophy and skin and vascular changes as well as hand posture. The hand and wrist are palpated to detect nodules, joint swelling, and tenderness. Strength testing is performed. Grip strength may be quantified with the use of a hand-held dynamometer. Sensory testing is performed. Range of motion is assessed passively and actively. Decreased passive and active range is indicative of joint pathology, tendon pathology, or contracture. Isolated loss of active range of motion may be a sign of a tendon disruption. Range of motion of the forearm (supination and pronation) should be assessed, as the distal radioulnar joint may be a source of limited range in these movements. In addition, a complete upper extremity and neck examination is important to rule out more proximal problems that may be causing hand or wrist symptoms. A number of specific tests may also be performed.

Weber's Two-Point Discrimination Test
It is important to document and follow loss of sensation during the clinical course, especially in compressive neuropathies. In Weber's two-point discrimination test, equal pressure is exerted using a two-pronged object with a known distance separating the two points. An unfolded paper clip may simply be used. Normal digital two-point discrimination should be 6 mm or less when measured longitudinally on either side of the distal digits. The pressure applied should not be enough to blanch the skin.

Froment's Sign
To detect Froment's sign, the patient is asked to hold a piece of paper between the thumb and hand in the first web space. An inability to do so without flexing the IP joint is considered a positive sign. It is indicative of weakness of the thumb adductor, a muscle innervated by the ulnar nerve.

Tendon Isolation Testing
The flexor tendons can be tested in isolation according to their function (Figure 10.7). The FDP, which inserts on the distal phalanx, is tested by stabilizing the PIP joint and having the patient flex the finger. If the FDP is intact, the distal phalanx should flex.

The FDS is isolated by having the examiner stabilizing the adjacent fingers, keeping them in full extension. The purpose of this stabilization is to remove the contribution of the FDP to PIP flexion. Because the FDP tendons arise from a common muscle, it is impossible to flex one DIP joint without also flexing the neighboring ones. Therefore, the examiner stabilizes the adjacent finger PIP and DIP joints and asks the patient to flex the finger being tested. Normally

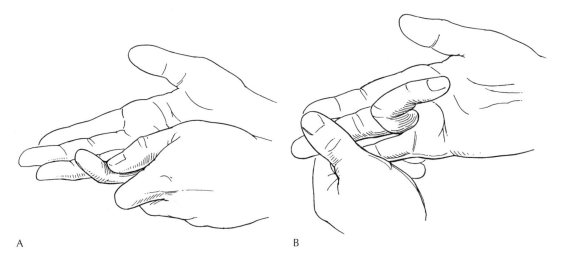

FIGURE 10.7   *A. Testing the flexor digitorum profundus. B. Testing the flexor digitorum superficialis. The profundus can easily be tested by checking for motion of the distal interphalangeal joint. Because the profundus usually flexes both the proximal interphalangeal and distal interphalangeal joints, it is more difficult to test the superficialis by itself. This is accomplished by stabilizing the adjacent finger distal interphalangeal joints in extension.*

the PIP (but not the DIP) flexes. If it does not, it indicates possible FDS rupture. It should be noted that some people without injury have an inability to flex the PIP joint in isolation—especially in the small finger, but also in some cases in the ring finger. This is usually a bilateral occurrence and may be inherited. Therefore, a positive test must be interpreted with caution.[1]

Intrinsic Muscle Flexibility Testing

The intrinsic hand muscles that insert on the extensor apparatus of the digits flex the MCP and extend the PIP and DIP joints. To test for tightness (which can occur with fibrosis or rheumatoid arthritis), the patient is asked to hyperextend the MCP and maximally flex the IP joints (putting the muscles at maximal stretch). The MCP joints are then flexed (relaxing the muscles). If this flexion allows the IP joints to flex further, it is a sign of intrinsic tightness or inflexibility.

Watson's Test

Watson's test is a useful test for scapholunate instability (a tear of the scapholunate ligament). The examiner places volar pressure on the scaphoid tuberosity (near the base of the thenar eminence). The wrist is moved from ulnar to radial deviation. If the patient experiences pain or a "clunk" with radial deviation, the test is positive and suggests scapholunate instability.

Finkelstein's Test

Finkelstein's test (Figure 10.8) checks for inflammation of some of the thumb tendons, specifically the extensor pollicis brevis and abductor pollicis longus. These two tendons form the volar border of the anatomic snuffbox. The patient holds the thumb clasped in a fist and then ulnarly deviates the wrist. Pain over the tendons at the wrist and distal forearm is a positive finding. It should be noted that a mild amount of pain is normal.

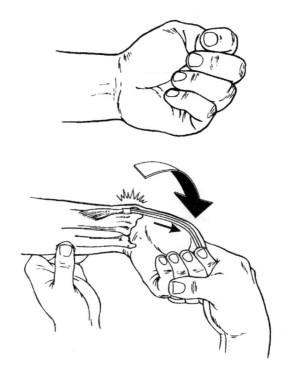

FIGURE 10.8   *Finkelstein's test for DeQuervain's tenosynovitis.*

Phalen's Test

Phalen's test (Figure 10.9) is a test for carpal tunnel syndrome (CTS). The patient is instructed to hold the hands together, back to back, for 1 minute. Pain or numbness in the distribution of the median nerve is a positive finding. The sooner these symptoms are produced, the worse the condition may be; but it must be noted that there is a high rate of false-positive and false-negative results.[2,3]

Side-to-Side Confrontational Strength Testing

Side-to-side confrontational strength testing (Figure 10.10) is a test for intrinsic hand muscle weakness.[4] Patients are told that this is a test to see "how strong your little fingers are." They are instructed to hold the hands with the fingers abducted and the little fingers touching, then to push the hands together while trying to resist this with the little fingers. If one side is weaker than the other, the little and ring fingers come together as depicted in the figure. This can be due to weakness from ulnar neuropathy or other nerve damage, or from muscle weakness, such as after an injury or period of casting.

Tinel's Test

Tinel's test, tapping over the median nerve at the wrist with either a finger or a reflex hammer, sometimes causes pain and numbness in the median

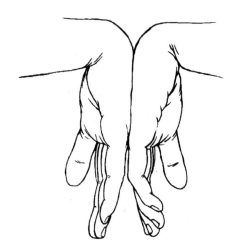

FIGURE 10.9   *Phalen's test.*

nerve distribution. This test is adjunctive in making the diagnosis of carpal tunnel syndrome, but it is insensitive and not of much clinical value.[3]

Edema Measurement

To quantify the extent of hand swelling, the fingers and wrist can be measured circumferentially. Another, more accurate, technique is to measure hand volume by water displacement. This allows serial measurement of the progression of edema.

Allen's Test

Allen's test evaluates the patency of the radial and ulnar arteries to the hand. The patient is asked to clench the hand in a fist while the examiner occludes one artery with firm pressure. When the patient opens the fist, the hand should quickly turn pink. If it remains pale, it is a sign that the opposite artery is occluded.

Ancillary Diagnostic Testing

Most ancillary radiographic studies involve plain x-ray films to evaluate for fracture and abnormal bone alignment, or to detect signs of degenerative joint or inflammatory disease. Computed tomography scanning is useful for detecting occult fractures and assessment of bone healing. Magnetic resonance imaging (MRI) is useful for evaluating the soft tissues as well as some osseous abnormalities, such as avascular necrosis. Bone scanning is also useful for detecting occult fractures and avascular necrosis. Cineradiography is useful for detecting carpal instability patterns, whereas arthrography aids in the diagnosis of intercarpal ligament tears and tears of the TFCC. Laboratory tests are commonly used to help diagnose connective tissue disease.

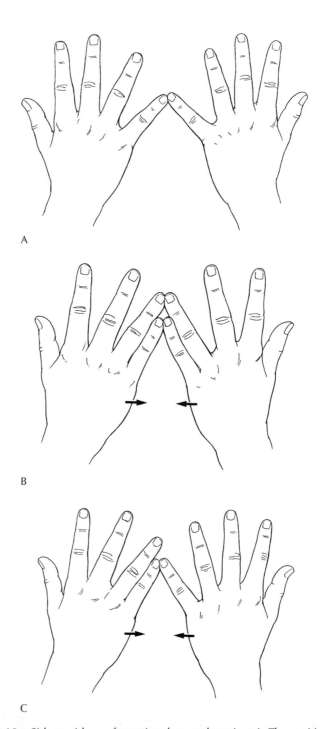

FIGURE 10.10 *Side-to-side confrontational strength testing.* **A.** *The position of the hands.* **B.** *The patient is asked to push the hands together while resisting this motion with the fifth digits. This is a negative result, indicating symmetry of strength.* **C.** *A positive test, indicating unilateral weakness.*

Diagnosis and Treatment of Specific Disorders

Carpal Tunnel Syndrome

CTS is a compression neuropathy of the median nerve as it passes under the transverse carpal ligament. This ligament is stout and unyielding, and any condition that results in increased pressure within the carpal tunnel space can compress the nerve, leading to damage or neuropathy. Patients with CTS have been shown to have greater pressures within their carpal tunnels than asymptomatic individuals.[5] This increased pressure can occur in metabolic conditions such as diabetes mellitus and hypothyroidism, in pregnancy, or in the presence of a mass in the carpal tunnel (e.g., a ganglion). Although CTS does appear to be related to certain activities and jobs that stress the wrist with repetitive motion (secretarial or computer work), awkward posture (e.g., that of a dental hygienist), cold environment (meat/fish packing), or vibration, this association is not as clear-cut as often assumed.[6] CTS does appear to be correlated with obesity and a squarer (as opposed to flat) wrist.[7,8] CTS can be caused by trauma to the wrist or by synovitis, such as in rheumatoid arthritis. Often the etiology is unknown.

Diagnosis
Patients typically complain of pain, numbness, or tingling in the median nerve distribution. This often occurs with certain activities or hand postures, such as those used during driving. It may progress from intermittent to constant, and is particularly common at night. Weakness and atrophy may eventually occur in the thenar muscles.

On examination, patients may have a positive Phalen's test and Tinel's sign (beware of a high rate of false-positive and false-negative results). They also may have a positive median nerve compression test, which is performed by placing constant pressure on the carpal tunnel: It is positive when pain or paresthesias are produced in the median nerve distribution (again, beware of the high rate of false-positive and false-negative results).[2,9] Patients may also have reduced two-point discrimination and decreased sensation to light touch.

Definitive diagnosis is made electrodiagnostically with an electromyogram (EMG), which reveals slowing of nerve conduction across the wrist or signs of axonal damage in the thenar muscles. Occasionally, patients may have CTS without objective EMG abnormalities.

When CTS is considered as a diagnosis, other conditions, such as diabetes mellitus, hypothyroidism, peripheral neuropathy, more proximal median neuropathy, radiculopathy, and inflammatory arthritis should be considered in the differential.

Treatment
The treatment of CTS includes both nonoperative and operative measures. Generally, patients are evaluated on a case-by-case basis. Patients with intermittent symptoms, mild or no EMG changes, and a clear cause of the condition may be treated nonoperatively. This treatment involves nonsteroidal anti-inflammatory drugs (NSAIDs), avoidance of exacerbating activity, and a wrist

control splint.[10] The splint should be in neutral or slight extension, as extreme flexion or extension increases the pressure within the carpal tunnel. If symptoms progress or persist, surgery may be considered. It is important not to avoid surgery for too long in persistent cases, as permanent nerve damage could occur. In severe cases in which irreversible damage has already occurred, surgery may not improve symptoms but could prevent progressive worsening of symptoms. Pregnant patients, or those with temporary causes of CTS, can usually be treated nonoperatively. A patient with severe symptoms and marked EMG abnormalities at initial evaluation should be treated operatively from the outset.

Operative treatment entails a complete division of the transverse carpal ligament. It is an effective procedure that can be done through an incision on the palm (with occasional extension across the wrist). Endoscopic carpal tunnel releases done through one or two very small incisions have been performed for years now, and have been proven to be safe and reliable in the hands of experienced surgeons.[11]

Some physicians inject the carpal tunnel with steroids to treat CTS. This offers transient relief to 80% of patients, but only 22% are symptom-free 12 months later. Those with mild presentations are the ones most likely to benefit.[2,12]

Patients with CTS should make appropriate workplace or activity modifications. In general, there is a poor prognosis for conservative management in patients older than 50 years of age, those who have had symptoms for more than 10 months, those with constant paresthesias, those with stenosing flexor tenosynovitis, and those with a Phalen's test that is positive in less than 30 seconds.

Ulnar Neuropathy at the Wrist

In ulnar neuropathy (which is less common than CTS), the ulnar nerve becomes compressed in Guyon's canal. It is most likely to occur in cyclists, weight lifters, and people who work with vibrating tools. It can also occur secondary to trauma.

Diagnosis

Ulnar neuropathy at the wrist has a similar presentation to CTS, except that the paresthesias are in the sensory distribution of the ulnar nerve. It often appears in conjunction with CTS (which can cloud the presentation). Motor weakness affects the hypothenar muscles, the intrinsic hand muscles (weak finger abduction/adduction), and the thumb adductors (Froment's sign may be positive). Side-to-side confrontational strength testing is very sensitive in detecting intrinsic hand muscle weakness; however, this is a nonspecific finding that does not identify whether the weakness is due to muscular or neurologic cause. In very advanced cases, the hand is flat and atrophic and intrinsic muscle weakness can lead to a "claw-hand" deformity. Electro-diagnostic testing is the best way to confirm an ulnar neuropathy, and can also rule out more proximal ulnar nerve damage, CTS, radiculopathy, or plexopathy. Due to variations in the innervation patterns of the hand, symptoms of nerve damage can be highly variable. Many patients thought to have an ulnar neuropathy actually have CTS and vice versa. EMG can help sort this out *before* surgery.

When a diagnosis of ulnar neuropathy at the wrist is made, it is useful to obtain MRI imaging of the wrist to ensure that there is no compressive lesion that needs to be addressed, especially if no other obvious cause of the condition is present.

Treatment

Often, by simply decreasing the offensive activity, ulnar compression symptoms will improve. For example, padding handlebars and making frequent changes in cycling position can be very helpful for the cyclist. In the workplace, grips can be modified with larger handles to reduce the compressive forces of a power grip. A period of rest from exacerbating activities is often helpful and usually indicated, along with occupational or recreational activity modifications. Adjunct nonoperative treatment includes splinting, NSAIDs, and, rarely, steroid injections.

In refractory cases, recurrent cases, or those secondary to a mass, surgical decompression should be considered. If ulnar neuropathy is present in conjunction with CTS, both the transverse carpal ligament and volar carpal ligament are released.

Rheumatoid Arthritis

Rheumatoid arthritis (RA) is one of many inflammatory arthritides. It commonly affects the hand and, in many cases, results in severe deformities. RA is a systemic soft tissue process that affects the bones and ligaments secondarily. Hypertrophic synovitis can result in cartilage and ligament destruction, disruption of tendons, nerve dysfunction, and erosion or dislocation of joints. The wrist and MCP joints are most often involved, followed by the PIP joints. Optimal medical management is mandatory to retard the disease's potentially devastating consequences.

Diagnosis

RA is diagnosed by clinical symptoms, connective tissue laboratory tests, x-rays, and synovial fluid analysis.

Acutely inflamed joints are boggy and warm to touch. Late manifestations of the disease result in several different deformities.

- *MCP ulnar drift* occurs at the MCP joints, with an ulnar shift of the extensor tendons. The digits are deviated in an ulnar direction.
- *Swan neck deformity* results from a combination of muscle imbalance, intrinsic muscle tightness, and disease of the capsule and ligaments at the PIP joints. The deformity describes hyperextension of the PIP joint and flexion of the DIP joint (Figure 10.11).
- *Boutonniere deformity* is caused by an extensor imbalance at the MCP, which leads to hyperextension. Synovitis at the PIP joint results in attenuation or disruption of the central slip and subluxation of the lateral slips of tendons called the lateral bands. The end result is flexion of the PIP joint with extension of the DIP joint (Figure 10.12).

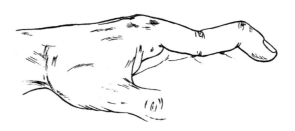

FIGURE 10.11   *Swan neck deformity of the finger.*

Treatment

Medical management of RA essentially consists of medications to reduce inflammation. This includes NSAIDs, oral steroids, gold salts, chemotherapeutic agents, and immunotherapy.

Rehabilitation begins with patient education on joint protection and energy conservation techniques to reduce inflammation and fatigue. A consultation with an occupational therapist helps patients and their families structure activities to place less stress on the joints. Assessment of daily activities is important, with the goal of reducing excessive flexor forces. The patient may be instructed in the use of large handled tools, cooking utensils, and doorknobs.

During acute flare-ups, resting hand and wrist splints may be used to reduce joint stress and inflammation. Passive and active range-of-motion exercises are avoided in acutely inflamed joints, as they increase the inflammation. Isomet-

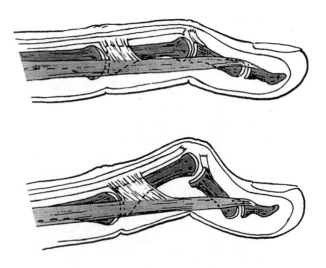

FIGURE 10.12   *Boutonniere deformity of the finger, caused by rupture of the central slip of the extensor tendon.*

ric exercises are acceptable to maintain strength.[13] Maintaining joint range of motion should be the goal in managing these patients (daily stretching routines can be useful, except during flare-ups).

Splinting of the hand and wrist may help to provide a more functional position and to prevent joint subluxation. Special splints are available to counteract the particular deformities present, such as ulnar drift, swan neck deformity, or boutonniere deformity.

Surgical intervention can be helpful for all deformities. There are numerous procedures, ranging from soft tissue reconstructions to implant arthroplasties to fusions. These procedures are beyond the scope of this chapter. However, successful surgical results depend on a close working relationship between the rheumatologist, physiatrist, orthopedic surgeon, and therapist.

Degenerative Joint Disease

Degenerative joint disease (DJD), also known as *osteoarthritis*, affects many joints, including those of the hand. DJD involves degeneration of the joint with a loss of articular cartilage and formation of bony spurs (called *osteophytes*) around the joint. Typically, the carpometacarpal joint of the thumb and the DIP joints in the hand are most affected. The PIP joints are less commonly affected.

Diagnosis
The primary complaints of DJD are pain and joint stiffness. Carpometacarpal involvement of the thumb is characterized by decreased pinch strength and a positive grind test (pain and crepitus with axial/rotatory forces applied across the thumb). The affected joints in the fingers have associated hard nodules (Heberden's nodes at the DIP joints and Bouchard's nodes at the PIP joints). The wrist has decreased and painful terminal range of motion. X-rays reveal characteristic findings such as joint-space narrowing, osteophyte formation, and subchondral sclerosis.

Treatment
Treatment focuses on maintenance of function, with protection against further stressors such as high-impact activities. NSAIDs, steroid injection, and splinting are mainstays of treatment. Surgical intervention is considered after exhausting nonoperative treatment. Operative procedures include arthroplasties (usually without the use of a joint implant) and fusions.

DeQuervain's Tenosynovitis

DeQuervain's tenosynovitis (Figure 10.13) is a stenosing tenosynovitis of the abductor pollicis longus and extensor pollicis brevis tendon sheath that causes radial-sided wrist pain. It is commonly an overuse syndrome, and is diagnosed by localized tenderness over the tendons, swelling, and a positive Finkelstein's test. Treatment involves rest, splinting, NSAIDs, ice, modification of activities, and steroid injection (if refractory to other measures). If the condition does not respond to nonoperative means, surgical release is indicated. This involves releasing the compartment around the tendons.

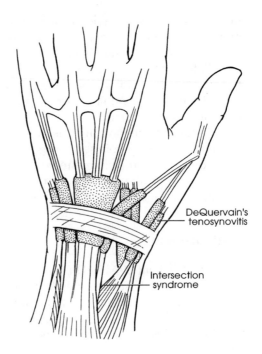

DeQuervain's
tenosynovitis

Intersection
syndrome

FIGURE 10.13   *Locations of DeQuervain's tenosynovitis and intersection syndrome.*

Tendonitis

There are multiple tendons crossing the wrist that are subject to inflammation. Any of these tendons can be affected by overuse. Diagnosis of a particular tendonitis is made by identifying a localized area of tenderness and swelling. Stress of the tendon in question should cause pain. On the volar wrist, tendonitis may affect the flexor pollicis longus in isolation (due to repetitive use of the thumb).[14] The flexor carpi radialis and ulnaris may also be affected. Intersection syndrome is an inflammation at the intersection of the first dorsal compartment (abductor pollicis longus and extensor pollicis brevis) and second dorsal compartment (extensor carpi radialis longus and brevis) just proximal to the extensor retinaculum (see Figure 10.13). This condition often causes audible crepitus, swelling, and pain in this region.

Treatment for all these forms of tendonitis involves rest, ice, NSAIDs, modification of activity, splinting, and, occasionally, injections. Surgical intervention is rarely necessary, although in refractory cases it may involve excision of the inflamed tissue.

Ganglion Cysts

Ganglion cysts are local mucoid outpouchings of joints. Most occur on the dorsal wrist and arise from degeneration of the scapholunate ligament.[15] They are probably caused by a one-way, valve-type structure that allows fluid to be pumped from the joint into the cyst. They are worsened by activity, especially repetitive wrist motion. Although they may be completely painless, symptomatic cysts can interfere with hand and wrist function. They often wax and wane in size, have a characteristic gel-like consistency on palpation, and transilluminate with a penlight.

In the past such cysts were often called *bible bumps* because they would be treated with vigorous compression, sometimes by rapping them with a bible. This can make the cyst disappear, but it often recurs. Treatment of ganglion cysts includes observation, rest, activity modification, NSAIDs, wrist splints, and needle aspiration or steroid injection. Ultimately, surgical excision is indicated for the persistently symptomatic ganglion.

Dupuytren's Contracture

Dupuytren's contracture is a progressive contracture of the palmar aponeurosis (fascia lying between the skin and flexor tendons). Histologically, it is a proliferative fibrodysplasia of the connective tissue. Nodules and cords, which progressively develop in the palmar aponeurosis, lead to contractures of the fingers and palm. It is seen most commonly in persons of Northern European descent, males, those older than 40 years of age, those with a positive family history, and those with a history of alcohol use, smoking, diabetes, or a seizure disorder.[16] It most frequently affects the ulnar part of the hand.

Treatment includes patient education, a home stretching program such as sitting on one's hands (although efficacy is not clear), and heating modalities as needed. Surgical release should be considered for significant contractures of the MCP joints and mild contractures of the PIP joints. Surgery involves resection of the offending palmar fascia.

Trigger Finger

In trigger finger, a localized swelling or nodule develops on the flexor tendon, usually in digits 2, 3, or the thumb. This disrupts the smooth gliding of the tendon within its sheath. The nodule gets caught in the sheath and has trouble moving through the sheath. It usually occurs in healthy persons, often middle-aged women, but may be seen in connective tissue disease states as well. It presents as a painful locking of the digit in flexion when the nodule becomes lodged within the tendon sheath (thus the "trigger finger"). The nodule is palpable and is felt to move with passive finger flexion and extension. Treatment includes splinting, NSAIDs, and steroid injections. Because the nodule often gets lodged within the tendon sheath during sleep (when the fingers are characteristically flexed), the patient may benefit from sleeping with a brace that keeps the fingers extended. X-ray may be obtained to rule out a bony block to movement. Refractory cases are treated with surgical release of the tendon sheath to allow more space for tendon gliding.

Raynaud's Disease

Raynaud's disease involves a painful vasoconstriction of the arteries of the digits. Such vasoconstriction usually occurs in response to environmental stimuli such as cold and repetitive trauma, or to central factors such as emotion and nicotine use. It may be seen in association with connective tissue diseases such as RA and scleroderma, and is sometimes the first sign of such a disorder; in this case it is termed *Raynaud's syndrome*. It may also present as a less severe form of vasoconstriction called *Raynaud's phenomenon*.

Patients typically complain of painful, pale digits, often after exposure to cold temperatures. Normal skin color does not return for some time (up to 20–30 minutes), even after entering a warm environment. Patients should be evaluated with an Allen's test to rule out arterial abnormality. In selected cases, a connective tissue examination may be indicated. Symptoms can sometimes be reproduced by placing the extremity in iced water. This may actually cause vasoconstriction in the digits of the contralateral extremity as well.

Treatment includes patient education about the need to keep the hands warm and protected. Pharmacologic treatment includes calcium channel blockers and calcitonin and serotonin antagonists. Surgical treatment in refractory cases entails digital sympathectomy.

Reflex Sympathetic Dystrophy

Reflex sympathetic dystrophy is covered in Chapter 15.

Trauma

Distal Radius Fractures
The most common type of distal radius fracture is the classic Colles' fracture. It usually occurs from a fall onto an outstretched hand. Treatment includes reduction of the fracture with casting and, in many cases, operative or external fixation.

Triangular Fibrocartilage Complex Tears
Tears of the TFCC are a common cause of ulnar-sided wrist pain. Patients usually have a history of a compression injury. Pronation and supination are most problematic for these patients, particularly with loading. Arthrography and MRI are helpful in the diagnosis, but arthroscopy is the definitive diagnostic measure. Nonoperative treatment involves NSAIDs, splinting, and activity modification. Operative treatment usually entails arthroscopy with débridement or repair of the tear.

Scapholunate Instability
Scapholunate instability is the most common intercarpal ligament injury. It results from a tear of the scapholunate ligament, usually caused by a fall with the wrist extended and supinated. Patients have anatomic snuffbox tenderness and tenderness directly over the scapholunate ligament region (directly distal to Lister's tubercle—a bony prominence on the distal radius). X-ray may show an increased gap between the scaphoid and lunate, or an increased angle between the scaphoid and lunate known as a *dorsal intercalary segmental instability deformity*. Early treatment is essential and includes operative repair

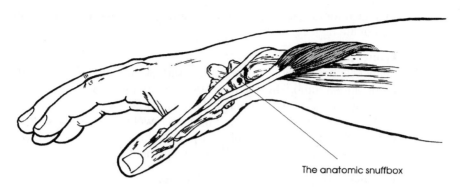

The anatomic snuffbox

FIGURE 10.14 *The anatomic snuffbox, bounded by the extensor pollicis brevis and abductor pollicis longus on the volar side and the extensor pollicis longus on the dorsal side. The scaphoid bone lies between these tendons at the wrist.*

of the ligament combined with pinning or internal fixation. Chronic instability leads to progressive arthritis.

Scaphoid Fractures
Scaphoid fractures are the most common carpal bone fractures. Because the vascular supply to the scaphoid enters this bone distally, proximal fractures have a high rate of nonunion and avascular necrosis. X-ray may initially be read as negative; therefore, if the patient has a history of injury to the wrist, and has anatomic snuffbox tenderness only (Figure 10.14), casting is indicated until the fracture is ruled out. Follow-up x-rays, bone scan, or computed tomography are helpful in ruling out a possible scaphoid fracture. For non-displaced fractures, casting is indicated. However, for athletes or patients who desire less casting, operative treatment is indicated. For displaced fractures, operative treatment is indicated initially.

Kienbock's Disease
Kienbock's disease is an avascular necrosis of the lunate. It is not clear whether it results from repeated microtrauma or from a single, traumatic event. Never-theless, the natural history is for the lunate to progressively collapse. X-rays may initially be negative, but MRI shows signal changes consistent with avas-cular necrosis. Later on in the course of the condition, x-rays become remark-able for sclerosis, cyst formation, and, eventually, collapse of the lunate. This condition is often associated with ulnar-negative variance (ulna is short relative to radius), and early stages can be treated with ulnar lengthening, radial short-ening, or revascularization procedures. Later stages (carpal collapse) are treated with limited carpal fusion, wrist fusion, or proximal row carpectomy (removal of the scaphoid, lunate, and triquetrum).

Metacarpal and Phalangeal Fractures
Many metacarpal and phalangeal fractures can be treated with closed reduc-tion (if displaced) and cast or splint immobilization. Operative intervention is

indicated for unstable fractures and for most fractures associated with malrotation of the digits.

Gamekeeper's Thumb

Gamekeeper's thumb is the result of a sudden stress to the ulnar collateral ligament of the thumb. Historically caused by an injury to the thumb during falconry, it is now more often caused by a ski pole while skiing (hence it is also called *skier's thumb*). Examination reveals swelling around the MCP joint of the thumb and laxity of the ulnar aspect of this joint. Treatment involves casting or operative repair of the collateral ligament.

Proximal Interphalangeal Joint Dislocations

Dorsal interphalangeal joint dislocations (base of middle phalanx is dorsal to head of proximal phalanx) are more common than volar dislocations (base of middle phalanx is volar to head of proximal phalanx). Immediate reduction is indicated. If not successful, open reduction is indicated. Most dorsal dislocations can be treated with buddy taping or splinting after successful reduction. Volar dislocations usually require immobilization in extension due to central slip injury.

Jersey Finger

Jersey finger is an avulsion of the flexor digitorum profundus from the distal phalanx (usually occurring with sporting activities, such as when a player grabs an opponent's jersey while pulling away). The ring finger is most commonly involved. The patient is unable to flex the DIP while the PIP joint is stabilized. Operative repair is indicated.

Mallet Finger

Mallet finger is an avulsion of the terminal extensor tendon of the distal phalanx. Forced flexion of the DIP while the finger is actively extended causes the injury, often when the extended fingertip is hit by a ball. Patients typically have a "drop" distal finger (giving the appearance of a mallet) and an inability to actively extend the DIP joint. Most of these injuries can be treated with extension splinting.

Central Slip Injury

Rupture of the central slip (part of the dorsal extensor apparatus) results in a boutonniere deformity (see Figure 10.12) if not recognized and treated early. Volar dislocations of the PIP joint are often associated with central slip tears. Early on, patients have a swollen and tender PIP joint and an inability to strongly extend the PIP joint. Prompt treatment is essential for good results and entails extension splinting of the PIP joint.

Points of Summary

1. The wrist and hand consist of a complex anatomic arrangement of osseous, ligamentous, cartilaginous, nervous, and musculotendinous structures.
2. The metacarpophalangeal (MCP) collateral ligaments are lax when the fingers are extended and taut when they are flexed. They are prone to contracture if immobilized in an extended position.

3. The carpal tunnel is a fixed space that contains the median nerve. The nerve is susceptible to a compression injury within this space. Carpal tunnel syndrome is best diagnosed by clinical symptoms and electromyogram.
4. DeQuervain's tenosynovitis is best diagnosed with Finkelstein's test.
5. Side-to-side confrontational strength testing can help in detecting intrinsic hand muscle weakness.
6. Hand and wrist symptoms may be the first signs of connective tissue disease.
7. Rheumatoid arthritis commonly affects the wrist and MCP joints.
8. Degenerative joint disease commonly affects the first MCP joint and the distal interphalangeal joints.
9. Ganglion cysts are mucoid outpouchings of the joint which are fed by a one-way, valve-type mechanism pumping fluid into the cyst.
10. Trigger finger is caused by a nodule on the tendon getting "stuck" in the tendon sheath.

References

1. Wilcox D, Buschbacher RM. Incidence of inability to flex the proximal interphalangeal joint in normal subjects. Arch Phys Med Rehabil 1998;79:1405–1407.
2. Rosenbaum RB, Ochoa JL. CTS and Other Disorders of the Median Nerve. Boston: Butterworth–Heinemann, 1993.
3. Gellman H, Gelberman RH, Tan AM, et al. Carpal tunnel syndrome: an evaluation of the provocative diagnostic tests. J Bone Joint Surg 1986;68A:735–737.
4. Buschbacher RM. Side to side confrontational strength testing for weakness of the intrinsic muscles of the hand. J Bone Joint Surg 1997;79A:401–405.
5. Gelberman RH, Hergenroeder PT, Hargens AR, et al. The carpal tunnel syndrome: a study of carpal canal pressures. J Bone Joint Surg 1981; 63A(3):380–383.
6. Nordstrom DL, Vierkant RA, DeStefano F, Layde PM. Risk factors for carpal tunnel syndrome in a general population. Occup Environ Med 1997; 54:734–740.
7. Gordon C, Johnson EW, Gatens PF, et al. Wrist ratio correlation with carpal tunnel syndrome in industry. Am J Phys Med Rehabil 1988;67:270–272.
8. Kuhlan KA, Hennessey WJ. Sensitivity and specificity of carpal tunnel syndrome signs. Am J Phys Med Rehabil 1997;76:451–457.
9. Kaul MP, Pagel KJ, Wheatley MJ, et al. Carpal compression test and pressure provocative test in veterans with median-distribution paresthesias. Muscle Nerve 2001;24:107–111.
10. Walker WC, Metzler M, Cifu DX, et al. Neutral wrist splinting in carpal tunnel syndrome: a comparison of night-only versus full-time wear instructions. Arch Phys Med Rehabil 2000;81:424–429.
11. Kerr CD, Gittins ME, Sybert DR. Endoscopic versus open carpal tunnel release: clinical results. Arthroscopy 1994;10:266–269.

12. Szabo RM. Nerve Compression Syndromes. In PR Manske (ed), American Society for Surgery of the Hand—Hand Surgery Update Vol 1 1994:21(1)–21(13).
13. Merritt JL, Hunder GG. Passive range of motion, not isometric exercise, amplifies acute urate synovitis. Arch Phys Med Rehabil 1983;64:130–131.
14. Buschbacher R. Overuse syndromes among endoscopists. Endoscopy 1994;26:539–544.
15. Angelides AC, Wallace PF. The dorsal ganglion of the wrist: its pathogenesis, gross and microscopic anatomy, and surgical treatment. J Hand Surg 1976;1:228–235.
16. Early PF. Population studies in Dupuytren's contracture. J Bone Joint Surg 1962;44B:602–613.

Suggested Readings

Kasdan ML (ed). Occupational Hand and Upper Extremity Injuries and Diseases (2nd ed). Philadelphia: Hanley and Belfus, 1998.

Rettig AC (ed). Hand and Wrist Injuries. Clin Sports Med 1998;17.

Watson HK, Weinzweig J, Zeppieri J. The natural progression of scaphoid instability. Hand Clin 1997;13:39–49.

11   Hips and Pelvis

Andrea R. Conti, Michael E. Berend, and Ralph M. Buschbacher

The hip joints and pelvis act to connect the axial skeleton (cervical, thoracic, and lumbar spine) to the lower extremities. They allow the transfer of kinetic energy from the upper body to the legs (and vice versa) during activity. Dysfunction within the pelvic girdle or the hips can cause significant pain. A careful physical examination, gait analysis, and specific tests to localize the pathology are often helpful in identifying pathologic conditions within the pelvis and hips.

Anatomy

Bones and Joints

The bony pelvis is an osseous ring formed by two os coxae that connect to each other at the pubis anteriorly and are joined to the sacrum and coccyx posteriorly. The os coxae consist of three parts, which fuse during development: the ilium, ischium, and pubis. At the confluence of these three bones is the acetabulum, a cup-shaped cavity that articulates with the head of the femur to form the hip joint.

There are four articulations within the pelvic girdle. These are the sacroiliac (SI) joints bilaterally, the pubic symphysis, and the sacrococcygeal joint.

Ligaments

A number of ligaments connect the pelvis to the surrounding structures (Figure 11.1). The iliolumbar ligaments connect the transverse processes of the fifth lumbar vertebrae (L5) to the iliac crests bilaterally. These ligaments provide a static restraint to forward translation of L5 on the sacrum. The sacrotuberous ligaments pass from the sacrum to the ischium, as do the sacrospinous ligaments. These ligaments act together to hold the sacrum in position and resist posterior rotation of the inferior sacrum. The interosseous and SI liga-

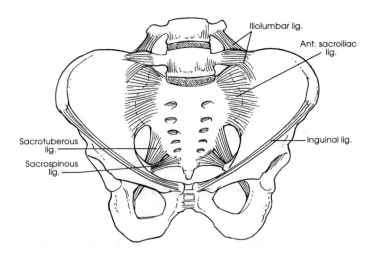

FIGURE 11.1   *The ligaments of the lumbosacral and pelvic region. (Ant. = anterior; lig. = ligament.)*

ments are composed of very strong short fibers that unite the sacrum and ilium. These are some of the strongest ligaments in the body, but may be disrupted in forceful trauma.

Muscles

The musculature of the pelvis (Figure 11.2) includes several large, strong muscles that act as prime movers for the lower extremities during ambulation. The iliacus and psoas (together iliopsoas) muscles are the chief flexors of the hip. Posteriorly the pelvis is covered by several layers of muscles. The superficial gluteus maximus extends the leg, whereas the deeper gluteus medius and minimus act to abduct the hip and rotate the thigh. During the stance phase of gait, these muscles exert their forces to control the trunk and pelvis.

Deep to the gluteal musculature are several short external rotator muscles. One of these, the piriformis, is particularly important. It originates on the anterior surface of the sacrum and passes through the greater sciatic notch to insert onto the greater trochanter (tuberosity) of the femur. It acts as an external rotator of the hip and as an abductor of the leg when the hip is flexed. The belly of this muscle passes over the sciatic nerve; in some people, the sciatic nerve actually passes through the muscle. Because of the anatomic relationship between the nerve and muscle, sciatic-type referral symptoms may be present with dysfunction in the pelvis or piriformis (Figure 11.3).[1–3]

Other muscles important to the function of the hip and pelvis are the hamstrings, hip adductors, and quadriceps. The hamstring group is made up of the semitendinosus, semimembranosus, and biceps femoris. The hamstrings have a common origin from the ischial tuberosity. One of the quadriceps muscles, the rectus femoris, also crosses the hip joint, as do the hip adductors.

While stabilizing and controlling the pelvis during movement, several of these muscles also act to compress the hip joint. Normally, during two-

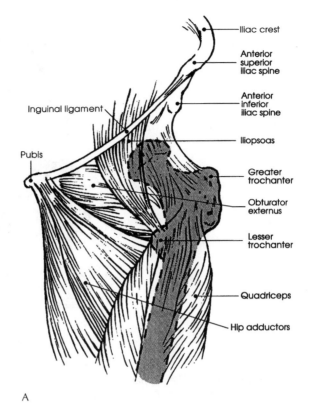

A

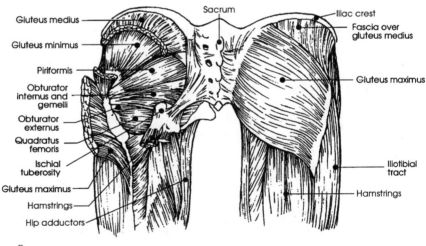

B

FIGURE 11.2 *Muscles of the pelvic girdle: anterior view (**A**), posterior view (**B**) (left-deep, right-superficial).*

legged stance, each hip joint must bear one-half of the weight of the body. When standing on one leg, the hip abductors contract to keep the pelvis from dropping. This joint compressive force plus body weight can equal four times body weight (Figure 11.4), and is a major reason why ambulation is painful in persons with hip joint pathology.

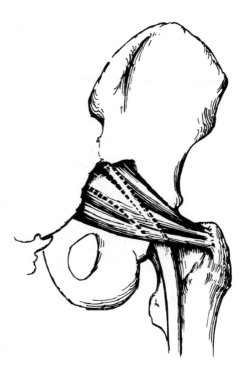

FIGURE 11.3 *The intimate relationship between the piriformis muscle and the sciatic nerve, which runs directly below the muscle.*

Examination and Testing Techniques

History and Physical Examination

Obtaining a clear and thorough history from the patient with musculoskeletal problems of the hip and pelvis is of primary importance. Musculoskeletal pain often stems from traumatic or overuse injury, and the specific nature of the motions involved in injury or the generation of symptoms is important in making the diagnosis. It is valuable to ask patients complaining of "hip pain" to point to the site of pain. Patients generally call the posterior or lateral buttock the "hip." True hip joint pain is usually felt in the anterior groin at the inguinal ligament. The history may also include questions about abdominal and urogenital problems, as these can cause pain to be felt in the hip and groin area.

General assessment begins with a static examination to compare the heights of the iliac crests, greater trochanters, and medial malleoli with the patient standing and supine. The alignment of the posterior superior iliac spine (PSIS) dimples should be observed to make sure they are level. Muscle mass and posture should be assessed as well. Special care should be taken to identify patterns of atrophy or malalignment that may result from leg length discrepancy, contracture of the hip capsule, or other deformities such as in the thoracic and lumbar spine.

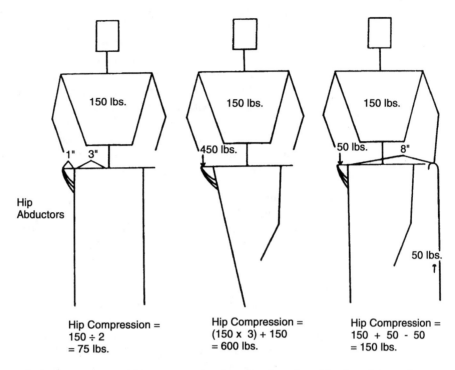

FIGURE 11.4 *Normal hip compression force is a function of body weight and muscular action. When standing on one leg, the hip abductors produce a compressive force of three times body weight (due to leverage effects). A cane held on the opposite side has great leverage and reduces joint compressive force many times more than the actual weight being carried on the cane.*

The bony landmarks and soft tissues should be palpated. The areas of the greater trochanter or ischial tuberosity are tender in bursitis of these locations. The iliac crest is tender in an apophysitis or avulsion fracture. The coccyx is tender in coccydynia. In conditions of SI joint dysfunction, the ligaments overlying this joint are often tender. The piriformis muscle is also often tender in SI joint dysfunction, as well as in piriformis syndrome. The gluteus medius and minimus sometimes have tender areas or trigger points from myofascial pain or overuse of these muscles. In conditions of sciatica the sciatic nerve is tender. It can be palpated halfway between the ischial tuberosity and the greater trochanter, especially when the hip is flexed, such as in a lateral decubitus position.

Range of motion (ROM) of the low back, pelvis, and legs should be assessed, as should muscle strength. Sensory and reflex testing of the lower extremities should be performed as well. It is important to realize that low back disease can cause pelvic, buttock, and hip pain, and thus the lower back should routinely be evaluated also. In addition, other, more specialized tests can be performed as follows.

Measuring Leg Length
A crude measure of leg length is to estimate the heights of the left and right iliac crests or the PSIS dimples of the standing patient. This is best done with the examiner seated behind the patient. With practice, the examiner can learn

to detect relatively minor leg length discrepancies. The pelvis can, however, also be tilted due to other causes, such as muscle splinting, scoliosis, or poor posture. In these cases, the leg lengths can seem to be unequal, when in fact they are not. True leg length is measured with the patient supine from the anterior superior iliac spine to the medial malleolus. Leg length may also be measured radiographically. Leg length discrepancies of 1 cm or less generally do not warrant correction with an orthosis. Discrepancies of greater than 1.5–2.0 cm may benefit from such intervention. For significant discrepancies, the shoe insert should gradually be thickened over the course of weeks or months, rather than the correction being made all at once. Surgical correction may be considered for more severe inequalities.

Hip Rotation
Flexing the hip and knee to 90 degrees in the supine position allows the examiner to assess internal and external rotation. These movements are often painful and restricted in degenerative joint disease and other painful conditions of the hip joints. The pain is worsened by applying pressure into the hip while testing ROM.

Thomas Test
The Thomas test is a physical examination maneuver to assess for hip flexion contracture. Patients are asked to lie supine and, with their hands, pull one knee to the chest to stabilize the pelvis and eliminate any extension of the back. The other leg can normally lie flat on the table. Patients with hip flexion contracture cannot lower their leg all the way to the table, and the hip remains in a flexed position.

Patrick's Test
In Patrick's test (Figure 11.5), the supine patient crosses the foot over the opposite knee, creating a so-called *figure 4* position. The knee of the upper leg is then gently pushed towards the table. Pain in the groin is indicative of hip joint pathology, whereas pain posteriorly in the SI joint area is a sign of dysfunction of this joint. This test is also called the *Faber test*, which stands for *f*lexion, *ab*duction, and *e*xternal *r*otation.

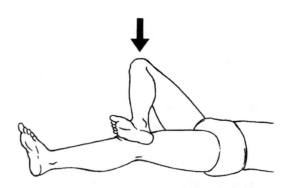

FIGURE 11.5 *Patrick's test (also known as the* Faber test—*stands for f*lexion, *ab*duction, *e*xternal *r*otation).

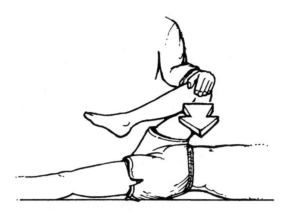

FIGURE 11.6   *Piriformis stretching.*

Piriformis Stretching and Test

To assess piriformis flexibility (Figure 11.6), the patient lies supine while the examiner flexes the hip and knee. The examiner adducts the leg (pushes it to the opposite side) to gauge flexibility on each side. If the patient resists this motion (the piriformis test), the piriformis muscle is stressed. Pain in the buttock is a positive sign.

Ober's Test

In Ober's test (Figure 11.7), the leg is passively extended and abducted with the patient lying in a lateral decubitus position, with the affected hip up. The knee is flexed to 90 degrees. When the examiner releases the leg, it should drop to the level of the lower leg. If the iliotibial tract or tensor fascia lata are excessively inflexible, the leg remains in an abducted position or the knee involuntarily extends. This test may be painful in trochanteric bursitis.

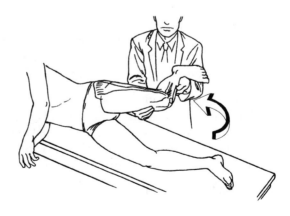

FIGURE 11.7   *Ober's test.*

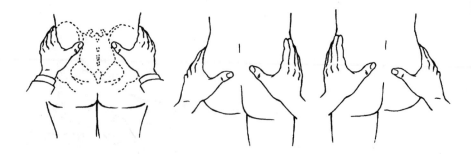

FIGURE 11.8   *The standing Gillette test. As the patient raises the leg, downward motion is felt over the posterior superior iliac spine. Asymmetry of motion is a sign of sacroiliac dysfunction.*

Passive Leg Extension (Modified Gaenslen's Test)

In passive leg extension the patient lies prone with the knee flexed at a 90-degree angle. The examiner passively extends the upper thigh at the hip (patients must be encouraged to relax and not actively extend the leg). Pain in the SI area is indicative of SI dysfunction.

Standing Gillette (Stork) Test

In the standing Gillette test (Figure 11.8), patients are asked to stand and raise first one knee and then the other toward the ceiling. If necessary they may steady themselves with a hand against a wall or other object, but they should not support any weight on this hand. The examiner sits behind the patient with the thumbs over the PSIS dimples and the fingers over the iliac crests. The motion of the SI joints is palpated with the thumbs. Normally, when the patient lifts a leg, the thumb on that side moves down (care must be taken that the patient is not guarding the back excessively, hiking the hip, or leaning). Asymmetric motion is indicative of SI dysfunction. Often, the thumb on one side does not drop, or even rises, in the person with SI problems.

Trendelenburg Test

In the Trendelenburg test, the patient stands on one leg. If the pelvis tilts downward excessively, it indicates that the gluteus medius and minimus on the supporting side are weak (see Chapter 5, Figure 5.4).

Abdominal Strength Testing

One simple way of assessing abdominal strength is to have the supine patient bring the knees to the chest, then straighten the knees and slowly lower the legs to the examination table. Inability to slowly lower the legs is a sign of abdominal muscle weakness.

Rectal Examination

Rectal examination should usually be performed in patients with back or pelvic pain of insidious onset. It may help to identify some tumors or an enlarged prostate. It also allows palpation of the undersurface of the piriformis muscle.

In persons with coccydynia, rectal examination and manipulation of the coccyx may be painful.

Ancillary Testing

Radiographs are often helpful in assessing for fractures, general deformities, arthritis, or other bony lesions. Computed tomography is useful in detecting bony pathology such as occult fractures, tumors, or traumatic injury to the SI joint. Magnetic resonance imaging (MRI) is helpful in evaluating lumbar disk disease, inflammation in the tendons and surrounding structures, and in evaluating the hip joints for evidence of stress fractures, osteonecrosis, or other lesions. Bone scans help detect stress fractures or infections.

Diagnosis and Treatment of Specific Disorders

Sacroiliac Joint Dysfunction

SI joint dysfunction is a relatively common occurrence, but is probably underdiagnosed. In most persons, SI pain lasts from a few moments to a few days and requires no intervention or treatment. In a small subset of persons, however, it can develop into a more troublesome condition that requires specialized treatment. Rarely, it can cause refractory and chronic low back pain.

It is unclear what causes SI joint dysfunction. The SI joint normally moves only a few degrees, and with age it becomes less mobile and actually fuses.[4] It is partly a fibrous joint and partly a synovial joint. Within the joint are ridges of bone. Surrounding the joint are very strong ligaments.

Because the SI joint loses mobility with age, SI joint dysfunction is a condition most commonly seen in young to middle-aged adults, although teenagers and older persons can get it as well. It is believed that the increased incidence of this condition in women versus men is at least partially due to the fact that the ridges of the SI joint are shallower in women. Pregnant women have hormonal changes that loosen the connective tissues of the joint (the hormone relaxin), which makes pregnant women particularly susceptible to SI joint dysfunction.

The biomechanics of the SI joint are complex. Although the two SI joints do not move much, they do move. When flexing or extending the back, these joints move symmetrically. When bending and twisting together or when asymmetric stresses are placed on the pelvis (e.g., golf swing, vacuuming, leg length discrepancy, poor work technique) the two joints must move independently.[5]

When asymmetric stresses are placed on the pelvis, the SI joints begin to cause pain. This may be precipitated by an acute forceful traumatic event such as a motor vehicle accident, especially in an offset collision or if there is rotation involved. In most cases, however, the joint is predisposed to injury by repetitive bending and twisting or by asymmetric motions (e.g., always turning to a computer monitor on one side of the desk, not the other). A forceful twisting motion may precipitate symptoms. An acute injury to the SI joint may be accompanied by a "popping" sensation in the low back. During recovery, continued aggravating activities delay healing. The SI joints may continue to pop intermittently. Sometimes these pops are associated with increased symptoms, at other times with decreased symptoms.

Because the SI joint is intimately associated with the piriformis muscle, SI joint dysfunction often occurs along with piriformis syndrome.

The SI joint may be involved in connective tissue diseases such as ankylosing spondylitis and Reiter's disease.[6] When there is an insidious onset of back pain and joint stiffness in persons (usually men) younger than 40 years of age that persists for more than 3 months, is associated with morning stiffness, is worse after inactivity, and improves with exercise, ankylosing spondylitis should be suspected, and appropriate x-ray and laboratory tests obtained. Reiter's syndrome is usually associated with other lower extremity joint involvement as well. When sacroiliitis appears in children, especially if the condition is unilateral, an infected joint should be suspected.[7] This usually is associated with fever and other signs of infection. Gout has also been described as a cause of SI pain.[8]

Diagnosis

Patients with SI joint dysfunction often present with a history of a bending and twisting injury or an asymmetric fall, such as on one side of the buttock. Young women commonly present with the condition (nurses, assembly line workers), but men get the condition also (bricklayers, rowers, packagers). Often there is an acute, moderately strenuous precipitating event, with worsening over the next few days. Symptoms wax and wane and are worsened with rotation, climbing stairs, and running. Occasionally the symptoms are associated with "popping" in the back. Commonly, there is radiation of pain into the buttock (94%), low back (72%), and leg (50%), but pain can also be felt in the groin (14%), distal to the knee (28%), and even into the foot (14%).[9]

On physical examination, these patients usually have a normal gait. They may have a mild to moderate decrease in back ROM, have asymmetric SI movement during back flexion, and are tender over the SI joint. In some cases, they are tender over the piriformis, and if a secondary myofascial pain has developed, they may be tender over the gluteus medius and minimus as well. Reflexes, sensation, and motor strength testing are normal, and the straight leg raise test is negative. They may have worsening of symptoms with the passive leg extension test and with Patrick's test. Asymmetry of SI movement on the standing Gillette test is common. They may have abnormal biomechanical factors such as hamstring inflexibility or leg length discrepancy. It should also be noted, however, that all the diagnostic tests do not have perfect sensitivity and specificity[10-12]; there is simply no "gold standard" for diagnosis, except for possibly a diagnostic anesthetic injection, which is rarely indicated. The clinician must take the totality of the history and examination findings into account when making the diagnosis. Lack of response to treatment may indicate that a reassessment of the condition should take place.

SI dysfunction can mimic muscular pain or radiculopathy. Electromyography may be necessary to rule out nerve root pathology: It is normal in uncomplicated SI dysfunction. MRI is not usually necessary. In some cases, SI problems can be secondary to a mild subclinical radiculopathy. Such radiculopathy, although causing minimal or no symptoms, may cause mild weakness, which alters the body biomechanics enough to cause SI symptoms. In SI cases refractory to treatment, electromyography or MRI of the lumbosacral spine may be useful to detect such radiculopathy. Unless the radiculopathy is treated, SI symptoms will persist.

Treatment

Patients with acute SI dysfunction frequently respond to a short period of rest, local heat, and nonsteroidal anti-inflammatory drugs (NSAIDs).

If symptoms persist, the initial treatment approach is to normalize movement and equalize the symmetry of the joint movement. Later, SI stabilization exercises are taught. In acute dysfunction, a number of techniques can be tried, and taught to the patient. The adductor squeeze involves having the patient, in a sitting position, put one hand outside each knee and push the knees apart while resisting this motion with the hands. This is done for approximately 10 seconds, after which the patient places the hands (as fists) between the knees and then briskly adducts the knees. This often causes a pop to be felt or heard, and rapidly relieves symptoms. The pelvic tilt technique is performed by having the patient stand with the back against a wall, feet shoulder width apart and one foot-length from the wall. They are told to contract the abdominal and buttock muscles for 10 seconds and repeat a few times. Finally, the patient can be taught to stand with feet shoulder width apart and with the hands on the hips, thumbs over the SI joints. They push the pelvis forward and from side to side and gently mobilize the joints in the direction in which they feel discomfort.

If these techniques are not successful at normalizing SI motion, the patient may benefit from muscle energy techniques. These exercises involve placing an asymmetric stress on the pelvis, such as forcefully flexing one leg while extending the other. This should be taught by a physician or therapist well-versed in these techniques.

When normal motion of the joints is attained, most people have a complete and permanent resolution of their symptoms. If not, they should be taught a stabilization program. This may consist of general back stabilization exercises (lifting one leg, one arm, or the opposite leg and arm in the quadruped position), Swiss ball exercises, and abdominal strengthening. Another exercise that is extremely useful, but which requires a major commitment from the patient, is exercise bicycling while standing up. Elliptical trainers, cross-country ski simulators, and sliding exercises (mimicking speed skating) may also be helpful.

Most persons respond to a week or two of exercises. Sometimes these need to be taught and guided by a physical therapist. If symptoms do not improve, patients may benefit from an SI joint injection.[13] One, two, or (rarely) three corticosteroid injections are beneficial as an adjunct to the exercise program. Heating modalities may be useful as well. Some persons also benefit from wearing an SI belt. This belt is different from other back braces. It is relatively narrow, fits under the iliac crests, and compresses the pelvis. Often there is a pad over the sacrum. Most persons with SI dysfunction do not get relief from such a belt, but in a subset of patients (20–30%) it provides dramatic relief, and thus should be tried relatively early.

Piriformis Syndrome

As described earlier, the piriformis muscle is closely associated with the SI joint, as well as the sciatic nerve. With spasm or inflammation of the piriformis, a pain referral pattern of sciatica is common, as are symptoms of sacroiliac joint dysfunction. Only rarely does piriformis syndrome present as an isolated entity. In some cases this can occur from overuse, isolated pressure on the muscle, or from buttock trauma.[1]

Diagnosis
Patients with piriformis syndrome complain of symptoms similar to those of SI joint dysfunction, as well as sciatic nerve–type symptoms. They may also have pain on walking, climbing stairs, and twisting their bodies. On examination, the muscle is exquisitely tender to palpation. Piriformis strength testing reveals weakness (or pain inhibition) and inflexibility of the muscle and reproduces the patient's pain. SI tests and the straight leg raise test may be positive. The tender muscle may also be palpated on rectal examination.

Treatment
Piriformis syndrome is managed by relaxing the overstressed and irritated muscle. Treatment includes rest, NSAIDs, ice massage, heat, and a piriformis-stretching program. Associated SI dysfunction may need to be treated as well. The muscle can be stretched by the patient flexing and adducting the leg (knee bent), in a position similar to that for the piriformis stretching test. Surgical sectioning of the muscle has been described, but is almost never necessary.[1]

Trochanteric Bursitis

The greater trochanter is a superficial structure on the proximal femur and the site of the attachments of the strong abductors of the hip. The iliotibial band (ITB) overlies the trochanter, with a bursa between them. The ITB is attached to the tensor fascial lata and gluteus maximus muscles. Direct trauma, prolonged pressure, or a tight iliotibial tract can be sources of irritation to the bursa, which can become inflamed. The ITB may be tight over the greater trochanter and be the cause of a "snapping hip" laterally.

Diagnosis
Patients often complain of pain "in the hip." When asked to point to the site of pain, they place a finger right behind or on the greater trochanter. They may experience pain when ascending stairs, during a one-legged stance on the side of the symptoms, when lying on the affected side, and at night. Pain may be worse when first arising from a seated position. The snapping can sometimes be recreated by having the patient stand, adduct the leg, and rotate the leg. The snap is palpated as the ITB passes over the greater trochanter. The area of the trochanter is very tender, and in some cases pain is referred down the leg with palpation.

Treatment
As in any bursitis, treatment consists of rest, ice massage, NSAIDs, and the removal of any irritating pressure. Later, ultrasound and stretching of the ilio-

tibial tract and hamstrings are helpful. Structural abnormalities, such as leg length discrepancies and inflexibility of other muscles, should be addressed. Aggravating activities must be modified or curtailed. The bursa may also respond well to steroid-anesthetic injection. In rare cases, surgical resection may be considered.[14]

Degenerative Joint Disease of the Hip

The most common painful condition of the hip joint is osteoarthritis, or degenerative joint disease. It involves a deterioration of the articular cartilage and subchondral bone and results in loss of ROM, decreased limb length, and osteophyte formation. The cause is not known, but it is associated with aging. Symptoms progress gradually; initially, they are only present with activity, but later their presence is constant. In severe cases, there is pain at night.

Diagnosis
Arthritis of the hip most commonly presents as pain in the groin area, although some persons feel it more laterally or in the buttock. Early on, symptoms occur with increased activity and are relieved by rest.[15] ROM of the hip is restricted, especially in flexion and internal rotation. Gait becomes abnormal, with the shoulders tilting to the side of the affected hip during ambulation. This tilt decreases the joint compressive force on the joint described earlier, because the patient in essence balances on the joint and requires less muscle contraction to keep the pelvis from dropping. There may also be a limp. Radiographs reveal a loss of joint space and the classic changes of arthritis.

Treatment
Conservative treatment of arthritis includes maintaining joint ROM through non-weight-bearing activities such as pool exercises. Bicycling also may help in maintaining an active lifestyle, but does not help stretch the hip flexors. Frequent rest periods with no weight-bearing exercise at all may help in controlling symptoms and in slowing the progression of the degeneration.[15] Weight loss decreases the joint compressive forces. NSAIDs are used judiciously.

A cane used on the opposite side helps to decrease the joint compressive force (see Figure 11.4). The length of the cane should be measured from the floor to the distal wrist crease of the standing patient (tip of cane 6 inches lateral to fifth toe) to give an elbow flexion angle of 20–30 degrees.[16] Surgical treatment with total joint replacement is the final stage of treatment.

Myofascial Pain and Muscle Strain

Leg length discrepancies, abnormal gait, or overuse can cause myofascial pain of the muscles of the hips and pelvis. The most commonly involved muscles are the hip abductors, the gluteus medius and minimus, and the tensor fascia lata. Tendonitis and tears of the hip abductors can also cause low back and pelvic pain.[17]

Treatment of overuse problems and myofascial pain consists of rest, heat, ice massage, and possibly tender or trigger point injection, as well as stretching and strengthening exercises. Orthotic shoe inserts are occasionally useful. Aggravating activities should be avoided, and modifications in work or sport technique may be helpful. If the muscles or tendons are torn, surgical re-attachment may be considered.[14]

Groin strains (adductor muscles) are common sports injuries. They can occur during forceful adduction or when the leg slips into abduction during weight-bearing exercise. Iliopsoas strains cause anterior hip and groin pain, which is worsened with resisted hip flexion. This can occur in sports injuries in which the leg is forced into extension or when vigorous flexion is blocked. Treatment of these strains is similar, with rest, ice, NSAIDS, and later, deep heat. Stretching and, later, strengthening activities are added as tolerated. Proper biomechanics and technique must be restored to prevent recurrence. These conditions are often slow to recover.

Nerve Entrapment

There are a number of nerves that can become entrapped or irritated about the pelvis, including the ilioinguinal, iliohypogastric, and genitofemoral nerves.[3] These conditions are rare, and are beyond the scope of this chapter.

Meralgia paresthetica is the most common nerve entrapment condition of the hip and pelvis. It involves compression or irritation of the lateral femoral cutaneous nerve at or near the inguinal ligament. It can cause pain, burning, and sensory loss in the anterolateral thigh. Because this is purely a sensory nerve, there is no associated muscle weakness. Meralgia paresthetica is related to trauma (seat belts), obesity, rapid weight gain or loss, tight clothing, or pressure during surgery or childbirth. Diagnosis is usually made clinically, although electromyography or evoked potential studies can also be helpful. Sometimes the nerve can be palpated as a swollen mass 1 cm medial to the anterior superior iliac spine, above or below the inguinal ligament.[18] Treatment is with the avoidance of aggravating factors, ice, transcutaneous electrical nerve stimulation, desensitization techniques, and time. NSAIDs, tricyclic antidepressants, gabapentin (Neurontin), and anticonvulsants can also decrease symptoms. Surgical treatment is rarely necessary.[3]

Hip Pain and Limping in Children

See Chapter 17.

Coccydynia

Pain in the coccygeal region may be a result of direct trauma to the coccyx. Referred pain from gastrointestinal or pelvic floor pathology should also be considered as causes of pain in this region. Treatment of acute coccydynia includes ice, pressure relief, relaxation training, proper sitting (on the ischial tuberosities, not on the sacrum and coccyx), and NSAIDs. In addition, ultrasound treatment may be useful. A program of steroid-anesthetic injection combined with coccygeal manipulation has been reported to be successful in approximately 85% of patients.[19]

Groin/Pelvic Pain

There are many other, less common causes of groin and pelvic pain, which can only be mentioned briefly here.

Sports hernia is an occult hernia or tear of the aponeurosis of the internal oblique muscle. It can cause chronic and refractory groin pain, especially with running and "cutting" type exercise. It is seen most frequently in soccer, rugby, and ice hockey players. There is tenderness at the superficial inguinal ring. Surgical repair may be necessary.[20]

Iliopsoas tendonitis or bursitis can cause a condition of an "internal snapping hip" as well as anterior groin pain. Bony avulsion of this muscle's insertion onto the lesser trochanter can also occur.

A hip pointer is a direct contusion to the iliac crest, usually seen in collision sports activities. Fracture should be ruled out. This injury results in local pain, tenderness, and swelling. Symptoms worsen with bending away from the side of injury. The injury responds to ice, rest, and, later, abdominal and trunk stretches. Padding should be used on return to sports activity.

Acetabular labral tear may present with chronic, deep, sharp hip pain with a catching or "giving-way" sensation. Symptoms are worsened with leg extension. There may be pain on internal rotation and a click on Thomas's test. It can be diagnosed on MRI arthrography and is treated surgically.[20]

There are various urogenital and rectal pain syndromes that can also cause pelvic pain. These syndromes are rare, and may be associated with psychiatric disorders in some (but not all) cases; they are beyond the scope of this chapter.[21] They can often be treated successfully, and an evaluation must rule out radiculopathy and intrapelvic adhesions. Specialized myofascial treatment techniques are often useful, but an experienced therapist is needed to perform these.

Some cases of lower abdominal or pelvic pain may be due to abdominal muscle myofascial pain. This is sometimes perpetuated by internal pathology such as adhesions, but may be treated successfully with stretching, heat, ice, and strengthening techniques. Steroid injections are particularly helpful, but must be done with particular care in this area so as not to puncture the abdominal cavity.

Other conditions to include in the differential diagnosis of pelvic and hip pain include intra-abdominal or intrapelvic pathology, hernias, torsion testes, connective tissue disease, osteitis pubis (suspect with pubic pain and bony erosion of the pubic symphysis), pubic instability,[22] stress fractures, aseptic necrosis of the hip joint, and congenital abnormalities such as a sacralization of lumbar vertebrae or vertebralization of sacral segments.

Points of Summary

1. The sacroiliac joint is a mobile joint.
2. Sacroiliac disease is a common cause of low back and buttock pain.
3. The piriformis muscle is often involved in sacroiliac dysfunction.
4. Trochanteric bursitis is a common cause of "hip" pain.
5. The symptoms of degenerative joint disease of the hip are often treated with good result with a cane, which, by virtue of the leverage it pro-

vides, relieves the hip joint of much more force than the weight it actually supports.

6. Pain in the pelvis and hip often radiates distally. Similarly, pain felt in this area may be attributable to primary back pathology.

References

1. Benson ER, Schutzer SF. Posttraumatic piriformis syndrome: diagnosis and results of operative treatment. J Bone Joint Surg 1999;81A:941–949.
2. Adkins SB, Figler RA. Hip pain in athletes. Am Fam Physician 2000;61: 2109–2118.
3. McCrory P, Bell S. Nerve entrapment syndromes as a cause of pain in the hip, groin, and buttock. Sports Med 1999;27:261–274.
4. Bowen V, Cassidy JD. Macroscopic and microscopic anatomy of the sacroiliac joint from embryonic life until the eighth decade. Spine 1981;6(6):620–628.
5. Marymont JV, Lynch MA, Henning CE. Exercise-related stress reaction of the sacroiliac joint. Am J Sports Med 1986;14(4):320–323.
6. Khan MA. Ankylosing spondylitis. In JH Klippel (ed), Primer on the Rheumatic Diseases. Atlanta, GA: Arthritis Foundation, 1997.
7. Reilly JP, Gross RH, Emans JB, et al. Disorders of the sacroiliac joint in children. J Bone Joint Surg 1988;70A(1):31–40.
8. Bastani B, Vemuri R, Gennis M. Acute gouty sacroiliitis: a case report and review of the literature. Mt Sinai J Med 1997;64:383–385.
9. Slipman CW, Jackson HB, Lipetz JS, et al. Sacroiliac joint pain referral zones. Arch Phys Med Rehabil 2000;81:334–338.
10. Slipman CW, Sterenfeld EB, Chou LH, et al. The predictive value of provocative sacroiliac joint stress maneuvers in the diagnosis of sacroiliac joint syndrome. Arch Phys Med Rehabil 1998;79:288–292.
11. Meijne W, van Neerbos K, Audemkampe G, et al. Intraexaminer and interexaminer reliability of the Gillet test. J Manipulative Physiol Ther 1999;22:4–9.
12. Dreyfuss P, Dreyer S, Griffin J, et al. Positive sacroiliac screening tests in asymptomatic adults. Spine 1994;19:1138–1143.
13. Slipman CW, Lipetz JS, Plastaras CT, et al. Fluoroscopically guided therapeutic sacroiliac joint injections for sacroiliac joint syndrome. Am J Phys Med Rehabil 2001;80:425–432.
14. Kagan A. Rotator cuff tears of the hip. Clin Orthop 1999;368:135–140.
15. McKeag DB. The relationship of osteoarthritis and exercise. Clin Sports Med 1992;11(2):471–488.
16. Kumar R, Cheng Roe M, Scremin OU. Methods of estimating the proper length of a cane. Arch Phys Med Rehabil 1995;76:1173–1175.
17. Kingzett-Taylor A, Tirman PFJ, Feller J, et al. Tendinosis and tears of gluteus medius and minimus muscles as a cause of hip pain: MR imaging findings. AJR Am J Roentgenol 1999;173(4):1123–1126.
18. Williams PH, Trzil KP. Management of meralgia paresthetica. J Neurosurg 1991;74:76–80.

19. Wray CC, Easom S, Hoskinson J. Coccydynia, etiology and treatment. J Bone Joint Surg 1991;73B(2):335–338.
20. O'Kane JW. Anterior hip pain. Am Fam Physician 1999;60:1687–1696.
21. Wesselmann U, Burnett AL, Heinberg LJ. The urogenital and rectal pain syndromes. Pain 1997;73:269–294.
22. LaBan MM, Meerschaert JR, Taylor RS, et al. Symphyseal and sacroiliac joint pain associated with pubic symphysis instability. Arch Phys Med Rehabil 1978;59:470–477.

Suggested Readings

Boyd KT, Peirce NS, Batt ME. Common hip injuries in sport. Sports Med 1997;24:273–288.

Bradshaw C. Hip and Groin Pain. In P Brukner, K Khan (eds), Clinical Sports Medicine (2nd ed). Sydney, Australia: McGraw-Hill, 2001.

O'Kane JW. Anterior hip pain. Am Fam Physician 1999;60:1687–1696.

Wesselmann U, Burnett AL, Heinberg LJ. The urogenital and rectal pain syndromes. Pain 1997;73:269–294.

12   Thigh and Knee

Michael E. Berend and Ralph M. Buschbacher

The knee is the most mobile joint in the lower extremity. It is structured to provide both mobility and stability, and this dual role is often challenged by movements that impose great stresses on the knee. The knee has both dynamic and static stabilizers. The dynamic stabilizers are the musculotendinous units that cross the knee, and the static stabilizers are the ligaments and menisci. Weight bearing also increases knee stability by increasing the congruency of the cartilaginous surfaces. Because of its great mobility, the knee is susceptible to a wide array of pathologies, both traumatic and overuse in nature.

The biomechanical demands on the knee joint are affected by the hip and ankle. Therefore, in evaluating disorders of the knee it is essential to possess a thorough knowledge of the anatomy and injury mechanisms of the entire lower extremity. As the origin of the major muscles that control the knee, the thigh must be understood as well.

Anatomy

The knee (Figure 12.1) is composed of three compartments: the patellofemoral articulation, the medial compartment, and the lateral compartment. Together, the medial and lateral compartments form the tibiofemoral joint. The femur's articular surfaces are the medial and lateral condyles. The lateral femoral condyle is relatively flat, whereas the medial condyle is convex. The medial and lateral tibial plateaus serve as the concave articulations for the femoral condyles. They are quite shallow. The incongruence of the articular surfaces causes the femur and tibia to move on each other in several planes. In addition to flexion and extension, the joint surfaces also glide on each other, and during the final degrees of knee extension, they rotate as well. This rotation (internal rotation of the femur during the last stages of extension) increases the stability of the joint.

Placed between the bony prominences of the femur and the tibia are two fibrocartilaginous disks called the *medial* and *lateral menisci*. These disks serve to deepen the interface between the two bones to enhance stability and act as shock absorbers during weight-bearing activities. The medial meniscus is held in place via its attachments to the deep medial joint capsule, the medial (tibial)

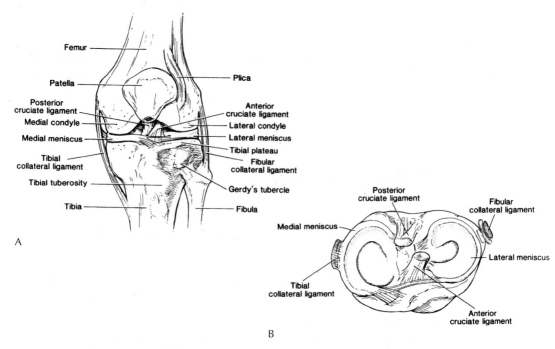

FIGURE 12.1 *The structures of the knee: (A) anterior view; (B) view looking down on the proximal tibia.*

collateral ligament, and the semimembranosus muscle. The lateral meniscus is more mobile. The menisci are vascularized only on their periphery.[1]

The patellofemoral joint is the articulation between the sesamoid patella and the trochlear intercondylar) groove of the femur. The patella tracks in the trochlear groove as the knee flexes and extends. The patella is connected to the fascia about the knee by the medial and lateral retinaculae, which are fibrous sheets of connective tissue (Figure 12.2).

There are several key supporting ligamentous structures that, in addition to the joint capsule, reinforce the stability of the knee. The medial knee is protected against valgus forces, such as a blow to the outside of the knee, by the medial (tibial) collateral ligament (MCL). A segment of this ligament blends with the joint capsule and attaches to the medial meniscus. Therefore, these structures can be injured with similar mechanisms. The lateral (fibular) collateral ligament (LCL) protects the knee against varus forces such as a blow to the inside of the knee. It is not connected to the lateral meniscus and is thus not particularly associated with injuries to this meniscus.

There are two crossed intra-articular ligaments of the knee, the cruciate ligaments. These ligaments provide the majority of static knee stability. The anterior cruciate ligament (ACL) runs from the anteromedial tibia to the posterolateral femur. This ligament prevents excessive anterior translation of the tibia on the femur, as well as hyperextension. It also plays an important role in rotation of the knee during flexion and extension. The posterior cruciate ligament

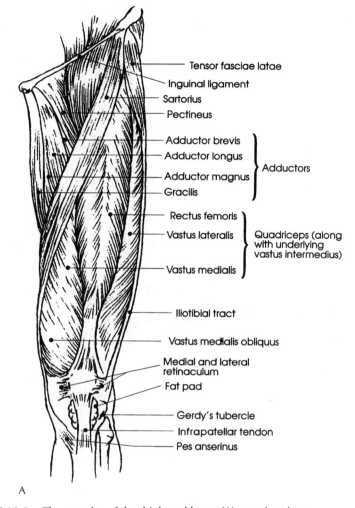

Tensor fasciae latae
Inguinal ligament
Sartorius
Pectineus

Adductor brevis
Adductor longus
Adductor magnus } Adductors
Gracilis

Rectus femoris }
Vastus lateralis   } Quadriceps (along
with underlying
vastus intermedius)
Vastus medialis }

Iliotibial tract

Vastus medialis obliquus

Medial and lateral
retinaculum
Fat pad

Gerdy's tubercle
Infrapatellar tendon
Pes anserinus

A

FIGURE 12.2   *The muscles of the thigh and knee: (A) anterior view.*

(PCL) extends from the posterolateral tibia to the anteromedial femur. It prevents excessive posterior movement of the tibia. These ligaments work in concert with the tibial plateau and the intracondylar roof of the femur to provide a four-bar linkage-type joint, which acts as a stabilizing force for the knee.

The muscles of the thigh also contribute to the dynamic stability of the knee joint (see Figure 12.2). The thigh muscles can best be divided into three compartments: the quadriceps, or anterior compartment; the adductors, or medial compartment; and the hamstrings, or posterior compartment. The quadriceps act to extend the knee, the adductors adduct the leg, and the hamstrings flex the knee. The hamstrings also decelerate the lower leg during running. Posteriorly, the knee joint is also crossed by the gastrocnemius and popliteus calf muscles.

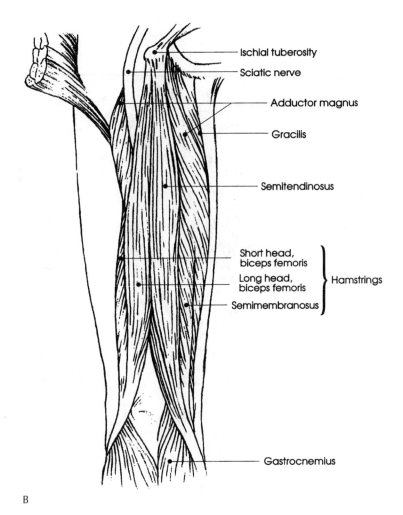

Ischial tuberosity

Sciatic nerve

Adductor magnus

Gracilis

Semitendinosus

Short head, biceps femoris

Long head, biceps femoris

Semimembranosus

} Hamstrings

Gastrocnemius

B

FIGURE 12.2 *Continued. B. Posterior view.*

The lateral knee has some additional support from the iliotibial band (tract) (ITB), which extends from the tensor fascia lata and gluteus maximus muscles to insert onto Gerdy's tubercle on the anterolateral aspect of the proximal tibia.

On the medial side of the knee is the pes anserinus ("goose's foot"). It is the combined tendinous insertion of the sartorius, gracilis, and semitendinosus muscles. It is located on the anteromedial knee at the level of the tibial tuberosity. It is surrounded by a bursa.

Examination and Testing Techniques

History

The most important aspect of injury evaluation is the history. If the patient can describe the mechanism of injury in a traumatic situation, this gives insight into the potential injury pattern. For example, a blow to the outside of the knee creates a valgus stress, which is most likely to injure the MCL.

In obtaining a history from patients with overuse injuries, questions should be asked about any potential causative factors. For example, changes in training duration, intensity, or footwear can precipitate knee pain. Consistent running on one side of the road can also cause an ITB irritation or foot injury by increasing stress on the lateral side of the knee, because most roads are crowned for drainage and the lower (outside) leg absorbs forces in a different pattern than the inside leg.

If the patient reports hearing or feeling a "pop" during the injury, it is most often suggestive of an ACL tear (in more than 90% of the cases). Other potential causes of a "pop" are a dislocation of the patella, osteochondral fracture, or meniscus tear.

The location of pain is important. Pain along the medial knee may indicate injury to the MCL complex or the medial meniscus, whereas pain on the lateral joint may be indicative of an injury to the LCL, lateral meniscus, or the popliteus tendon insertion. Pain at the patellofemoral joint may be suggestive of patellar subluxation or abnormal tracking, whereas pain at the infrapatellar tendon (patellar ligament—between the patella and the tibial tubercle) or quadriceps tendon (insertion of quadriceps onto the superior patella) may be indicative of tendonitis of these structures. A number of other factors are also important in the history. They include the following.

Swelling

Acute swelling is usually due to a peripheral meniscal tear (in the vascular zone of the meniscus), ligament tear (usually ACL), or intra-articular fracture of the knee. Swelling within a few hours is generally due to cartilaginous injury, such as a meniscal tear in the non-vascular zone, but can also be due to ligamentous injury.

Swelling on the sides of the infrapatellar tendon (below the patella) is a sign of an infrapatellar bursitis. Swelling around and above the patella is indicative of knee joint effusion. Superficial swelling over the patella is a sign of prepatellar bursitis.

Knee Catching and Locking

The patient may report that the knee becomes "stuck" in certain positions. This can be seen with displaced meniscal tears, loose osteochondral fragments, patellofemoral joint dysfunction, or plica syndromes. Locking, with the inability to reach full extension, most often results from meniscal bucket handle tears displaced into the intercondylar notch.

Examination

The examination should begin with an assessment of both of the lower extremities, and perhaps even the spine. This gives information about atrophy, neurovascular status, range of motion (ROM), and strength of the entire leg, as well as other potential injuries or predispositions to injury. It is helpful to examine the uninjured knee first to establish a baseline for alignment, swelling, stability, range of motion, and strength, as well as to reassure the patient about the examination.

Inspection

Observation of the patient's mobility during gait and during independent movement within the examination room serves as a guide to the severity of the injury. The muscles of the injured and uninjured sides should be assessed for atrophy. The position of the patella should be noted to detect whether it is high-riding (patella alta), or low-riding (patella baja). Patella alta predisposes to patellar instability because the patella is less stabilized in the trochlear groove of the femur. Because it provides less leverage in knee extension than a normally situated patella, it also makes the quadriceps more susceptible to overuse as they compensate for this deficit. A patella baja, due to greater com-pressive forces being exerted on it, is involved in more degenerative problems. A laterally positioned patella may be associated with patellofem-oral tracking abnormalities.

The patella should be observed with the patient sitting and the knee flexed to 90 degrees. The patellar surface should normally face straight forward, with an upward angle.

The knees should be assessed for valgus or varus positioning. The feet can be examined to assess any alignment abnormalities that may predispose to injury or overuse. If needed, the thigh and calf can be measured for circumference at a fixed distance (usually 10 cm) above and below the patella. This allows the tracking of muscle mass over time.

Palpation

Palpation of the injured area should begin with the structures least likely to have been injured. Once patients feel pain during the examination, they become apprehensive, and it is difficult to continue palpation.

Palpation should be used to determine the point of maximal tenderness in relation to the anatomic structures that have been described. Soft tissue swelling, crepitus, and knee joint effusion can also be assessed.

Palpation of the patellofemoral joint is best done with the patient in the prone position with the leg extended off the edge of the bed. This allows testing of this joint for medial and lateral translation of the patella, ROM, crepitus, tenderness along the medial and lateral retinaculae, and swelling of the infrapatellar region. The infrapatellar tendon and quadriceps tendon can also be examined.

The medial part of the vastus medialis, also called the vastus medialis obliquus (VMO) should be palpated during active muscle contraction to assess its muscle mass, especially in relation to the opposite side. Weakness of this part of the muscle often results in abnormal patellar tracking.

The lateral knee is best palpated in the so-called *figure-4* position, with the patient's heel resting on the contralateral thigh. This allows excellent differentiation of pain coming from the lateral condyle, the lateral joint line, the lateral meniscus, the popliteus tendon, the LCL, Gerdy's tubercle, and the ITB. This position puts the LCL under stress and makes it a defining landmark in the evaluation of this area.

The medial knee is most readily evaluated in the seated position with the knee flexed to 90 degrees to differentiate tenderness along the medial condyle, medial joint line, or pes anserinus.

Range of Motion and Muscular Strength

Joint ROM (active and passive) and muscular strength should be assessed. The uninvolved side of the body can be used as a control to determine normal range and strength. Active, pain-free ROM is an effective indicator as to the severity of knee and thigh injuries. The clinician should determine whether pain, spasm, or mechanical obstruction limits ROM.

Squatting can be used to assess knee flexion range as a screening technique. If the patient is unable to fully extend the knee, it can be a sign of meniscal injury, ACL tear, or arthrofibrosis.

Stability Testing

Varus and valgus stress testing should be performed with the knee fully extended and in 30 degrees of flexion (Figure 12.3).[2] During full extension the anterior and posterior cruciate ligaments, as well as the medial and lateral joint structures, are taut. Thus, if valgus or varus stress at full extension reveals abnormal laxity in any direction, it is indicative of significant soft tissue damage. When valgus and varus stress is applied at 30 degrees of knee flexion, the cruciate ligaments become lax and the medial and lateral stabilizing structures are tested in isolation. Thus, if only the collateral ligaments are damaged, varus and valgus stress testing at 30 degrees of flexion is more likely to be abnormal.

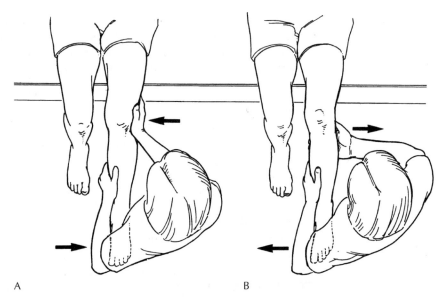

A   B

FIGURE 12.3   *Valgus (A) and varus (B) stress testing at the knee. This should be performed with the knee fully extended and in 30 degrees of flexion.*

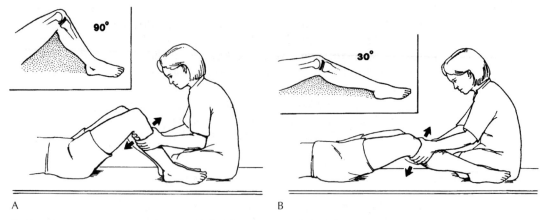

FIGURE 12.4   *A. Anterior and posterior drawer testing. B. The Lachman's test.*

Special Tests

Anterior and Posterior Drawer Tests

Anterior and posterior drawer tests (Figure 12.4) are performed at 90 degrees of knee flexion. The patient is usually supine, and the examiner may sit on the patient's foot to stabilize the lower leg. In this position, either an anterior or posterior force is applied to the proximal tibia. Excessive anterior movement is indicative of a deficient ACL. Excessive posterior movement is indicative of a torn PCL. When the patient is in this position with the quadriceps relaxed, a sagging of the proximal tibia may be present, which is also indicative of a PCL tear. This sagging is best viewed from the side. Pulling forward on a sagging tibia may give the impression of a false-positive anterior drawer test.

In addition to excessive movement or translation, the firmness of the end point of the drawer test may indicate ligament injury if it is "softer" than the uninjured side.

Lachman's Test

The Lachman's test (see Figure 12.4) is a more sensitive test of the ACL than the anterior drawer test. The posterior tibia has a lip that projects upward. This, as well as the meniscus, creates a wedge that may stabilize the knee during anterior drawer testing (see inset on Figure 12.4). The Lachman's test removes this wedge by placing the knee in 30 degrees of flexion. The lower leg again is stabilized, and an anterior force directed on the proximal tibia. Excessive anterior translation is indicative of an ACL tear. This test has been found to more closely test the stability of the ACL.[3,4] The firmness of the end point of movement is again of importance.

The Lachman's test is usually described with the patient lying supine, with the knee flexed 20–30 degrees. This position makes it difficult to grasp the lower leg while stabilizing the thigh, especially in large individuals. One easier method of performing the test (in patients who can sit on the edge of the examination table) is to have them sit in this position while the examiner sits in front of them and traps their ankle between his or her knees, which allows the use of both hands to perform the test.

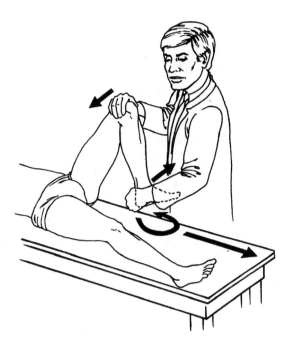

FIGURE 12.5 *McMurray's test for meniscus tears. The examiner passively flexes the patient's knee, applies valgus stress to the knee, and externally rotates the lower leg. The leg is then slowly extended. The same procedure is repeated with the lower leg internally rotated while applying varus stress.*

Pivot Shift Test

The pivot shift test is also a test of the ACL. The patient is supine with the leg extended. The examiner applies a valgus force to the knee, internally rotates the lower leg, and then brings the knee into flexion. A shift of the tibia at approximately 30 degrees of flexion is considered a positive finding.

McMurray's Test

A torn meniscus often produces a click or a catch in the knee during flexion and extension. McMurray's test (Figure 12.5) is designed to elicit this click or catch more readily during the physical examination. The patient is supine. The examiner passively flexes the knee while holding the knee in one hand and the foot in the other. The lower leg is externally rotated while applying a valgus stress, then slowly extended. A palpable or audible click over the joint line is indicative of a probable meniscal tear. The test is also performed with a varus stress and internal rotation to the knee. It is important to realize that the majority of meniscal tears will not have a positive McMurray's test. A negative test does not rule out such a tear.

Patellar Apprehension and Grinding

Patellar apprehension testing is best performed with the patient prone, and can be assessed by applying a lateral force to the patella while the knee is flexed from full extension to 30–40 degrees of flexion. If this maneuver produces a feeling that the patella is going to dislocate, the test is positive.

The patellar grind test involves applying pressure onto the patella to push it into the trochlear groove in full extension. Pain is a positive finding. However, this test is often uncomfortable even in asymptomatic patients, and is therefore relatively nonspecific.

Quadriceps Angle Measurement

The quadriceps angle (Q-angle) (Figure 12.6) is the angle formed between the quadriceps (measured from the anterior superior iliac spine to the center of the patella) and the infrapatellar tendon (center of patella to center of tibial tubercle). An excessive Q-angle is felt to predispose individuals to patellofemoral joint dysfunction because the quadriceps tend to pull the patella laterally. In women, the Q-angle should be less than 22 degrees with the knee in extension and less than 9 degrees with the knee in 90 degrees of flexion. In men, the comparable angles are 18 and 8 degrees.[5]

Functional Tests

A number of additional tests can be performed to assess knee and thigh function. These include tests such as squatting, single-legged squatting, and duck walking (in a squat). These movements are usually severely limited in persons with intra-articular pathology, ligamentous instability, or meniscal tears. Persons who are able to perform these maneuvers may very well not have an internal derangement of the knee. Care must be taken not to have patients injure themselves while performing these tests.

Ancillary Diagnostic Testing

X-Rays

The standard x-rays that should be obtained in knee disorders are standing anteroposterior, lateral, and sunrise (of the patella). Another possible view is the tunnel view (also known as *notch view*), which is made to view the intercondylar notch of the femur. X-ray reveals most fractures, degenerative changes, and the subacute to chronic changes of myositis ossificans.

Joint Aspiration

In conditions of effusion or suspected hemorrhage into the joint, a joint aspiration is often helpful. Obviously, bloody fluid helps make a diagnosis. If there is fat within this fluid, it may be indicative of an osteochondral fracture. Analysis of joint fluid also reveals signs of chronic inflammation or infection as well as many metabolic and connective tissue diseases.

Magnetic Resonance Imaging and Computed Tomography

Magnetic resonance imaging (MRI) is useful in assessing the soft tissues of the knee and allows excellent visualization of the ligaments and menisci. It also clearly shows effusions and subchondral bone injury such as bone bruises, which are almost always seen in the first week or two after ACL injury.[6] Muscle injuries such as hamstring strains can also be well visualized at the myotendinous junction.[7]

Computed tomography scanning is used to identify periarticular fractures about the proximal tibia and distal femur. It is not useful for determining ligamentous or soft tissue injuries about the knee.

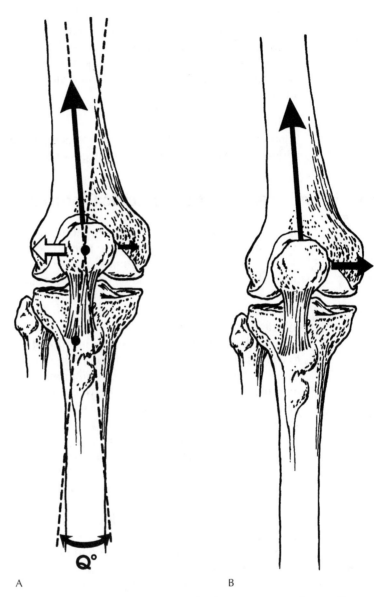

A   B

FIGURE 12.6   *The Q-angle and the muscular forces acting on the patella. Because the bulk of the quadriceps pulls along the line of the femur (long black arrow), it tends to pull the patella laterally out of place (open arrow). This is counteracted by the fibers of the vastus medialis, especially the vastus medialis obliquus (small black arrow).* **A.** *A weak vastus medialis obliquus cannot counteract the stronger bulk of the quadriceps. This results in a net lateral force vector (open arrow).* **B.** *The vastus medialis obliquus is strong and counteracts the lateral force to achieve neutral patellar tracking.*

Arthrography

Arthrography involves injection of radiopaque dye into the knee joint and can be used to detect ligamentous or meniscal tears. It has largely been replaced by MRI.

Arthroscopy

Diagnostic and therapeutic arthroscopy involves insertion of a fiber-optic viewing scope into the knee. It can be used to detect ligament damage, meniscus tears, and cartilaginous injury, among other injuries. It is used to débride meniscal tears, remove loose bodies, and aid in the reconstruction of the intra-articular ligamentous structures.

Bone Scans

Bone scans can be used to detect stress fractures, tumors, infections, and (with a triple-phase bone scan) the early stages of myositis ossificans.

Diagnosis and Treatment of Specific Disorders of the Knee

In an acute knee injury, the lower leg should not be allowed to dangle, which would cause the weight of the leg to pull on possibly damaged ligaments. Before a definitive diagnosis is made, especially if there is a possibility of an internal derangement of the knee or significant ligament sprain, the patient may benefit from wearing a knee immobilizer or hinged brace. Crutch walking and protected weight-bearing status may also be indicated, depending on the severity of the injury.

Immediate evaluation of knee injuries should begin with an assessment as to whether there is neurovascular compromise (which may be a surgical emergency), ligamentous injury (thereby compromising the stability of the joint), muscular injury (which may lead to weakness and atrophy), or intra-articular injury such as to the menisci or articular cartilage. Unless contraindicated, gait should be observed.

The location and nature of the knee complaint may direct the examiner to certain diagnoses. Anterior knee pain is often caused by patellofemoral joint problems. If there is tenderness at the upper pole of the patella, there may be a quadriceps tendonitis or a partial tear of the quadriceps insertion. Tenderness at the lower pole of the patella can be a sign of infrapatellar tendonitis. Weakness of knee extension can be indicative of a ruptured patella, infrapatellar tendon, or quadriceps.

Medial joint line tenderness is seen in meniscal pathology and in degenerative joint disease (DJD). Medial knee pain above the joint line is a sign of MCL injury, whereas pain below the joint line is indicative of either MCL damage or pes anserine bursitis.

Lateral knee pain can be due to ITB problems. If the pain is over the lateral joint line it can be a sign of meniscal pathology or DJD.

Posteromedial knee pain can be due to medial meniscal problems. If associated with a posterior fullness it may be due to a Baker's cyst. Popliteal pain can be seen in a popliteal aneurism.

A "locking" or "catching" sensation can be due to meniscal pathology, patellofemoral joint dysfunction, plica, or DJD.

If the patient complains of "stiffness," it may be indicative of a knee joint effusion or DJD.

It should also be remembered that complaints of knee pain might be due to referred pathology, such as from hip DJD or radiculopathy. Night pain can be due to tumor. Concomitant signs of infection may be indicative of a septic joint.

Proprioception is affected by injury.[8] Therefore, balance exercises should begin as soon as the patient can bear weight comfortably. Persons with knee injury may have long-term balance deficits.[9]

Ligamentous Injury

Injuries to the ligaments of the knee are quite common in athletic events. Most commonly injured is the MCL, followed by the ACL (possibly in common with the MCL), the PCL, and the LCL.

The MCL is injured with the application of a valgus force to the knee. This usually occurs in traumatic injuries, such as during collision sports, but can also result from repetitive forceful activities such as breaststroke swimming.[10] The LCL is injured with varus force. ACL injury usually occurs when the athlete stops abruptly or changes direction with the foot planted. Approximately half the time it is associated with meniscal damage. Often the athlete describes a "pop" felt in the knee and is unable to continue to play. There is usually an acute hemarthrosis. ACL injury may be associated with an anatomically narrow intercondylar notch of the femur.[11] PCL injury occurs when the proximal tibia is pushed posteriorly with the knee flexed; for example, when hitting the dashboard in a car accident or falling onto a flexed knee. PCL injuries usually do not result in clinical instability, and may even heal without surgical intervention.

Due to the relationship between the MCL and the medial meniscus, more complex injuries such as the "unhappy triad of O'Donoghue" can result. This triad includes MCL sprain, ACL sprain, and medical meniscus lesion (although the lateral meniscus is actually more commonly injured). Ligamentous injury can be graded as I (sprain with no laxity), II (sprain with some laxity and with a firm end point), or III (complete rupture with no end point).

Diagnosis

The history is important in focusing the examination on the aspect of the knee that was injured. The mechanisms described above can lead to the specific ligament injuries listed.

It is valuable to examine the knee as soon as possible after injury, before hemarthrosis, effusion, or a pain response has developed. Later it is much more difficult to properly examine the knee.

In ACL injury the anterior drawer and pivot shift tests may be positive and the Lachman's test is usually positive. There is usually a significant effusion. MRI confirms the diagnosis.

In PCL damage there may be posterior sagging of the proximal tibia, and posterior drawer testing should be positive (care must be taken not to view this as a false-positive anterior drawer test). With the knee flexed, active quadriceps contraction may make the proximal tibia move forward. With the patient supine and the examiner holding the relaxed leg up by the heel, the knee may go into hyperextension. There may be an effusion. Again, MRI confirms tearing of this ligament.

Collateral ligament injuries do not result in a tense joint effusion unless the intra-articular vascularized structures are damaged as well. The patient does, however, experience pain and tenderness along the joint line and along the affected ligament. Complete active and passive ROM of the knee is usually not possible, as the injury results in a loss of motion that increases with injury severity. Depending on the severity of the injury, ligamentous stress tests may reveal laxity of the joint. All stress testing must be done bilaterally to determine if a difference in laxity exists.

Treatment

Treatment for acute anterior and posterior cruciate ligament injuries should be performed, in most cases, by an orthopedic surgeon. Acute ACL injury, especially in a young or active patient, is usually treated surgically. The majority of athletes can return to pre-injury function within 9–12 months. Postoperative rehabilitation should focus on closed kinetic chain quadriceps strengthening exercises to minimize stress on the ACL. Nonsurgical treatment, when pursued, involves strengthening the muscles surrounding the knee, possible bracing, and activity modification.

PCL injury is usually treated nonoperatively. It can be treated with nonsteroidal anti-inflammatory drugs (NSAIDs), rest, ice, compression, early elevation, and quadriceps strengthening to improve knee function.

Treatment of MCL and LCL injury depends on the severity of the injury. The severity also affects prognosis and time to recovery.

For grade I injuries, early treatment involves NSAIDs, ice, compression, and elevation. Crutches may be needed for a brief period. It is important to achieve full ROM as quickly as possible. Once proper ROM has been established, exercise bicycling and an isometric and isotonic strengthening program for the quadriceps and hamstrings should be pursued. Recovery usually takes a few days to a few weeks.

Grade II sprains can be treated similarly to grade I injuries, but with a longer treatment period. Grade II injuries may take 4–6 weeks to heal enough for the patient to return to activity; in some cases, a hinged knee brace may be used to prevent valgus or varus forces during the early healing period. Bracing is typically for a 3–6 week period, and is also used during the return to sporting activities.

Grade III MCL sprains are usually managed nonoperatively. Treatment includes a hinged knee brace (for up to 3 months), early non-weight-bearing status with crutches, and early ROM exercise, followed by quadriceps and hamstring strengthening. Full weight bearing is usually achieved in 4 weeks. Such injuries usually require a brace during the early return-to-function phase. Grade III LCL sprains usually require surgical repair.

MCL and LCL sprains may leave the patient with some minor residual laxity; however, this is rarely clinically significant. Resumption of normal activity, especially athletic activity, should resume only when normal ROM, strength, and function are regained.

Meniscus Injuries

Injury to the meniscus usually involves a twisting injury to a flexed knee. Because the medial meniscus is less mobile than the lateral meniscus (due to its attachment to the joint capsule and MCL), it is more frequently damaged than the lateral meniscus. Injury to the medial meniscus is often associated with MCL or ACL damage. Tears of the meniscus are often traumatic; however, repetitive trauma (e.g., from running) may also cause a gradual separation of collagen fibers, resulting in a tear. Tears may result from rotatory forces being superimposed on weight bearing.

In older patients, degenerative meniscal tears may develop in the posterior horns of the menisci. These cannot usually be attributed to any specific traumatic event and may become symptomatic with minor trauma, such as arising from a squatting position.

Diagnosis

In an acute meniscus injury, patients usually complain of pain around the joint line of the knee. They may have knee stiffness and locking or clicking of the knee, which is worsened by twisting and squatting activities. Occasionally, with displaced meniscal tears, there can be locking of the knee in one position. Effusions tend to be mild to moderate with meniscal tearing (after the acute hemarthrosis resolves), and patients with larger effusions may have osteochondral loose bodies rather than meniscal tears. On examination the joint line is generally tender. There may be pain on passive forced knee flexion, especially with rotation. Knee extension is often incomplete. The diagnosis can be confirmed by MRI or arthroscopy. Overuse-type tears may be associated with intermittent pain and swelling.

Treatment

Early conservative treatment following acute meniscal injury includes rest, ice, compression, and elevation. ROM is re-established as tolerated, followed by a strengthening and functional exercise program (avoiding extreme knee flexion). If this fails, MRI evaluation to assess associated injuries and surgery may be considered.

Over the past 40 years, the trend in surgical treatment of meniscal tears has gone from total meniscectomy to meniscal preservation. Small asymptomatic tears are treated conservatively. If they become symptomatic with pain, mechanical (blocking) symptoms, or recurrent effusions, then a partial meniscectomy can be done on an outpatient basis. Larger tears (which are often displaced), especially if associated with mechanical symptoms, may require partial meniscectomy earlier on.

The meniscus has a blood supply only on the outer third of its circumference. This leads to limited healing potential, with the majority of tears being in the so-called *white zone* in the inner two-thirds of the circumference, which has a limited blood supply. Tears about the periphery, which are associated with ACL injuries, have a higher chance of healing with surgical repair.

Degenerative tears in the 40- and 50-year age groups can initially be treated with a period of rest, immobilization, NSAIDs, and a functional rehabilitation program. A knee sleeve is often helpful to provide warmth and compression to the knee. If a nonoperative treatment program is unsuccessful, partial meniscectomy may be considered.

Patellar Instability

The patella is a sesamoid bone within the extensor mechanism of the knee. It connects the quadriceps tendon to the infrapatellar tendon (patellar ligament) to provide greater leverage in extension. It lies in the trochlear groove of the femur. In patients who have a greater than normal Q-angle or patella alta, or a shallow or hypoplastic trochlear groove, the patella may slip out of the groove laterally. This is normally prevented by the vastus medialis, especially the VMO.[12] In patients with a weak VMO, it is believed that lateral subluxation or dislocation is more likely to occur. Other factors that predispose an individual to lateral displacement of the patella include external tibial torsion, laxity in the medial retinaculum, a tight lateral retinaculum, pes planus, and excessive foot pronation.

Instability of the patella can result in acute dislocation, acute subluxation, or chronic dislocation and subluxation.

Diagnosis

An acutely dislocated patella can usually be detected by observation or palpation; however, it is often relocated by the time a physician examines the knee. The patient usually has a history of a "pop" and has a feeling that the knee went "out of joint." This usually occurs with the foot planted and with a turning away from the side of injury. There is marked pain and decreased ROM. The majority of dislocations occur laterally.

Examination reveals an effusion and tenderness medially along the patella and medial retinaculum. Lateral translation of the patella may produce a feeling of apprehension. There may also be crepitus of the patella, as dislocation causes chondral injury as well. Palpating the undersurface edges of the patella reveals tenderness.

When the patella has subluxated, the patient may again report that the knee went out of joint. Knee locking, catching, or a feeling of weakness at the knee is also common. Examination of the knee may reveal swelling and tenderness along the medial patella. There may be lateral hypermobility of the patella, and passive movement of the patella in this direction may cause acute pain and apprehension.

Patients with a history of dislocation or subluxation may have lateral patellar movement towards the end of extension. They often have a poorly developed VMO. Apprehension testing is positive.

Treatment

Acute dislocation of the patella can easily be reduced with extension of the leg. This results in a rather pronounced movement of the patella back into the trochlear groove. Both dislocation and subluxation are treated with ice and by splinting in extension. X-rays should be obtained, as osteochondral fractures may be associated with this condition.

After an initial acute dislocation, the leg can be held extended (the position of least pressure on the patella) in a knee immobilizer (with crutch walking and partial weight bearing) for several weeks to facilitate healing. In subluxation, a lesser period of extension positioning is warranted. In recurrent dislocations, the patient may be put in a knee immobilizer until symptoms resolve. This is followed by a strengthening program emphasizing the quadriceps, especially the VMO [see the next section, Patellofemoral Dysfunction (Chondromalacia)]. A knee sleeve brace with a patellar cutout may be worn in this early period. Special knee braces with lateral buttresses and strapping systems help prevent lateral translation of the patella and can also be considered.

In cases refractory to conservative treatment, a lateral retinacular release may be necessary. If an excessive Q-angle is causing abnormal patellar alignment, a realignment osteotomy of the tibial tubercle can be performed.

Patellofemoral Dysfunction (Chondromalacia)

Chondromalacia is a term that has been used—and abused—widely in the past. It implies that there is a degeneration of the patellofemoral joint, and is not actually a clinical, but rather a pathologic, diagnosis. Patients with patellofemoral joint pain may have chondromalacia. However, many patients with obvious degeneration by arthroscopy or x-ray have no joint pain. Consequently, the cause of the pain is not clear.

Patellofemoral dysfunction occurs because of abnormal tracking of the patella,[13] usually due to muscular imbalance in the quadriceps.[12] This may be associated with some of the abnormalities described earlier for patellar instability. There may be a patella alta, an increase in Q-angle, foot hyperpronation, pes planus, genu valgum, external tibial torsion, or femoral anteversion, as well as inflexibility of the hamstrings, gastrocnemius, and iliotibial tract.[14] Patients suffering from patellofemoral dysfunction are often active young women in their teens or 20s.

Diagnosis

Patellofemoral dysfunction generally has an insidious onset. Pain and discomfort first appear following activities such as climbing stairs. Later there are characteristic complaints of knee pain (especially while running up or down hills), aching of the knees after sitting for long periods of time (theater sign), or occasional painful catching or locking of the knee. Physical examination may reveal tenderness of the medial patella, pain on patellar compression, a positive apprehension sign, and often, patellofemoral joint crepitus. This crepitus can usually be elicited with the patient sitting and performing ROM actively with the examiner's hand over the patella. There may be atrophy of the VMO. A prone examination of the patellofemoral joint may reveal contracture of the medial or lateral retinaculae.

Treatment

Early treatment includes relative rest and the application of ice after activity.[13] A patellar tracking brace with a lateral buttress to improve patellar tracking can also be used.[14,15] Later treatment involves strengthening the quadriceps, especially the VMO.[14] Because the patellofemoral joint reactive force is greater in knee flexion,[16] the strengthening program is performed with the knee in relatively greater knee extension. The VMO is also preferentially exercised in this position. This can be done with a number of exercises, including quadriceps setting exercises, straight leg raising, terminal extension exercises, and exercise bicycling.

Quadriceps setting exercises are isometric exercises performed to strengthen the muscles without irritating the joint structures. Patients lie supine with the knee extended. They slowly contract the quadriceps, hold this position for 10 seconds, relax, and repeat the sequence. This exercise can be performed throughout the day and in positions other than supine, and with the knee at various angles.

When quadriceps setting has been mastered, patients may progress to straight leg raises. In this exercise, they lie supine with the opposite leg flexed. The quadriceps should be contracted, as when doing the setting exercise, and the foot dorsiflexed. The injured leg is then lifted to the height of the opposite leg, slowly lowered, and the muscles relaxed. The sequence is then repeated. Ankle weights may be added as tolerated.

Terminal extension exercises are isotonic knee contractions done over the final 30 degrees of extension only. These can be performed with special weight machines (found at many health clubs), with ankle weights, or by rolling a blanket under the knee to allow the foot to be lifted.

Bicycling with the knee in excessive flexion aggravates patellofemoral dysfunction. Therefore, the bicycle seat should be kept a bit high (but not too high) to keep the knees relatively extended during this exercise.

In addition to this strengthening program, hamstring and gastrocnemius flexibility, NSAIDs, ice, shoe orthotics, and avoidance of exacerbating activities are important. Manual stretching of the lateral retinaculum or taping of the patella may be attempted in conjunction with strengthening.[17,18] Conservative care is usually successful. Only rarely is a lateral retinacular release or a tibial tubercle osteotomy required to correct underlying malalignment or contracture.

Patellar Tendonitis and Quadriceps Tendonitis

Patellar tendonitis, known as *jumper's knee*, is an overuse syndrome of the infrapatellar tendon. It is most often seen in running, jumping, climbing, and kicking activities such as basketball and soccer. If the tendonitis persists without treatment, the tendon may rupture. It the tendonitis occurs at the upper pole of the patella it is called *quadriceps tendonitis*.

Diagnosis
The history and location of the pain are clues to these disorders. Tenderness may be present along the insertion of the infrapatellar tendon or the quadriceps tendon onto the patella. The patient often describes pain during the landing phase of jumping and may complain of the knee becoming stiff and sore with prolonged periods of sitting. Symptoms are made worse by extreme knee flexion, which stretches these structures.

Treatment
Treatment consists of rest (a few days to a few weeks), ice, and NSAIDs. The use of an infrapatellar tendon circumferential strap may help alleviate pain. A strengthening program of the quadriceps and flexibility exercise for the hamstrings and gastroc-soleus musculature helps. Activity modification is also important. Eccentric exercise may be valuable.[19]

Osgood-Schlatter's Disease

See Chapter 17.

Iliotibial Band Inflammation

Iliotibial band inflammation, also known as *runner's knee*, involves irritation and inflammation of the ITB as it crosses the lateral femoral epicondyle. It is aggravated by running, especially running downhill.[20] The ITB rubs over the lateral femoral epicondyle as the knee is flexed to approximately 30 degrees. When this flexion is performed repeatedly, especially in distance runners, it can develop into a friction syndrome, with bursitis beneath the tract. It may be more common in runners who supinate their feet excessively.

Diagnosis

When the knee is slowly flexed, the ITB can be felt to slip over the femoral epicondyle. Pain and tenderness of the tract as it slips over the epicondyle are indicative of irritation of this structure.[20] Occasionally, the tensor fascia lata is inflexible, and stretching of this muscle may reproduce the symptoms of knee pain (see Ober's test in Chapter 11). Palpation of the lateral knee in the figure-4 position can help in differentiating tenderness over the lateral epicondyle from joint line tenderness.

Treatment

Treatment consists of ice, stretching, NSAIDs, and rest. Avoiding running on hills and slopes, new shoes, and shoe orthotics, which prevent excessive supination or pronation, may be helpful as well. Corticosteroid injection into this area occasionally may provide some relief of pain.

The hip abductors, tensor fascia lata, and ITB can be stretched by having the patient stand sideways approximately a foot from a wall, hand against the wall. The foot farthest from wall is crossed over towards the wall and the pelvis is stretched towards the wall. A similar stretch can also be done facing a table, with the hands on the table, by crossing one foot to other side and pushing the pelvis in that same direction. Leaning away from the foot increases the stretch.

Inflamed Plica

The medial plica is a redundant fold of synovial membrane situated in the medial knee. It is present in some persons as a vestigial embryonic fold of the membrane.[21] Because it can be entrapped in the patellofemoral joint or medial compartment on the femoral condyle, the plica is sometimes inflamed, producing anterior knee pain. This can occur due to trauma or overuse.

Diagnosis

Patients complain of anterior or anteromedial knee pain. This is exacerbated by running, especially running hills. Characteristically, the patient reports that knee pain occurs with prolonged sitting, and that after getting up and taking a few steps, it resolves. This most likely occurs because the plica slips back out of the patellofemoral joint. An inflamed plica may cause knee clicking, swelling, catching, and weakness. It is sometimes confused with meniscal tears or patellofemoral dysfunction. It can sometimes be differentiated from these conditions if the inflamed plica is palpable at the anteromedial knee.

Treatment

Treatment consists of rest, NSAIDs, and strengthening of the quadriceps. A small muscle called the *articularis genu* pulls the synovial membrane out of the joint during knee extension, and quadriceps-strengthening exercises may help develop this muscle to pull the plica out of the area in which it is being compressed. Corticosteroid injection may also help. Conservative care usually gives good results, although arthroscopic resection of the plica is occasionally necessary.

Degenerative Joint Disease

DJD occurs in the knee as in many other joints of the body. It is associated with aging, although aging is probably not the sole cause. There is some element of "wear and tear" involved in its progression, and it can be precipitated by previous injury, abnormal biomechanics, or total meniscectomy. It is associated with obesity and family history and has an insidious onset.

Diagnosis

DJD of the knee is characterized by increasing pain with activity, especially weight-bearing activity. Early on, pain occurs only with activity. Later it occurs constantly. The pain can occur at night and after rest and is sometimes relieved by gentle activity. There may be loss of ROM, a feeling of stiffness, difficulty rising from a chair, and difficulty with stairs and walking long distances. Occasionally, there are symptoms of locking of the knee.

On physical examination, there is joint crepitus with knee motion. There are prominent osteophytes palpable on the medial and lateral knee. X-ray reveals the characteristic signs of DJD with asymmetric joint-space narrowing and periarticular bone erosion. Patients may have a limp, as well as joint effusions. It is important to examine the hip, as hip conditions can cause symptoms of knee pain.

Treatment

Treatment is with rest, ice, and NSAIDs. Water aerobic exercises or exercise bicycling can be quite helpful. Regular exercise of moderate intensity may help to decrease the symptoms and improve functional endurance. A cane can be used on the opposite side. In early DJD of the medial compartment of the knee in active patients, special braces can be used that slightly alter the alignment of the knee to apply a valgus stress, which allows more weight bearing in the lateral compartment. This reduces pain in certain individuals.[22] In severe cases, joint replacement may be necessary.

Bursitis

There are numerous bursae distributed throughout the knee. These fluid-filled sacs can become inflamed following direct impact or overuse.

The most prevalent site of bursitis in the knee is the prepatellar bursa on the surface of the patella. This injury is caused by a fall directly onto the knee or by persistent kneeling, and is often referred to as *housemaid's knee*. Prepatellar bursitis is common in wrestlers and in persons who kneel frequently.

Inflammation in the bursa can be treated with ice, compression, and NSAIDs. Corticosteroid injection is performed in refractory cases. Occasionally, aspiration of the bursa is necessary to rule out infection.

Another relatively common bursitis is pes anserine bursitis. This is generally an overuse problem and responds well to rest, ice, NSAIDs, and, in some cases, a corticosteroid injection.

Extensor Mechanism Rupture

The extensor mechanism can be torn at either the quadriceps tendon or the infrapatellar tendon. This can occur in sedentary individuals who engage in unaccustomed activity, or in younger patients, while jumping or doing heavy lifting. The patella can also fracture. In the case of an infrapatellar tendon tear, there may be upward displacement of the patella. Knee extension is weak. These problems should be evaluated by an orthopedic surgeon. They are usually treated surgically.

Baker's Cyst

Baker's cyst is a swelling at the posteromedial knee. The cyst communicates with the knee joint, is often associated with meniscus tears, and occasionally originates from the medial hamstring tendons. Patients complain of pain, fullness, and aching in the posterior knee. The cyst may be detected by observing posterior swelling, and can sometimes be felt lateral to the medial hamstring tendons. MRI confirms the diagnosis.

Treatment is through avoidance of aggravating activity, reassurance, and treatment of any associated conditions.

Patients with rheumatoid arthritis often have a large Baker's cyst. It can dissect into the calf and cause neurovascular compromise or deep venous thrombosis. If the cyst ruptures, there can be a bruising in the calf and below the lateral malleolus (called a *crescent sign*).

Other Conditions of the Knee

Knee pain can be caused by referred pain from the hip or back. It can also be due to tumor, infection, connective tissue disease, stress fracture, or other fractures.

Diagnosis and Treatment of Specific Disorders of the Thigh

Quadriceps Contusion

Quadriceps contusion is a frequently encountered athletic injury. Its severity is often underestimated early on while the athlete is active and the muscle is "warmed-up." After a brief rest, however, the symptoms worsen. Any continued activity may exacerbate the injury and result in more significant hemorrhage.[23]

Diagnosis
This condition is diagnosed by a history of trauma, thigh pain and swelling, and decreased ROM, especially of knee flexion.

Treatment
Early treatment for a quadriceps contusion is essential. This includes protection from further aggravation or injury to control additional hemorrhage. Crutches

may be necessary if walking is painful. Ice should be applied for 20–30 minutes while a comfortable stretch is applied. No vigorous or assisted stretching should be attempted. Compression in the form of a foam pad and elastic wrap is then applied. The patient is encouraged to minimize activity and to maintain lower extremity elevation whenever possible. Activity or exercise that may cause rebleeding should be avoided in the first week after injury.

Heat modalities, including hot whirlpools and ultrasound, are not indicated until the individual starts to show good progress in knee ROM. Massage is also contraindicated in the acute and subacute stages of the quadriceps contusion. Only active stretching exercises should be done by the patient—no assistance should be attempted. Functional rehabilitation and a gradual return to activity are instituted as tolerated.

A serious complication of severe or repeated contusion to the anterior thigh is myositis ossificans, a form of heterotopic ossification. In this condition, the hemorrhagic tissue is gradually replaced by an island of bone. This complication may severely limit an athlete's sports participation.

Quadriceps Strain

Delayed-onset muscle soreness occurs frequently in the quadriceps when a new activity is initiated, especially if it is an eccentric activity. Soreness progressively worsens over a 24 to 48-hour period and then begins to resolve. A strain is suspected if pain, stiffness, and spasm continue beyond this time. Strains are often seen in sprinting, jumping, and kicking activities. Muscle strain injuries in the anterior thigh occur most commonly in the rectus femoris muscle, which crosses two joints. They are usually not the result of contraction alone, but of contraction plus stretch. The damage occurs near the muscle-tendon junction.[24]

Diagnosis
The symptoms associated with a muscle strain can range from a perception of tightness to generalized pain radiating down the anterior thigh. Localized tenderness is usually palpable at the site of injury. Manual muscle tests help isolate the injured structure. The degree of injury is best determined by the amount of functional restriction the athlete has and by the limitation in knee ROM.

Treatment
Ice and *gentle* stretching in the pain-free ranges are recommended initially. When ROM is regained, a progressive strengthening program is instituted. It is important to regain bilaterally equal strength and flexibility before returning to strenuous activity to avoid the common problem of re-injury. Because of the potential complications that exist with a thigh contusion, any strain that presents with a significant hematoma should be treated very carefully.

Hamstring Strain

Injuries to the hamstrings have been categorized into two types: acute and insidious onset. The acute onset hamstring injury is commonly associated with sprinting, hurdling, or long-jumping, whereas insidious onset strains are associated with a progressive lack of flexibility of the hamstrings.[25]

Diagnosis

In an acute strain, the athlete experiences a sudden, severe pain that results in marked functional restriction. A "pop" or tearing sensation is often described during the history. Generalized pain occurs, but typically localized tenderness can be palpated. Swelling may occur, making the palpation of any defects difficult to appreciate.

Insidious onset strains are associated with less well-localized hamstring pain. The muscles are usually lacking in normal flexibility.

It is important to distinguish between avulsion of the hamstring from the ischium (tenderness at the gluteal fold) from a strain, which occurs at the myotendinous junction more distally in the thigh. In avulsion, there may be lack of strength in hip extension.

Treatment

Hamstring strains are often debilitating injuries because they seem to recur when a rehabilitation program is not followed. Acute strains should be treated with ice, compression, and gradual (pain-free) stretching, with the goal of achieving full ROM before starting a strengthening protocol. The addition of physical therapy modalities such as ultrasound and massage in the subacute phase may help increase flexibility. Later on, strengthening of the hamstrings and their antagonists, the quadriceps, as well as the gluteals, helps prevent recurrence. Intramuscular corticosteroid injection can also be performed.[26]

Other Conditions of the Thigh

Other conditions that can cause thigh problems include metabolic or connective tissue disease, stress fractures, ischial bursitis, hernias, nerve compression, infection, and tumors, among many others.

Points of Summary

1. Most knee injuries can be treated conservatively using rest, ice, compression, and elevation.
2. Radiographs should be obtained to rule out associated fractures or osteochondral injuries.
3. Magnetic resonance imaging scanning helps in the diagnosis of injuries to the soft tissues, ligaments, and cartilage, as well as bone contusions.
4. In injuries to the knee in which major ligament damage or meniscal tears are suspected, or when there is a rapid onset of swelling, orthopedic surgery consultation should be obtained.
5. Injuries to the anterior cruciate ligament or menisci may be suspected if there is a rapid onset of swelling.
6. Overuse injuries can be caused by postural and strength imbalances, and evaluation should include all aspects of the kinetic chain, from the foot to the hip.
7. Eliminating the source of overuse injuries, rather than just treating the symptoms, is imperative for long-term success.

8. Thigh injuries are commonly perceived as being insignificant. However, they can result in serious sequelae and must be properly addressed.

References

1. Arnoczky SP, Warren RF. Microvasculature of the human meniscus. Am J Sports Med 1982;10(2):90–95.
2. Johnson MW. Acute knee effusions: a systematic approach to diagnosis. Am Fam Physician 2000;61:2391–2400.
3. Noyes FR, Grood ES, Butler DL, et al. Clinical laxity tests and functional instability of the knee: biomechanical concepts. Clin Orthop 1980;146: 84–89.
4. Butler DL, Noyes FR, Grood ES. Ligamentous restraints to anterior-posterior drawer in the human knee. A biomechanical study. J Bone Joint Surg 1980;62A:259–270.
5. Snider RK (ed). Essentials of Musculoskeletal Care. Rosemont, IL: American Academy of Orthopedic Surgeons, 1997.
6. Speer KP, Spritzer CE, Bassett FH, et al. Osseous injury associated with acute tears of the anterior cruciate ligament. Am J Sports Med 1992;20: 382–389.
7. Speer KP, Lohnes J, Garrett WE. Radiographic imaging of muscle strain injuries. Am J Sports Med 1993;21:89–95.
8. Laskowski ED, Newcomer-Aney K, Smith J. Proprioception. Phys Med Rehabil Clin N Am 2000;11:347–358.
9. Holder-Powel HM, Rutherford OM. Unilateral lower-limb musculoskeletal injury: its long term effect on balance. Arch Phys Med Rehabil 2000; 81:265–268.
10. Rodeo SA. Knee pain in competitive swimming. Clin Sports Med 1999; 18:379–387.
11. Huston LJ, Greenfield MLVH, Vojtys EM. Anterior cruciate ligament injuries in the female athlete. Clin Orthop 2000;372:50–63.
12. Eisele, SA. A precise approach to anterior knee pain. Physician Sports Med 1990;19(6):127–139.
13. Juhn MS. Patellofemoral pain syndrome: a review and guidelines for treatment. Am Fam Physician 1999;60:2012–2022.
14. Baker MM, Juhn MS. Patellofemoral pain syndrome in the female athlete. Clin Sports Med 2000;19:315–329.
15. Garrick JG. Anterior knee pain (chondromalacia). Physician Sports Med 1989;17(1):75–84.
16. Hungerford DS, Lennox DW. Rehabilitation of the knee in disorders of the patellofemoral joint: relevant biomechanics. Orthop Clin N Am 1983;14(2):397–402.
17. Walsh WM, Helzer-Julin M. Patellar tracking problems in athletes. Prim Care 1992;19(2):303–330.
18. Shelton GL. Conservative management of patellofemoral dysfunction. Prim Care 1992;19(2):331–349.
19. Fyfe I, Stanish WD. The use of eccentric training and stretching in treatment and prevention of tendon injuries. Clin Sports Med 1992;11(3): 601–624.

20. James SL. Running injuries of the knee. AAOS Instructional Course Lectures. 1998;47:407–417.
21. Calvo RD, Steadman JR, Sterling JC. Managing plica syndrome of the knee. Physician Sports Med 1990;18(7):64–74.
22. Kirkley A, Webster-Bogaert S, Litchfield R, et al. The effect of bracing on varus gonarthrosis. J Bone Joint Surg 1999;81A:539–548.
23. Bull CR. Soft Tissue Injuries to the Hip and Thigh. In JS Torg, RP Welsh, RJ Shephard (eds), Current Therapy in Sports Medicine—2. Toronto, BC: Decker, 1990.
24. Garrett WE. Muscle strain injuries. Am J Sports Med 1996;24:S2–S8.
25. Garrett WE, Rich FR, Nikolaou PK, Vogler JB. Computed tomography of hamstring muscle strains. Med Sci Sports Exerc 1989;21(5):506–514.
26. Levine WN, Bergfeld JA, Tessendorf W, et al. Intramuscular corticosteroid injection for hamstring injuries. A 13-year experience in the National Football League. Am J Sports Med 2000;28:297–300.

Suggested Readings

Brotzman SB, Head P. The Knee. In SB Brotzman (ed), Clinical Orthopaedic Rehabilitation. St. Louis, MO: Mosby, 1996.

James SL. Running injuries of the knee. AAOS Instructional Course Lectures.1998;47:407–417.

Macnicol MF. The Problem Knee. Oxford, UK: Butterworth–Heinemann, 1995.

13   Lower Leg, Ankle, and Foot

Michael J. Stonnington

There are multiple conditions that can affect the lower leg, ankle, and foot. Many of these conditions are very common but are nevertheless misunderstood, owing to the complexity of this area of the body. This chapter explores the fundamentals of diagnosing and treating this important anatomic region.

Anatomy

Bony Anatomy and Articulations

The lower leg bones, the tibia and fibula, are depicted in Figure 13.1. The tibia articulates with the femur proximally at the knee joint. Distally, both the tibia and fibula contribute to the ankle mortise, which, along with the talus, forms the tibiotalar (ankle) joint. The fibula articulates with the tibia at the proximal and distal tibiofibular joints.

The ankle joint is composed of articulating surfaces between the superior, medial, and lateral talus and the distal tibia and fibula. The joint allows mainly dorsiflexion and plantarflexion, but also some inversion and eversion. The talus is wider anteriorly than posteriorly, and dorsiflexion brings the wider part of the bone into the ankle mortise. This "wedging" effect makes the ankle more stable and less prone to injury in dorsiflexion than in plantarflexion.

The subtalar joint is the articulation formed by the inferior talus and superior calcaneus. Motion at this joint occurs in the three planes of flexion/extension, abduction/adduction, and inversion/eversion.

The bones of the foot and ankle are divided into four groups (Figure 13.2): the tarsals, metatarsals, phalanges, and sesamoids. The sesamoid bones are small, rounded masses of bone found within the tendon of the flexor hallucis brevis. They are located on the weight-bearing surface of the first metatarsophalangeal joint.

The midtarsal joint (transverse tarsal) joint is composed of two joints, the talonavicular and calcaneocuboid joints. Motion at the midtarsal joint occurs on

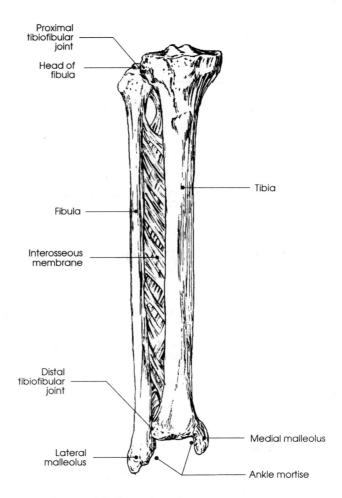

Proximal
tibiofibular
joint

Head of
fibula

Tibia

Fibula

Interosseous
membrane

Distal
tibiofibular
joint

Medial malleolus

Lateral
malleolus

Ankle mortise

FIGURE 13.1   *The bones of the lower leg.*

the longitudinal and the oblique axes, allowing for movement in all three planes.

In addition, there are joints between all the adjacent tarsals, between the tarsals and metatarsals, and between the phalanges. Of these, the first metatarsophalangeal joint is most often involved in foot dysfunction.

Ligaments

The fibula is held closely to the tibia via the strong and thick interosseous membrane (see Figure 13.1). The proximal and distal tibiofibular joints are supported by anterior and posterior ligaments, which allow some gliding and longitudinal rotation of the fibula to occur. Because the superior portion of the ankle joint, the so-called *ankle mortise,* is formed by the tibia and the fibula, it is very important that these two bones be held together. Any widening of their alignment is called a *diastasis* and disrupts the integrity and proper biome-

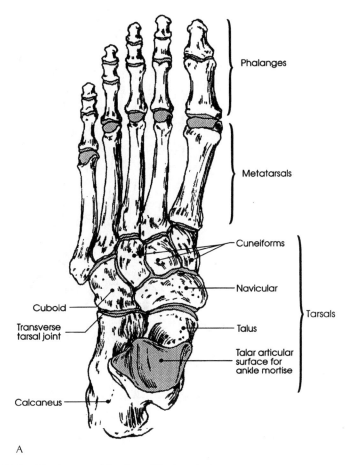

Phalanges

Metatarsals

Cuneiforms

Navicular

Cuboid

Talus

Transverse
tarsal joint

Talar articular
surface for
ankle mortise

Calcaneus

Tarsals

A

FIGURE 13.2   *The bones of the foot:* **(A)** *dorsal view.*

chanics of the joint. The tibia and fibula are held together tightly by what is called a *syndesmosis*, which in this case is a complex of supporting structures of the ankle. It includes the interosseous membrane, the anterior and posterior inferior tibiofibular ligaments, and the inferior transverse ligament.

Other important ligamentous structures at the ankle joint (Figure 13.3) are the medial deltoid ligament and the lateral ankle ligaments (anterior talofibular, calcaneofibular, and posterior talofibular ligaments). The deltoid ligament lies over the medial ankle joint. It is typically divided into four parts (tibionavicular, tibiocalcaneal, anterior tibiotalar, and posterior tibiotalar) and prevents excessive eversion of the ankle. The anterior talofibular (ATF) ligament passes from the anterior fibula to the lateral talus. This ligament prevents excessive inversion and anterior translation of the talus and is the most frequently injured ligament in ankle sprains. The calcaneofibular (CF) ligament passes from the inferior lateral malleolus to the lateral calcaneus. It prevents excessive inversion, particularly when the ankle is dorsiflexed. The posterior talofibular ligament is located on the posterior aspect of both the talus and fibula. It prevents excessive inversion of the rearfoot complex.

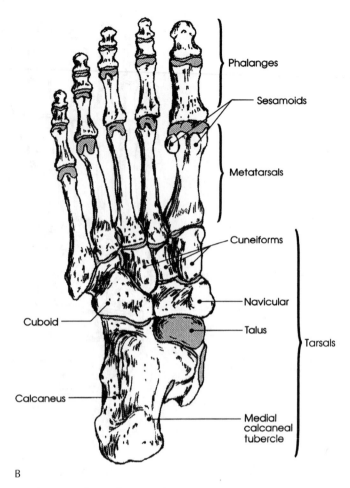

Phalanges

Sesamoids

Metatarsals

Cuneiforms

Navicular

Cuboid

Talus

Tarsals

Calcaneus

Medial
calcaneal
tubercle

B

FIGURE 13.2 *Continued.* **B.** *Plantar view.*

The midtarsal joint is supported from below by the plantar calcaneonavicular ("spring") ligament, a thick band of fibers whose primary function is to maintain the medial longitudinal arch.

Compartments and Muscles of the Lower Leg

There are four compartments in the lower leg: the anterior, superficial posterior, deep posterior, and lateral (Figure 13.4). The anterior compartment contains muscles that predominantly dorsiflex the foot and extend the toes. The superficial posterior and deep posterior compartments contain the calf muscles and flexors of the ankle and toes. The lateral compartment contains muscles that predominantly evert the foot.

The plantar fascia originates from the calcaneus and inserts onto the five heads of the metatarsal bones. It supports the longitudinal arch of the foot. Fascial bands also separate the muscles of the leg compartments, and some (the

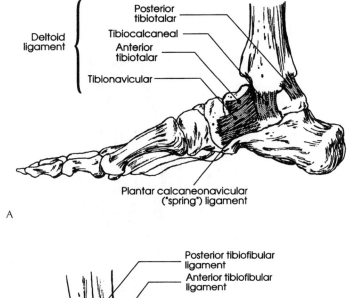

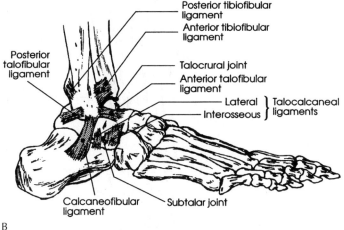

FIGURE 13.3   *The ligaments of the ankle: medial (**A**) and lateral (**B**) views.*

retinacula) anchor the tendons of the leg muscles where they pass by the ankle to the foot.

Normal Gait

The foot plays an important and complex role in gait. While it is being planted on the ground it must be flexible, yet during push-off it must be rigid to act as a lever. During normal gait, initial heel contact is on the lateral aspect of the calcaneus with the foot in a slightly supinated (adducted, inverted) position. The contact phase is characterized by pronation (abduction, eversion). Pronation is an important component of the contact phase for two reasons. First, it allows the foot to become a loose adapter to uneven terrain, and second, it assists in shock absorption. Because the foot pronates during the contact phase, the lower extremity rotates internally.

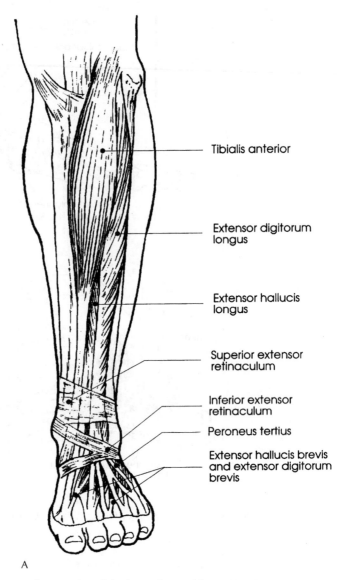

Tibialis anterior

Extensor digitorum longus

Extensor hallucis longus

Superior extensor retinaculum

Inferior extensor retinaculum

Peroneus tertius

Extensor hallucis brevis and extensor digitorum brevis

A

FIGURE 13.4   *The muscles of the lower leg and foot: (**A**) anterior view; (**B**) posterior (superficial) view.*

The mid-stance period is characterized by the foot being in full ground contact and beginning to supinate. This motion continues throughout the mid-stance and propulsive phases. The initiation of supination allows the foot to become a rigid lever in preparation for propulsion. Additionally, because the mid-stance phase is characterized by the onset of supination, the lower extremity begins to rotate externally.

During the mid-stance of the gait cycle, the tibia migrates anteriorly over the talar dome by approximately 10 degrees. Therefore, this amount of motion

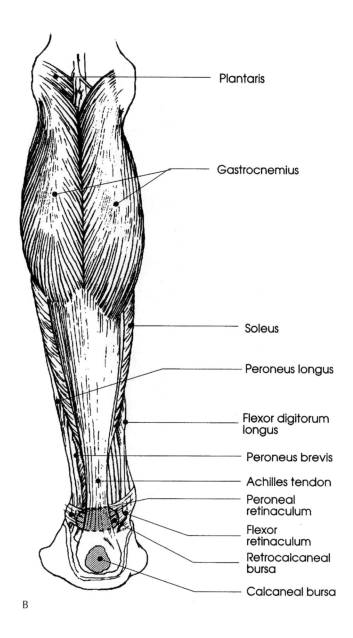

Plantaris

Gastrocnemius

Soleus

Peroneus longus

Flexor digitorum longus

Peroneus brevis

Achilles tendon

Peroneal retinaculum

Flexor retinaculum

Retrocalcaneal bursa

Calcaneal bursa

B

must be present in the ankle joint to allow for normal gait.[1] If this 10 degrees is not present, whether due to a tight gastrocnemius-soleus complex or osseous deformity, the foot must compensate for the deficit.

During the push-off (propulsion) phase of gait, increased tension is developed in the plantar fascia of the foot. This helps to elevate the medial longitudinal arch, which in turn facilitates supination and stabilizes the foot. At the same time, the sesamoid bones allow the first metatarsal head to glide posteriorly, which makes propulsion more efficient by providing proper metatarsophalangeal extension.

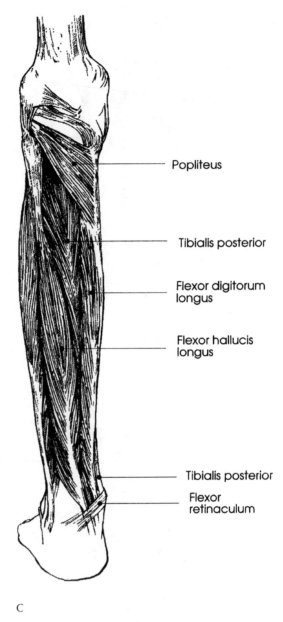

Popliteus

Tibialis posterior

Flexor digitorum
longus

Flexor hallucis
longus

Tibialis posterior

Flexor
retinaculum

C

FIGURE 13.4   *Continued.*   *C. Posterior (deep) view.*

The motion of the first toe and metatarsal are particularly important in gait. If the metatarsal were rigid, the toe would extend only approximately 30 degrees, thus significantly limiting foot motion during push-off. Instead, during push-off, the metatarsal moves in a plantar direction, gliding over the sesamoids and allowing 60 degrees of great toe extension. This motion is controlled by the flexor tendons of the toe in what is called the *Windlass mechanism.*

Examination and Testing Techniques

History and Physical Examination

The history should include questions about the mechanism of injury, past medical history, whether the onset was sudden or gradual, ability to continue sports participation after the injury occurred, the duration of symptoms, and the patient's general health status. It is useful to differentiate overuse problems from traumatic events. Questions should be asked about exacerbating or relieving factors (especially exercise) and any associated symptoms. Inquiring about training techniques and schedules, equipment (especially shoes), and changes in training surfaces helps identify causes of overuse injury.

The examination begins after the onset of injury or as the patient enters the room. Observing for a limp, limited motion, or any gait deviations serves as the basis of the examination.

Observations should include looking for signs of edema, ecchymosis, deformities, or scars. Clinical signs of hyperpronation include callus formations, clawing or splaying of the toes, and hallux valgus deformities. Retrocalcaneal exostoses or bursitis ("pump bumps") are signs of abnormal shearing forces occurring at the calcaneus due to hyperpronation.[1] The alignment of the calcaneus with respect to the lower leg should be evaluated to detect varus or valgus deformity of the hindfoot (Figure 13.5).

Palpation of the injury should begin away from the injured site or on the uninvolved extremity. Initial palpations, which do not produce pain, improve the patient's relaxation and trust.

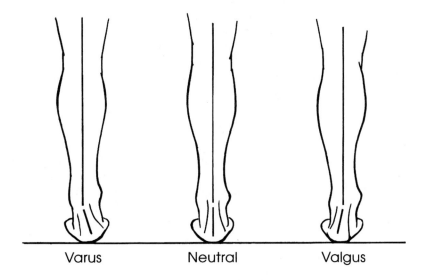

Varus | Neutral | Valgus

FIGURE 13.5 *Hindfoot position in relation to the lower leg: valgus, varus, and neutral posture (of left leg).*

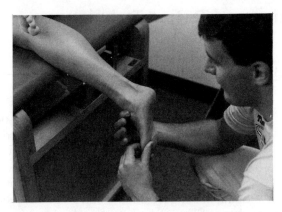

FIGURE 13.6 *Locating the neutral position of the subtalar joint. The foot is inverted and everted until the talus is equally prominent on either side of the ankle. Passive dorsiflexion "locks" the foot in this position.*

Because all parts of the lower extremity are components of a "kinetic chain," it is important to examine the joints above and below the injured area. A thorough examination helps to differentiate between musculoskeletal and referred pain.

Range-of-motion (ROM) and muscle-strength testing are also important in evaluating the foot and ankle. The unaffected side can usually be used as a comparison. Pain or laxity on inversion and eversion ROM stress testing are signs of ankle ligament injury. A number of specific examination techniques are also helpful and are described in the following text. In addition to these tests, it is helpful to observe the patient's gait and to examine the shoes to detect abnormal patterns of wear.

Subtalar Neutral Foot Positioning

The alignment of the foot and ankle is best evaluated with the subtalar joint in the neutral position (Figure 13.6). This position is located by the examiner passively inverting and everting the foot, finding that position in which the talus is equally palpable, or not palpable at all, on either side of the ankle. Slight dorsiflexion "locks" the foot in this position. Once the neutral position is attained, the ankle and foot can be assessed for varus or valgus deformity (compared to the lower leg). Alignment is also assessed with the patient standing. Any changes in varus or valgus deformities compared to the non-weight-bearing examination should be noted.

The ankle joint is examined by placing the subtalar joint in the neutral position and passively dorsiflexing the foot. A minimum of 10 degrees of dorsiflexion is required for normal gait. If this amount of motion is absent, the knee is flexed to eliminate the influence of possible gastrocnemius contracture. An increase in dorsiflexion after flexing the knee is indicative of a tight gastrocnemius muscle. No such change might be indicative of a shortened soleus muscle, contracture of the joint capsule, or an abnormal osseous "block" at the ankle.

First Metatarsophalangeal Joint Motion

Passive motion of the first metatarsophalangeal (MTP) joint is affected by the position of the first metatarsal. If the metatarsal is allowed to move freely, the joint should extend 60–70 degrees to allow for normal gait. If the examiner stabilizes the first metatarsal, the amount of motion obtained by passively extending the great toe is less, approximately 30 degrees.

Alignment of the First Ray
The examiner grasps the first metatarsal head between the thumb and index finger of one hand (thumb on plantar surface), while holding the remaining metatarsal heads with the other hand. The thumbs should be level. If the thumb holding the first metatarsal head rests below (caudal to) the other thumb, the first ray is in an abnormal plantar flexed position. Passive dorsiflexion and plantarflexion of the first metatarsal bone should be equal in both directions.

Thompson's Test
A special test to detect a rupture of the Achilles tendon, Thompson's test is performed with the patient lying prone and feet resting over the edge of the table. Gently squeezing the calf musculature normally causes the foot to plantarflex. The absence of plantarflexion is considered a positive finding.

Anterior Drawer Test
The anterior drawer test (Figure 13.7) is used to detect laxity of the anterior talofibular ligament or calcaneofibular ligament. The distal tibia and fibula are stabilized with one hand while the other cups the heel and exerts pressure anteriorly. If the foot is placed in approximately 20 degrees of plantarflexion,

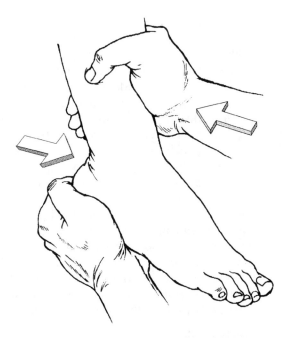

FIGURE 13.7   *The anterior drawer test. The foot is in 20 degrees of plantarflexion to test the anterior talofibular ligament. The examiner pulls the foot anteriorly. If the foot is dorsiflexed, then this primarily tests the calcaneofibular ligament.*

then excessive anterior translation of the talus is indicative of ATF ligament injury. If this test is done in dorsiflexion and there is excessive translation, then the CF ligament may be predominantly injured.

Inversion/Eversion Stress Test
In the inversion/eversion stress test, the patient lies supine with feet over the edge of the table (or remains sitting). Then the lower leg is stabilized while the talus is tilted from side to side, and inversion/eversion stress is applied. This tests the integrity of the lateral (mainly calcaneofibular) and deltoid ligaments.

Ancillary Diagnostic Testing

Plain radiographs are commonly used to evaluate bony alignment and joint condition and to detect fractures. They are indicated in all but the simplest ankle sprains to rule out associated fractures. Occasionally they are supplemented by stress testing or arthrography to help diagnose ligamentous injury. Bone scans are useful to detect stress fractures. Magnetic resonance imaging (MRI) is useful to assess for osseocartilaginous injury or avascular necrosis (particularly in the talus), and soft tissue pathology. Computed tomography (CT) is useful for assessing some complex fractures, such as those in the calcaneus.

Diagnosis and Treatment of Specific Disorders

General Approach

When dealing with traumatic conditions of the lower leg, ankle, and foot, the diagnosis and treatment is usually relatively straightforward. When dealing with overuse or biomechanical problems or trauma that was precipitated by biomechanical factors, the diagnosis and treatment is more complex. The evaluation must include the entire kinetic chain. Training errors, footwear, and pre-existing anatomy are of great importance. Although many structural abnormalities or variants can be corrected or compensated for, not all can, especially not for persons desiring to be elite athletes or hyperendurance participants. Although we all strive to return people to the activity and functional level they desire, this is simply not always possible when it comes to the foot and ankle, and patients should be told this fact before they worsen their condition.

In the disorders described in this section, a stretching program is often recommended. In general, this should include the entire kinetic chain, usually encompassing the hamstrings, gastroc-soleus, and foot (and occasionally the hip flexors and abductors). The gastrocnemius is stretched with the knee straight. Because it crosses two joints, the ankle and knee, this optimally stretches the muscle. The soleus crosses only the ankle joint, so it is best stretched with the knee bent. The muscles and fascia of the plantar foot can be stretched by raising the heel or by squatting.

Ankle Sprains
Ankle sprains range from mild to severe. In mild sprains, the functional integrity of the ligament is intact. In moderate sprains there is some disruption of the lig-

ament, whereas in severe sprains, there is complete rupture of the ligament. The exact ligament(s) injured is dependent on the mechanism of injury. Typically, three mechanisms cause ankle sprains: inversion, eversion, or rotation. These can occur in isolation or in combination with one another. The following descriptions of ankle sprains assume that isolated injury mechanisms have occurred. Combinations of injury mechanisms add to the damage and symptoms described.

In all ankle sprains it is important to perform the physical examination as early as possible. Edema forms rapidly and hampers the exact localization of the site of injury. Also, pulses and sensation in the foot should be checked in all ankle sprains to rule out associated neurovascular compromise. Radiographic studies may be obtained to rule out fracture.

Inversion Ankle Sprains

Inversion ankle sprains are the most common type of ankle sprain. Most sprains are to the ATF ligament, although they may involve damage to any of the three lateral ligaments. The CF ligament is often injured as well, but it is usually damaged along with the anterior ligament, and rarely by itself. With the ankle in the plantarflexed position, the ATF ligament is stretched and the ankle joint is at its least stable position. Thus, this ligament is at risk of injury. With the ankle in the neutral position, the CF and posterior talofibular ligaments are more likely to be damaged.

Diagnosis

The ankle may be forcefully inverted by running on uneven surfaces, by landing on someone's foot while jumping, or by having the foot stabilized and forced into inversion. On inspection immediately after injury, there may be swelling over the injured lateral ligament. If not treated immediately with ice, compression, and elevation, diffuse forefoot and ankle swelling develop. Palpation elicits point tenderness over the injured ligament. ROM and strength may be limited by pain, swelling, and possible injury to the peroneal tendons.

Special tests to evaluate the ligamentous structures include the anterior drawer test, plantarflexed inversion, and neutral inversion. Radiographs help rule out an associated fracture.

Eversion Ankle Sprains

The eversion ankle sprain causes damage to the deltoid ligament. Eversion sprains often occur in combination with a rotational mechanism of injury.

Diagnosis

The history may be of forced eversion caused by running or landing on an uneven surface, or from another person falling on the lateral leg while the foot is stabilized. Inspection and palpation reveal swelling and point tenderness over the injured medial ligament. ROM and strength are limited due to pain, swelling, and possible muscular injury to the inverters of the ankle. Testing should include passive eversion.

Syndesmosis Sprains

Syndesmotic injuries are most frequently caused by external rotation or hyperdorsiflexion of the ankle. They are often associated with injury to the deltoid ligament. The syndesmosis complex becomes injured or frankly disrupted.

Diagnosis

Patients usually describe twisting of the body with the foot planted and stabilized. They may also describe falling forward with the foot planted so as to cause hyperdorsiflexion. Patients often have tenderness over the distal tibiofibular ligaments and possibly over the deltoid ligament as well. Pain frequently occurs with forced external rotation or dorsiflexion of the foot. The "squeeze test" is a maneuver whereby the examiner compresses the fibula to the tibia at midleg level. If the patient complains of pain around the syndesmosis, then the test is positive and suggests a syndesmosis injury. Patients also complain of pain with weight bearing. X-rays are required to rule out diastasis at the syndesmosis.

Treatment of Ankle Sprains

The immediate treatment for all ankle sprains is rest, ice, compression, and elevation (RICE). Regardless of the mechanism of injury, these steps help to control secondary damage caused by swelling and bleeding into the soft tissues. Elastic wrap or tape application may help to provide compression. Air stirrups or lace-up supports are also useful and may provide enough stabilization to allow the patient to ambulate within a day or two of injury (or immediately, in some cases). Intermittent compression may also help to reduce edema formation. Ankle supports can be useful throughout the treatment of ankle sprains[2]; timing and rationale of application is summarized in Table 13.1.

Rehabilitation begins with relative rest to control swelling and encourage healing (Table 13.2). For most patients, controlled ambulation is allowed as long as it does not stress the damaged ligaments. During the subacute period, gentle non-weight-bearing exercises in an elevated position maintain joint ROM, and nonsteroidal anti-inflammatory drugs (NSAIDs) reduce inflammation and pain. Gentle exercises to maintain plantarflexion and dorsiflexion without stressing the injured structures are indicated. Those exercises include passive heelcord stretching with a towel, isometric exercises for dorsiflexion and plantarflexion, seated multidirectional tilt board ROM exercises, and elevated active ROM. The period of rest is kept to a minimum to eliminate the deleterious effects of immobilization.

Crutches may be used early on for a partial-weight-bearing gait. In some cases, a neutral foot orthotic device is effective at enabling patients to progress to weight-bearing status more comfortably and at a faster rate of return. The orthotic device holds the subtalar joint in its neutral position, the optimal position for function, and eliminates any extra stress to the healing tissue. Lace-up braces, continued taping, or an air stirrup application may also be used to provide support during early return to activity. Isometrics should begin as tolerated to promote strengthening of the ankle musculature.

As soon as possible after the injury, the patient is encouraged to ambulate, at first for limited periods of time. As tolerated, more walking, strengthening exercise, complex drills, and sports-specific activities are added. Total recovery time can last from a few weeks to 6 weeks or so, depending on the severity of the injury. Ice, compression, elevation, and wrapping/bracing may be useful throughout the acute and subacute phases of recovery.

TABLE 13.1   Various forms of ankle support and their potential uses

Type of support	When to use	Rationale	Advantages	Disadvantages
Taping	Acute sprain	Support	Good support	Requires skill
	Early rehabilitation	Compression	Can be left in place for a few days	Loses support rapidly
		Proprioception		Expensive
Elastic wrap/bandages	Acute sprain	Compression	Reduces edema	Circulatory compromise
				Poor support
Air stirrup	Acute sprain	Support	Wear under shoes	Decreases performance
	Early rehabilitation	Compression	Good support	Cumbersome
		Proprioception		
Lace-up support	Early rehabilitation	Good support	Can be retightened	Uncomfortable break-in
	Chronic instability	Proprioception	Maintains support	Non-uniform compression
	Prophylaxis		Wear under shoes	

TABLE 13.2   Functional progression after ankle sprain

Partial weight bearing

Weight shifting from side to side

Assisted heel raises

Full weight bearing

Proprioception drills

Strengthening drills

Single leg heel raises

Step-ups

Slow walking

Walk-jog

Two foot jumping drills

Single leg hopping

Faster running—straight, level surface

Running on uneven surfaces

Coordination drills—figure-8 running, small circle running, carioca/cross over, cutting

Activity-specific exercise

Return to full activity

The patient progresses from the activities at the top of the list and moves down as tolerated.

Proprioception has been shown to be impaired after an injury to the ankle.[3] It is theorized that joint nerve receptors are damaged and must be retrained before one may safely return to activity. Exercises to improve proprioception begin with balancing on one foot and multidirectional board balancing, and eventually progress to tubing-resisted hip motions while bearing weight on the involved ankle (standing on the injured leg forces this ankle to respond to the resistance applied to the other leg) (Figure 13.8). Functional activity is added when tolerated. Long-term bracing or taping is rarely necessary, but may be considered in some athletes. Such support may help by increasing proprioception more than any mechanical support being offered. Rarely, patients with complete ligamentous rupture and unstable joints require surgical treatment.

Syndesmosis sprain injuries need to be thought of differently from standard ankle sprains, mainly because surgical intervention is not unusual and prolonged recovery time from these injuries is expected. Treatment with immobilization, and next a functional brace, is indicated. However, if there is diastasis at the syndesmosis on x-ray, operative intervention with screw fixation across the syndesmosis is necessary.[4] The patient is generally kept non-weight-bearing until the ankle is pain free.

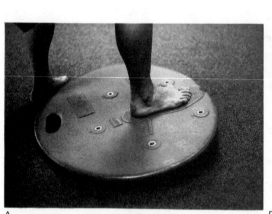

A

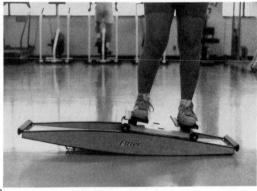

B

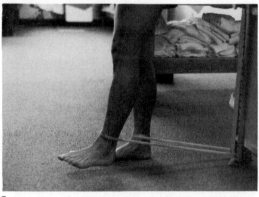

C

FIGURE 13.8 *Proprioceptive exercises: **(A)** balance board; **(B)** slide board; and **(C)** rubber tubing resistance exercise. The patient is weight bearing on the involved extremity with the tubing around the opposite leg. This strengthens the involved leg and stimulates proprioception.*

Achilles Tendonitis, Achilles Tendon Rupture, and Retrocalcaneal Bursitis

The Achilles tendon is the common tendon of the gastrocnemius and soleus muscles, which insert onto the posterior calcaneus. This tendon serves as a primary plantarflexor and secondary supinator. Located between the tendon and the upper calcaneus is the retrocalcaneal bursa. Located posterior to the calcaneus (under the skin) is the calcaneal bursa.

The Achilles tendon possesses a "zone of avascularity," which is the most common site of tendon microtrauma or rupture. Located 2–6 cm above the tendon insertion, this avascular zone is also an area in which the collagen fibers of the tendon tend to rotate and are more prone to overuse and injury.[5]

Causes of Achilles tendonitis and rupture include overuse, excessive forced dorsiflexion (causing an eccentric contraction), an inflexible gastroc-soleus complex, and hyperpronation (which may be caused by tibia vara or varus foot deformities).[5] Achilles tendonitis is fairly common, especially in runners and jumpers, and particularly in athletes who have recently increased their mileage or changed their training. A rupture of the tendon is much less common than tendonitis.

Achilles tendonitis is sometimes associated with retrocalcaneal bursitis. The retrocalcaneal bursa may become inflamed as a result of direct trauma, compressive forces (poor-fitting footwear), or abnormal biomechanical stresses. Long-standing cases can result in Haglund's deformity, which is a markedly prominent posterosuperior tuberosity of the calcaneus. Some patients also get a calcaneal bursitis between the tendon and the skin, a so-called *pump-bump* because it is often caused by shoe irritation.[6]

Diagnosis

Evaluation of an inflamed Achilles tendon reveals swelling (although not always), point tenderness, and discomfort with passive dorsiflexion or active plantarflexion. A thorough examination should be conducted to identify any ankle, hindfoot, midfoot, or forefoot abnormalities.

If the retrocalcaneal bursa is inflamed, the examiner may elicit tenderness by palpating anterior to the distal tendon, directly superior to the calcaneus. Palpating on either side of the tendon may reveal "fullness" in the area of the bursa. If insertional tendinitis is present, the patient will be tender directly on the posterior Achilles tendon over the posterosuperior tuberosity of the calcaneus.

With an Achilles tendon rupture, the patient often reports a sensation of being kicked in the calf. Palpation reveals a defect at the rupture site and Thompson's test is positive. These patients cannot walk "on their toes."

Patients with calcaneal bursitis are tender over the posterior calcaneus and have local swelling in this area.

Treatment

The treatment program for Achilles tendonitis should address any abnormal alignment in the foot or ankle while pursuing anti-inflammatory management. Rest, ice, anti-inflammatory medications, and cold whirlpools are all indicated treatments for acute tendonitis. A heel lift may be helpful because it reduces the tension on the injured structures and allows ambulation with reduced discomfort. It should not be used indefinitely so that a permanent shortening of the gastroc-soleus does not develop. A medial heel wedge or a semirigid orthotic device may help control excessive pronation.

Long-term treatment focuses on restoring proper flexibility to the gastroc-soleus structure (and the entire kinetic chain of the lower extremity). This is followed by strengthening exercises, including eccentric training. High-heeled shoes should be avoided.

Patients with a retrocalcaneal bursitis are treated basically the same as for Achilles tendonitis, with NSAIDs, ice, heelcord stretching, rest, and proper footwear. In some cases the bursa may be injected with a steroid-anesthetic solution, but as this may weaken the tendon and lead to rupture, it should be done with extreme caution, and only by a specialist in this area. In refractory cases of bursitis, exostectomy of the posterosuperior tuberosity of the calcaneus, excision of the bursa, and localized débridement of diseased tendon should be considered.

Partial tears of the tendon are treated with a period of immobilization with a cast or Achilles tendon boot, followed by the use of a heel lift and rehabilitation program as outlined in the previous section. Surgical intervention is most often indicated in neglected partial tears because there is painful scar and granulation tissue that may need to be excised. Exostectomy of the calcaneal tuberosity may also be helpful in some of these cases (if the tear is near the insertion of the Achilles tendon). For complete tears, there are numerous studies that advocate either operative or nonoperative treatment. Generally, in athletes and very active people, acute repair is indicated. The rerupture rate for nonoperative treatment is higher in many (but not all) of these articles.[7,8]

Plantar Fasciitis

Common etiologic factors of plantar fasciitis include overuse, training errors, repetitive trauma, and biomechanical factors (i.e., hyperpronation, pes cavus/pes planus). It is usually an overuse injury and may be aggravated by increased body weight, poor shoe support, or a change in running surface. In chronic cases, the insertion of the fascia may form a heel spur.

Diagnosis

Plantar fasciitis usually presents as an insidious onset of plantar heel pain. The patient typically reports pain with combined passive dorsiflexion of the ankle and extension of the great toe. Palpation is remarkable for tenderness over the plantar fascia and, in particular, over the medial calcaneal tubercle (see Figure 13.2). Patients classically report severe pain on taking their first few steps in the morning, followed by relief as they get moving. The reason for this is that people sleep with their feet plantarflexed. At night, the connective tissue of the foot shortens. Standing up in the morning stretches this already irritated tissue, causing pain.

Treatment

Treatment and rehabilitation of plantar fasciitis should focus on reducing inflammation and controlling exacerbating forces. Ice immersion or ice massage, performed 3–4 times per day (especially after exercise), helps reduce the inflammation. Flexibility exercises of the calf and foot musculature, hamstrings, and the first MTP joint should also be performed 3–4 times a day. Strengthening exercises for the gastrocnemius and arch musculature, such as towel curls, marble pick-ups, and towel-gathering exercises, can also be incorporated into the rehabilitation program. NSAIDs help reduce pain and inflammation; occasionally, steroid-anesthetic injections are necessary. However, these injections are extremely painful and can cause thinning of the plantar fat pad.

Comprehensive management should also address proper footwear, and possibly the implementation of an orthotic device. An in-shoe heel cup helps in two ways. First, it provides medial and lateral compression on the heel, preventing medial and lateral redistribution of the heel fat pad. By doing this, it increases the thickness of the heel pad directly over the plantar fascia. Second, it provides a slight heel lift, which can be beneficial as well (by not stretching the gastroc-soleus as much). However, such a heel cup should not be used indefinitely, as it allows the gastroc-soleus to shorten. A night-time splint (ankle–foot orthosis) that maintains the foot in a position of dorsiflexion may also be helpful.

If there are alignment abnormalities such as hyperpronation, an orthotic device such as a semirigid in-shoe orthotic device needs to be considered to help control abnormal biomechanical stresses. Shock wave treatment has been advocated for treatment of plantar fasciitis and has shown some relatively successful results.[9]

Heel spurs commonly occur in persons with plantar fasciitis. They develop as a secondary response to the fasciitis and are not the primary cause of the pain. The presence of a heel spur is not an indication for surgery, and the patient should be reassured of this. If a spur is removed without addressing its underlying biomechanic causes, it often recurs.

In rare refractory cases, plantar fasciotomy can be considered in treating plantar fasciitis. One study shows an 84% satisfactory rate in fasciotomy patients who had a complete trial of conservative treatment without improvement.[10]

Shin Splints

The currently accepted term for shin splints is *medial tibial stress syndrome* (MTSS). Typically, MTSS is a result of periostitis at the origin of the tibialis posterior. The differential diagnosis includes posterior tibial tendonitis, anterior tibial tendonitis, exertional (chronic) compartment syndrome, and tibial stress microfractures.[11] These conditions all result from cumulative trauma and are considered overuse injuries.

The tibialis posterior muscle provides arch support to the foot. Abnormalities, such as a forefoot varus, which leads to compensatory subtalar joint pronation, increase the stress placed on the muscle. It contracts eccentrically in an effort to slow the compensatory pronation, thereby placing its tendon under additional stress. This can contribute to the MTSS.

Diagnosis

With tibialis posterior irritation, the patient reports discomfort along the medial border of the tibia. Palpation reveals tenderness along the middle and distal thirds of the tibia. Manual muscle testing of plantarflexion and inversion may elicit a report of pain or weakness. The evaluation should also include looking for possible hyperpronation.

Symptoms occurring in the leg are typically related to overuse (i.e., performing too much, too soon, too fast). Other etiologic factors include a change in running terrain, poor flexibility, poor footwear, and alignment abnormalities.

Treatment

The management program for MTSS should focus on controlling inflammation, improving flexibility of the heelcord and first MTP joint, strength training, and reducing excessive pronatatory forces (possibly with different shoes, or orthotics). Strengthening exercises, such as toe raises with tubing resistance and towel gathering exercises, strengthen the plantarflexors and invertors of the foot. Foot abnormalities and training errors should be addressed if they are a problem. Rarely, in refractory cases, posteromedial fascial release may be performed.

Stress Fractures
Stress fractures of the foot and lower leg are frequently seen as a result of training errors or improper lower extremity biomechanics. Training errors include improper footwear and running surfaces. An excessively rapid progression of training intensity or duration may lead to stress fractures as well. In addition, excessive pronation is a biomechanical factor that can lead to increased torsion stress on the tibia. Common sites for stress fractures are the metatarsals, calcaneus, tibia, and tarsal navicular.

Diagnosis
Diagnosis is made through palpation, plain radiographs, bone scans, and occasionally, CT scan or MRI. Palpation may reveal local tenderness. Percussion of the bone, even at sites distant from the stress fracture, may cause pain to be felt at the fracture site. Plain x-ray may not detect the stress fracture in its early stages. Bone scan usually makes the definitive diagnosis. However, if the diagnosis is equivocal, a CT scan or MRI may be very helpful. For example, CT scans are particularly helpful in talus stress fractures.

Treatment
Stress fractures are managed with a period of prolonged rest to allow adequate healing of the fracture. If activity is resumed too early, the fracture will recur or not heal. In some cases, operative fixation is indicated. After rest and healing, training is resumed at a slowly graduated pace.

Exertional Compartment Syndrome
Also termed *chronic compartment syndrome*, this condition needs to be differentiated from acute compartment syndrome. Acute compartment syndrome is an increase of pressure within tissue compartments of any of the extremities to an injurious level. A compartment pressure elevation typically occurs after significant injury to an extremity. Pressures in the extremity can be measured with a catheter device; if they are above 30 mm Hg or within 10–30 mm Hg of diastolic blood pressure, an acute compartment syndrome is likely present. Pain (particularly on passive stretch of the involved compartments) is the earliest and most reliable indicator of a compartment syndrome. Pallor, paralysis, paresthesias, and pulselessness are later findings. In the lower extremity, the leg is most often involved. The acute compartment syndrome typically involves all four compartments of the leg (anterior, lateral, superficial posterior, and deep posterior), and all compartments need to be emergently released with fasciotomies. If not treated, permanent nerve damage and muscle necrosis occurs.

This is, however, in stark contrast to an exertional compartment syndrome, which is not an emergency situation. An exertional compartment syndrome is usually associated with sports participation such as running and weightlifting. The anterior and deep posterior compartments are most frequently involved. Exercise results in an increase in compartment pressures, thus resulting in symptoms.

Diagnosis

Patients with exertional compartment syndrome often go undiagnosed for a long time, as most physicians are not familiar with this condition. Patients typically complain of a gradual onset of pain with exercise; the pain eventually reaches a level that precludes further exercise. Occasionally, patients complain of associated paresthesias and weakness. The diagnosis is made by taking a thorough history of the patient and measuring compartment pressures before, during, and after exercise. Most agree that resting pressures greater than 15 mm Hg, pressures greater than 30 mm Hg during exercise, or a failure of pressures to decrease to less than 20 mm Hg 5 minutes after exercise, are all very suggestive of exertional compartment syndrome.[11] The differential diagnosis includes stress fractures, medial tibial stress syndrome, peripheral vascular disease (in older patients), popliteal artery entrapment, and radiculopathy.

Treatment

Nonoperative treatment, which involves activity modification and NSAIDs, can be successful in milder exertional compartment cases. Unfortunately, patients usually do not respond to conservative measures, simply because they are unwilling to modify their activities (most of these patients are avid athletes and very exercise-conscious). In these patients, fasciotomy of the involved compartment is indicated.[11]

Metatarsalgia

Metatarsalgia refers to foot pain in the proximity of the metatarsal heads. It is most commonly caused by abnormal foot biomechanics and repetitive forces, which cause increased stress to the transverse metatarsal arch. It is more common in the pes cavus foot, but many abnormal foot alignments of the hindfoot, midfoot, or forefoot can contribute to a metatarsalgia.

Diagnosis

Palpation reveals point tenderness over the plantar surface of the metatarsal heads, usually the second and third. Compression of the metatarsal heads elicits pain. Differential diagnoses include a metatarsal stress fracture or a neuroma.

Treatment

Metatarsalgia is treated with correction of abnormal biomechanics. Metatarsal arch pads, orthotics, a change in training techniques, and strengthening and flexibility exercises are all useful. The metatarsal pads or "bar" can be inserted in the patient's shoes just proximal to the metatarsal heads to relieve some of the weight from the painful area. Care must be taken not to place the pad or bar directly under the metatarsal heads, as this worsens the symptoms. If needed, such a support can be built into a custom-made shoe. If all other measures fail, surgical correction may be considered.

Morton's Neuroma

Morton's neuroma refers to a localized entrapment of an interdigital nerve, usually between the third and fourth metatarsals and deep to the transverse metatarsal ligament. There is localized enlargement and swelling of the interdigital nerve. A causal factor may be narrow shoes, especially high heels.

Diagnosis

The patient may complain of a shooting pain or paresthesias in the forefoot, which worsens with activity. Side-to-side forefoot compression or palpation between the metatarsals elicits pain or paresthesias if a neuroma is present. Sometimes, local swelling may be detected.

Treatment

Treatment consists of NSAIDs, modalities to control pain and inflammation, wider shoes, metatarsal pads, and injections. If the neuroma is refractory to conservative treatment, surgical excision is usually successful.

Hallux Valgus

Hallux valgus is a progressive deformity of the MTP joint of the great toe. It results in a bunion (localized prominence) to form medial to the metatarsal head.

Diagnosis

A hallux valgus deformity is present if there is lateral deviation of the great toe and the hallux valgus angle (angle formed by the metatarsal and proximal phalanx) is greater than 15 degrees.

Treatment

Several etiologic factors may lead to hallux valgus, so the treatment program should focus on the cause of the deformity. In most cases, abnormal biomechanics are the contributing factor. Therefore, a treatment program that addresses any flexibility, strength, or biomechanical deficits is helpful. Wide shoes with orthotic supports, NSAIDs, and taping or toe spacers may decrease symptoms. In many cases, surgical correction is indicated.

Hallux Rigidus

Hallux rigidus, as its name implies, involves a loss of ROM of the first MTP joint. It is caused by trauma and degenerative joint disease. There are usually bony spurs adjacent to the joint. The result is pain and restricted first MTP motion. It is more common in persons who stress their toes, such as dancers.

Diagnosis

Pain and limited motion of the first MTP joint are the main complaints. X-ray usually reveals formation of osteophytes on the dorsal aspect of the first metatarsal head and at the base of the proximal phalanx.[12] There is a decrease in ROM, especially of extension, at the joint.

Treatment

Conservative management includes NSAIDs, ice, and taping. A rigid sole with a rocker bottom may decrease symptoms. Steroid injection into the joint may occasionally be helpful, but is often just temporary. In refractory cases, cheilectomy (excision of osteophytes around the metatarsal head and proximal phalanx) is the most common surgical procedure, and is relatively efficacious.[13]

Turf Toe

Turf toe is an injury of the first MTP joint, typically caused by acute or chronic forced extension of the joint. This condition involves joint capsule irritation with secondary trauma to the musculotendinous structures. In some cases, dorsal osteocartilaginous impaction of the metatarsal head and proximal phalanx may occur. Artificial turf has increased its frequency. Differential diagnoses include a flexion sprain of the first MTP joint and sesamoiditis.

Diagnosis
Evaluation reveals tenderness (at a minimum, it is dorsal), redness, swelling, and limited MTP motion. Gait analysis reveals an inability to perform push-off motion efficiently during gait.

Treatment
Treatment consists of controlling the pain and swelling. Several methods of treatment are useful. The first is taping of the joint to decrease the motion at the MTP joint and provide stability during the propulsive period of gait. Also, rest, ice, elevation, progressive joint mobilization, and NSAIDs are indicated. Stiff-soled shoes may be helpful. For athletes, the stiff-soled shoe can also incorporate a spring-steel that extends from distal heel to distal insole. This further restricts extension. In severe injuries, it is not uncommon for an athlete to miss several weeks of playing time. Rarely, surgery to remove MTP joint loose bodies or repair of an avulsed plantar capsule may be indicated.

Sesamoiditis
Located on the inferior aspect of the first MTP joint, the sesamoid bones are located within the flexor hallucis brevis tendon. Sesamoiditis is an inflammation of the tissues that surround the sesamoid bones.

Diagnosis
The patient reports discomfort during gait, especially with propulsion. Palpation reveals point tenderness over the sesamoid bones. Passive great toe extension coupled with palpation over the plantar aspect of the MTP joint elicits pain. In some cases the sesamoids may fracture, and x-ray study or bone scan may help to make the diagnosis.

Treatment
Treatment may include metatarsal pads or a metatarsal bar placed proximal to the metatarsal heads to relieve pressure on the sesamoids. An orthotic insert with metatarsal extension relieves stress on the bones. Flexibility exercises for the first MTP joint and heelcord, as well as NSAIDs and modalities to control pain and inflammation, promote tissue healing.

Pes Planus
Pes planus is often referred to as a *pronated foot* or *flat foot*. The cause may be congenital or due to muscle weakness (especially of the tibialis posterior), ligamentous laxity (plantar "spring" ligament), trauma, paralysis, or postural deformity. There are two types of pes planus—flexible and inflexible. In flexible pes planus, the foot is flat only during weight bearing. When the patient stops standing, the foot returns to a normal alignment. Flexible pes planus may respond to orthotic treatment to prevent it from turning into an inflexible pes planus, in which the foot stays flat even without bearing weight.

Diagnosis

Examination reveals that the pes planus foot is either rigid or flexible. Depending on the severity of the deformity, there may be an associated calcaneovalgus or foot varus deformity. The foot must be evaluated during non-weight-bearing as well as standing and walking. Comparison should be made to the opposite side.

Treatment

Strengthening exercises for the intrinsic muscles of the foot, as well as flexibility exercises for the calf musculature, are indicated. The patient with a pes planus deformity may benefit from a semirigid orthotic device to provide arch support and calcaneal control. Patients with a flexible flat foot are more likely to benefit from an arch support. A rigid pes planus cannot be corrected by an orthosis. In cases of refractory, painful pes planus or in feet with significant deformity not correctable with nonsurgical means, surgical treatment should be considered.

Pes Cavus

The cavus (high-arched) foot may also be either rigid (maintaining a high arch on weight bearing) or flexible (arch height decreases on weight bearing). This foot type may predispose the individual to problems caused by a lack of shock absorption (i.e., stress fractures, metatarsalgia).

Diagnosis

Depending on the severity of the deformity, biomechanical analysis may reveal clawing of the toes, a hindfoot varus, or a forefoot valgus deformity. In addition, because it could be the result of a neuromuscular disease (e.g., Charcot-Marie-Tooth, polio), patients with a cavus foot should have a complete neurologic examination.

Treatment

Patients with pes cavus should tolerate a rigid orthotic device with a forefoot valgus post. In addition they should be placed on a thorough flexibility program of the lower extremity. Surgery is a consideration in some cases, but the types of surgical corrections are many and often very complex.

Tarsal Tunnel Syndrome

Tarsal tunnel syndrome is an entrapment neuropathy of the posterior tibial nerve as it passes beneath the lacinate ligament (flexor retinaculum) behind the medial malleolus. It is uncommon, and most cases are post-traumatic in nature. It can be worsened by overpronation or a "fallen" arch, as this stretches the nerve.

Diagnosis

The diagnosis is confirmed with electrodiagnostic testing. Patients describe pain, burning, and paresthesias in the distribution of the tibial nerve branches to the sole of the foot. Percussion of the tibial nerve in its tunnel may reproduce symptoms.

Treatment

Avoidance of aggravating activity, orthotics, and NSAIDs are the usual methods of nonoperative treatment. In refractory cases, surgical release of the tunnel has been shown to be successful.[14] However, surgical release alters the foot biomechanics, and because this is a weight-bearing structure, such altered biomechanics may be worsened by a lot of walking or running. Because this nerve is stretched with pronation, the patient may benefit from strengthening the tibialis posterior or from wearing antipronation footwear or orthotics.

Acknowledgments

The author would like to acknowledge the contributions from this chapter's previous edition authors: John Leard, Denise L. Massie, Jack Brautigam, and Ralph Buschbacher. Significant portions of their chapter were maintained and unaltered for this current edition.

Points of Summary

1. Ankle inversion sprains are more common when the foot is plantarflexed. This is due to the loosening of the talar "wedge" in the ankle mortise.
2. Inversion ankle sprains are the most common ankle sprains. Syndesmosis sprains are often under-diagnosed and typically require a longer recovery period.
3. Proprioception is impaired after ankle sprain. Treatment should include proprioception exercise.
4. Anterior drawer testing isolates the anterior talofibular ligament.
5. Great toe abnormalities can often be treated with in-shoe orthotics with first metatarsal extensions to provide support.
6. Achilles tendonitis is treated with rest, ice, nonsteroidal anti-inflammatory drugs, orthotics or heel cup, and stretching of the foot, gastrocsoleus, and hamstrings.
7. Plantar fasciitis causes foot pain on first standing up in the morning. It usually responds to ice, stretching, and an orthotic device, especially a heel cup.
8. Acute compartment syndrome is a medical emergency that requires immediate surgical fasciotomy.
9. Exertional compartment syndrome is not a medical emergency, but often requires fasciotomies for resolution of symptoms.
10. Thompson's test detects a ruptured Achilles tendon.
11. Stress fractures can often be detected early with a bone scan.

References

1. Subotnick SI. Podiatric Sports Medicine. Mt. Kisco, NY: Futura Publishing, 1975;37,42,60.
2. Buschbacher RM. Ankle Sprain Evaluation and Bracing. In RM Buschbacher, RL Braddom (eds), Sports Medicine and Rehabilitation: A Sport Specific Approach. Philadelphia, PA: Hanley and Belfus, 1994;221–240.
3. Freeman MAR, Dean MRE, Hanham IWF. The etiology and prevention of functional instability of the foot. J Bone Joint Surg 1965;47B:678–685.

4. Miller CD, Shelton WR, Barrett GR, et al. Deltoid and syndesmosis ligament injury of the ankle without fracture. Am J Sports Med 1995;23:746–750.
5. Clement DB, Taunton JE, Smart GW. Achilles tendinitis and peritendinitis: etiology and treatment. Am J Sports Med 1984;12:179–184.
6. Myerson MS, McGarvey W. Disorders of the Achilles Tendon Insertion and Achilles Tendinitis. In JD Zuckerman (ed), Instructional Course Lectures, Vol 48, 1999;211–218.
7. Helgeland J, Odland P, Hove LM. Achilles tendon rupture: surgical or non-surgical treatment. Tidsskr Nor Laegeforen 1997;117:1763–1766.
8. Cetti R, Christensen SE, Ejsted R, et al. Operative versus nonoperative treatment of Achilles tendon rupture: a prospective randomized study and review of the literature. Am J Sports Med 1993;21:791–799.
9. Zingas CN, Collon D, Anderson K. Shock wave therapy for plantar fasciitis. Presented at the 16th Annual Meeting of the American Orthopaedic Foot and Ankle Society, Vail, CO: July 13–15, 2000.
10. Davis WH, Watson T, Anderson RB. Distal tarsal tunnel release with partial plantar fasciotomy for chronic disabling heel pain syndrome: outcome study of 85 patients. Presented at the 16th Annual Meeting of the American Orthopaedic Foot and Ankle Society, Vail, CO: July 13–15, 2000.
11. Rorabeck CH, Fowler PJ, Nott L. The results of fasciotomy in the management of chronic exertional compartment syndrome. Am J Sports Med 1988;16:224–227.
12. Donatelli R. The Biomechanics of the Foot and Ankle. Philadelphia, PA: FA Davis, 1990;258–259.
13. Mann RA, Clanton TO. Hallux rigidus: treatment by cheilectomy. J Bone Joint Surg 1988;70A:400–406.
14. Cimino WR. Tarsal tunnel syndrome: review of the literature. Foot Ankle 1990;11:47–52.

Suggested Readings

Digiovanni BF, Gould JS. Achilles tendonitis and posterior heel disorders. Foot Ankle Clin 1997;2:411–428.

Frey C. Ankle Sprains. In FH Sim (ed), Instructional Course Lectures 2001;50:515–520.

Nicholas JA, Hershman EB. The Lower Extremity and Spine in Sports Medicine (2nd ed). St. Louis, MO: Mosby, 1995.

Porter DA, Clanton TO. Primary care of foot and ankle injuries in the athlete. Clin Sports Med 1997;16:435–466.

Ranawat CS, Positano RG. Disorders of the Heel, Rearfoot, and Ankle. New York: Churchill Livingstone, 1999.

III Special Issues

14   The Occupational Medicine System

Ralph M. Buschbacher

Occupational medicine is a subset of medicine that presents unique challenges and circumstances to the clinician. In addition to treating the patient appropriately, the primary goal of occupational medicine is to return the injured worker to work as quickly as possible. The clinician who understands the intricacies of the system will have better outcomes with less frustration when treating the injured worker.

History

The worker's compensation system in the United States was developed in the early 20th century, and has its roots in 19th century Germany and in English common law. Before its development, an employer was not obligated to provide for the treatment of a person injured on the job. The injured worker had to sue the employer in civil court. In some cases this resulted in large awards to the worker, in others, none. This inequality led various states to enact statutes to create a no-fault system in which employers were obligated to provide for lost wages and medical treatment and to compensate for any permanent loss or disability. In return, workers lost the right to sue employers, along with the ability to collect awards for pain and suffering or punitive damages. There can still, in some cases, be lawsuits related to a work injury—for instance, for product liability, negligence, wrongful firing—but these are rare.[1–3]

Worker's compensation law across the United States is a patchwork of individual state systems, as well as a few federal programs for federal workers, merchant marine and railway workers, and longshore and lumber workers, among others. These systems are constantly being adjusted by the legislatures, so that it is impossible, in this chapter, to give a comprehensive overview of the various systems in place. Instead, some of the principles common to the treatment of injured workers are discussed.

Definitions

In worker's compensation cases, the physician is often called on to answer various medicolegal questions. The questions are often phrased in specific terms, and therefore it is important to know exactly what these terms mean. The following are some definitions of commonly used terms[1]:

Significant describes any contribution that is weighty, has a notable effect, and is at least partly responsible for an outcome.

Substantial includes elements that are worthy of note and that may have had an effect that should not be ignored.

Possible describes a concept or event that is "conceivable." Although broad, it should be used to describe outcomes or events that are reasonably anticipated.

Probable means "more likely than not" (i.e., a greater than 50% probability).

Major contribution describes an element that, depending on a state's definition, may be more than 50% of the total cause, or the largest proportionate share of the cause.

Aggravation may describe both symptomatic and pathologic worsening of the worker's condition, depending on the state's definition.

Unique Features of Occupational Medicine

The worker's compensation system is different from other medical treatment systems in that it deals with (obviously) injured workers only. This means that to receive treatment under the system, the workers must prove (1) that they were injured, and (2) that the injury was related to their employment. Workers generally fill out an injury report claim to receive entry into the system. Sometimes physicians are specifically asked to comment on whether they feel the injury was work-related.

Most employers use some sort of insurance to cover their worker's compensation cases. Otherwise, a particularly bad or costly injury might well bankrupt a small company. Larger companies are often self-insured.[4]

The clinician's relationship to a worker's compensation patient is somewhat different than that to other patients. Because the entity paying for the services is the company (or the company's insurance), the clinician is, in essence, acting as the representative of the company. There is some obligation (constrained by confidentiality issues) to open the medical findings to the worker's compensation insurance carrier,[2,4] and the company, in many states, has great latitude in determining who the treating physician is.[4] In some sense, the clinician is acting as a "company doc," although of course ethical treatment requires an honest, unbiased, and medically sound evaluation and treatment plan.

Just as when submitting a claim to an auto insurance company, each worker's compensation case is assigned to a claims adjustor of the insurance company. The claims adjustor reviews the case and approves or denies coverage for treatments and tests ordered by the physician. At times, the claims adjuster may assign a case manager. Case managers are often nurses. They review the prescribed tests and treatment and advise the claims adjustor on which should be covered. They offer a greater degree of medical expertise to assist the claims adjustor in making decisions. Although claims adjustors and cases managers at times seem like adversaries to the physician, they can also be tremendous aids, often expediting the scheduling of tests, second opinions,[5] treatments, and other patient services. When a good working relationship is developed between the physician and the case manager and claims adjustor, it can greatly expedite patient care.

When a worker is injured and a worker's compensation case is opened, the patient is usually initially seen by a generalist, often an occupational medicine doctor. Complex or refractory cases are referred to specialists. Depending on the nature of the injury, this might be an ophthalmologist (in the case of chemical exposure to the eye), a surgeon, or almost any medical specialist. Nonoperative musculoskeletal problems are referred to physical medicine and rehabilitation doctors, orthopedic surgeons, or other physicians specializing in musculoskeletal care. During the treatment period the patient might be placed on light duty. If no light duty is available or if the patient is taken off work completely, the injured worker receives wage replacement. This replacement wage varies from state to state and is generally a fairly minimal amount. This makes it relatively attractive to a minimum wage worker, who may be getting close to usual pay without having to work, but it is very unattractive to more highly paid employees.

After patients are finished with treatment, they are discharged. If completely restored to normal function, they are released without restrictions. If they need permanent restrictions, these are given at the time of discharge. In general, in the worker's compensation system, "permanent" restrictions may be lifted in 6–12 months if the patient improves and no longer needs them. Alternatively, they may indeed be permanent.

At discharge the physician (in most states) may be asked to give the patient a permanent partial impairment (PPI) rating. This is based on the principle that the worker is not and cannot be restored to the pre-injury state. PPI ratings are derived in a number of ways. Usually, they are determined using the American Medical Association's (AMA) *Guides to the Evaluation of Permanent Impairment.*[6] In this book, a whole host of different conditions, losses of function or range of motion, and impairments are listed in various tables and charts. The physician looks up the impairments, adds or combines them, and comes up with a global impairment rating. This rating is used by the insurance company, according to state statutes, to determine a monetary compensation for the patient.

Not all states require that the latest version of the *Guides* be used.[2] These guides are also just that—guides, not mandates. The physician can deviate from them or use a totally different rating system; however, it is useful to offer some sort of justification for the rating given.

If the patient or insurance company disagrees with the rating, they can ask for a second rating and, in some cases, a tie-breaking rating. When a patient is released and the case is closed, but the patient disagrees with this closure, he or she can appeal the decision to the state worker's compensation board. Usually, a second opinion is ordered by the board. Depending on this independent physician's recommendations, the case may be re-opened and further treatment provided.

In the worker's compensation system there is no financial incentive for patients to limit the amount of medical treatment they receive. It has been shown that as wage replacement rates rise, the duration and frequency of claims rise as well. Patients are, in essence, "rewarded for failure."[7]

Many physicians are frustrated when treating worker's compensation patients. Such patients are often unhappy with their jobs and become even unhappier after their injury (or the perceived poor handling of the injury). They may be poorly motivated to return to work early, or have secondary gain issues, such as wishing to be permanently transferred to lighter duty (which is often a problem in union shops). They also tend to experience poorer outcomes to treatment than those who are injured outside of work.[7] Depending on the personality of the treating physician, this can be a problem; but when it is kept in mind that most injured workers are decent, motivated people, and when it is understood how to use the system to advantage, such frustration can often be minimized. Others elect not to accept worker's compensation cases at all.

Treatment Approach

The actual treatment plan for injured workers is not that different than it would be for other persons. It is helpful to use a sports medicine approach, viewing the patient as an "occupational athlete." The patient needs to be actively involved in the treatment, and not just show up to "let the doctor fix me." It is particularly important not to reinforce illness behavior by providing secondary gain.

A small number of workers injured on the job account for a disproportionately large share of the costs of care.[8] This makes it important to identify difficult or refractory cases early. Although the ultimate outcome in a seriously injured or difficult patient may not be changed, getting the case to an earlier closure, rather than letting it drag on for 6 months or more (or even for years), greatly reduces the costs associated with that injury. A close working relationship with referring physicians allows both the referring physician and the specialist to identify injury and time parameters that facilitate transfer of appropriate patients. It is not always beneficial to refer patients too early, as many heal on their own, but waiting too long can adversely affect the outcome. As a general rule, it is appropriate to refer patients within 2–4 weeks of injury or at any time that recovery is slower than expected. In most cases, the specialist should see the patient every week, or at the most every other week, to ensure timely adjustment in the treatment. Longer delays allow the less motivated patient's progress to stagnate.

Factors that may delay recovery are listed in Table 14.1. The focus of treatment should be an increase in function, not necessarily a decrease in pain. Function is easier to measure objectively.

When workers have been off their regular duty for long periods of time they may become deconditioned. Returning them to regular duty all at once may cause re-injury or a new injury. In these cases, a course of work conditioning or work hardening may be indicated. Although the definitions of these two treatment protocols are not used uniformly, and the differences between the two may be nebulous at times, work conditioning generally involves basic

TABLE 14.1   Factors that may delay or negatively impact the recovery course in worker's compensation cases

Severe injury

Delay in initiating appropriate treatment

Poor job satisfaction

History of poor recovery from previous injuries

Poor cardiovascular fitness

Inadequate exercise

Dispute over whether the injury is work-related

Poor relationship with employer

Lack of modified duty availability

Return to work too soon or too late

Poor English proficiency

Disabled spouse

History of substance abuse

Anger or blame

Previous or ongoing litigation

Worker convinced that he is disabled

Lack of alternative job opportunities

SOURCE: *From RD Rondinelli, JP Robinson, SJ Scheer, SM Weinstein. Industrial rehabilitation medicine. 4. Strategies for disability management. Arch Phys Med Rehabil 1997;78:S21–S28.*

strengthening exercises, whereas the work hardening program adds job simulation.[9] On-site job evaluations and ergonomic assessment or modification may also aid in returning the injured worker to the job.

In cases that have gone on for a long time, especially if permanent work restrictions are indicated, it may be helpful to use the services of a vocational rehabilitation counselor. Vocational rehabilitation may help match the worker to an appropriate job and may also include training for such a job. Such programs may be available through state agencies.

Helpful Hints

Documenting on the First Visit Whether the Injury Is Work Related

Documenting if the injury is work related on the first visit helps in getting approval for further tests and treatments and shows the insurance company that the treating physician is attuned to the special requirements of the worker's compensation system. Sometimes workers make claims that non-work-related problems are due to their jobs; for instance, although fibromyalgia may be worsened by many kinds of activity, including work, it is not generally felt to be *caused* by work. It may very well require treatment, but not through the occupational medicine system. The same is true for

TABLE 14.2 Components of the initial report that may be of particular interest in worker's compensation cases*

Chief complaint
History of present illness
    Aggravating/relieving factors
    Treatment to date
    Tests to date
Current medications—for this and other problems
Past medical history
    Previous injuries, especially to same area
    How long it took to recover from previous injury
    Drug allergies
Social history
    Current job duties
    Smoking
    Hobbies, especially those that might contribute to injury
    Second jobs
    Vocational history
    Exercise history
Physical examination
    Pain behavior
    Biomechanics
Diagnosis
    Work related or not
Plan
    Estimated date of release from care

This is obviously not an all-encompassing list.

some cases of carpal tunnel syndrome; work is not always the cause. Table 14.2 lists some items that may be of importance in the initial report.

Give Feedback

Claims adjustors and case managers are usually quite reasonable about going along with the recommended treatment plan, as long as they are kept informed of the plan and the rationale for the plan. Physicians who do not communicate with the worker's compensation carrier are at risk of having the case "pulled."

Pulled Cases

In some states, when claims adjustors are not happy with the treatment plan, progress, or communication, they may "pull" a case from a given doctor and assign it to another. Such practice often has merit, but it sometimes seems arbitrary or capricious. It is best for the practitioner not to take it personally; it happens to everyone. Similarly, everyone experiences a situation sooner or later in which a case that has been pulled from another doctor is assigned to him or her. This is not cause for inflating the ego—it just happens. Explaining to the claims adjustor why this may not have been necessary is rarely useful, and getting angry is probably counterproductive. A good attitude to foster is that these people are trying to do their best, and at times they are simply going to disagree with you.

Expedite the Case

Healing takes time, but the time of treatment in worker's compensation cases is particularly costly to the insurance company. They lose money not just by paying for treatment, but even more so by having the patient off work. Added to this is the problem that the longer a person is off work, the less likely he or she is ever to return to the job.[8] While staying within the bounds of proper treatment, it is certainly advisable to try to expedite the care of the injured worker. This improves outcomes, as well as relations with the insurance company and employer.

Try Not to Keep Patients Off Work Completely

It is rare that an injured worker cannot do at least some work. Certainly in some cases of severe trauma, or in the postoperative period, the patient may need to be taken off work completely, but in most cases it is better to prescribe appropriate restrictions and light duty. Some patients argue that they can't work on such restrictions, that no such work is available, or that their employer is not adhering to the restrictions. These issues, even if they have merit, do not change the medical fact that the patient can work safely with restrictions. It may be helpful to call the employer to explain the restrictions. It is not helpful to let the employee manipulate the physician into giving unjustifiable restrictions. If the employer is unable to accommodate the restrictions, and if light duty is not available, then it is the employer's duty to send the patient home, not the doctor's.

Malingerers Are Rare; Symptom Magnifiers Are Not

Malingering is the conscious fabrication of signs and symptoms of a disorder to receive some benefit. Fortunately this is rare. Much more common is the patient who has a kernel of truth as the basis of his or her presentation and then magnifies this to an extreme. It is easy to become frustrated or disgusted by such behavior, but it may be helpful to view it as "they are simply trying too hard to convince me their pain is real."

In such cases it can be beneficial to engage in more counseling than usual or even to seek the assistance of a psychologist well-versed in treating injured workers. Many large companies also offer an employee assistance plan for the counseling of workers with emotional problems or difficulties. Fortunately, such patients usually do respond to treatment, although possibly more slowly than usual. In general, it is helpful to give the patient the benefit of the doubt, especially early in the treatment course. There are numerous success stories of patients who would have been easy to dismiss on their first presentation. It is helpful to remember that discharging them as "behavioral cases" early on may consign them to a lifetime of perpetuating such behaviors. "Holding their hands" a bit while treating their condition may return them to gainful employment.

TABLE 14.3   Waddell signs (for low back pain)*

Tenderness—nonorganic.

> Superficial—the skin is tender to light pinch over a wide area of lumbar skin.

> Nonanatomic—deep tenderness is felt over a wide area, is not localized to one structure, and often extends to the thoracic spine, sacrum, or pelvis.

Simulation—simulation of a test, when no test is being performed.

> Axial loading—low back pain is reported on vertical loading of the standing patient's skull by the examiner's hands.

> Rotation—local non-radiating back pain is reported when shoulders and pelvis are passively rotated in the same plane, as the patient stands relaxed with the feet together.

Distraction—a positive physical finding is demonstrated in the routine manner; this finding is then checked while the patient's attention is distracted. This distraction must be non-painful, non-emotional, and non-surprising.

> Straight leg raising—the patient whose back pain has a nonorganic component shows marked improvement in straight leg raising on distraction as compared with formal testing.

Regional—disturbances of a widespread region of neighboring body parts, such as the leg below the knee, the entire leg, or a quarter or half of the body.

> Weakness—"giving way" of many muscle groups that cannot be explained in a localized neurologic basis.

> Sensation—sensory disturbances fitting a "stocking" rather than a dermatomal pattern.

Overreaction—disproportionate verbalization, facial expression, muscle tension and tremor, collapsing, or sweating.

---

*The patient is given one point for each nonorganic physical examination sign (one point possible in each category, with a maximum score of 5 possible). A score of three or more is suggestive of a behavioral component to the patient's symptoms.
SOURCE: *From G Waddell, JA McCulloch, E Kummel, et al. Nonorganic physical signs in low back pain. Spine 1980;5:117–125.*

The Waddell Scale Is Often Useful in Documenting a Behavioral Component to the Patient's Condition

The Waddell scale is a five-point scale (Table 14.3) that helps to objectify symptom magnification.[10] It can help screen for difficult patients, may explain some poor outcomes, and may be a red flag for surgery.

Use Functional Capacity Evaluations Appropriately

The functional capacity evaluation (FCE) is a special test that is generally performed by physical therapists or exercise physiologists. It involves putting patients through a series of tasks to determine the maximal amount of activity they can safely perform in lifting, standing, sitting, and other activities. This might result in a report that states the patient can lift 15 lb from waist to shoulder frequently and 25 lb from floor to waist occasionally. The FCE includes tests of validity and also gives a composite impression that the patient can safely perform at one of the following physical demand levels of duty: sedentary, light, medium, heavy, and very heavy (Table 14.4).[11] Although the FCE may contain a disclaimer that it is not to be used to determine permanent work

TABLE 14.4 Activity demands for various physical demand levels of duty

Sedentary

  Exerting up to 10 lb of force occasionally, and/or a negligible amount of force frequently, to lift, carry, push, pull, or otherwise move objects; sitting most of the time.

Light

  Exerting up to 20 lb of force occasionally, and/or up to 10 lb of force frequently, and/or
  a negligible amount of force constantly to move objects. A job should be rated as light
  work when it (1) requires standing or walking to a significant degree, or (2) requires
  sitting most of the time but entails pushing and/or pulling of arm or leg controls, and/
  or (3) requires working at a production rate pace entailing the constant pushing and/
  or pulling of materials, although the weight of those materials is negligible.

Medium

  Exerting 20–50 lb of force occasionally, and/or 10–25 lb of force frequently, and/or
  greater than negligible up to 10 lb of force constantly to move objects.

Heavy

  Exerting 50–100 lb of force occasionally, and/or 25–50 lb of force frequently, and/or
  10–20 lb of force constantly to move objects.

Very heavy

  Exerting in excess of 100 lb of force occasionally, and/or in excess of 50 lb of force frequently, and/or in excess of 20 lb of force constantly to move objects.

SOURCE: *From Dictionary of Occupational Titles (4th ed, revised). Washington, D.C.: U.S. Department of Labor, 1991.*

restrictions, it certainly can be used, along with other factors and the judgment of the physician, in determining such restrictions. An invalid FCE must be interpreted with caution.

Determine the Time of Maximum Medical Improvement

An impairment is considered to be permanent and to have reached maximum medical improvement (MMI) when it is well-stabilized and unlikely to change substantially within the next year, with or without treatment.[6] Before a case can be closed, the patient must be determined to have reached MMI. It is helpful for the physician to use this exact wording in the discharge note. Otherwise, the claims adjustor usually writes a letter asking for clarification on this point. When seeing a patient for a second opinion, especially under the direction of the worker's compensation board, it is also important to state whether the patient is at MMI. If so, the case can be closed; if not, further treatment may be indicated. A PPI rating cannot be given until the person has been determined to be at MMI; the same holds for permanent restrictions.

Document and Explain the Permanent Partial Impairment Rating

An *impairment* is the "loss, loss of use, or derangement of any body part, organ system, or organ function."[6] The AMA *Guides* emphasizes objective factors in the determination of PPI, but also takes some subjective symptoms into account. Impairment ratings reflect the severity of the medical condition and the degree to which the impairment decreases an individual's ability to perform activities of daily living, excluding work.[6] Thus the PPI rating reflects a functional limitation, not disability. Impairment is not always directly corre-

TABLE 14.5   Components of the permanent partial impairment report that may be particularly relevant

Purpose of the examination
Narrative history of the condition
   Current clinical status
   Diagnostic test results
Work history
Review of medical record
Diagnosis and impairments
   If needed, address causation and apportionment
   Discuss impact of impairment on activities of daily living
State whether any further treatment is anticipated and what prognosis is
State whether person is at maximum medical improvement
Discuss permanent partial impairment rating criteria
Calculate permanent partial impairment and describe how it was calculated

SOURCE: *From L Cocchiarella, GBJ Andersson. Guides to the Evaluation of Permanent Partial Impairment (5th ed). Chicago: AMA Press, 2001.*

lated with disability, which implies an inability to perform various personal, social, and occupational demands. A given functional limitation can result in a vastly different disability, depending on the person's occupation. Table 14.5 lists some items that may be important in the PPI rating report.

Physicians actually have wide latitude in determining a PPI rating, as long as they explain their reasoning in determining the rating. Most physicians use the latest edition of the AMA *Guides*. Some states mandate that other rating scales be used. In some cases the categories in the *Guides* do not correspond with the exact clinical picture. In other cases the physician may determine that the *Guides* do not accurately reflect the impact on the patient. In these cases the physician may give a different rating. It is helpful to explain the reasoning behind this deviation from usual procedure, so that reviewers understand the rating given. In some cases, the PPI rating may seem inherently unfair. For instance, the actual functional loss of a digit may be drastically different in a concert pianist and a construction worker, yet the rating is the same. Also, a person with a well-healed injury may qualify for the same rating as a person who has chronic persistent pain after multiple operations. The rationale for this is that it is not wise to pay people more if they have greater pain complaints; if you pay people for pain, you will get more pain complaints.

When giving PPI ratings it is important to read the *Guides* carefully. Because this is a confusing book, it is best to read the applicable chapters numerous times before actually rating patients. Various courses on impairment rating may also be helpful. It cannot be overemphasized that giving proper ratings is imperative, and rating patients is not easy. When multiple impairments are present, they are sometimes added and sometimes "combined," using tables in the *Guides*. The reason for this is that adding impairments could give an impairment of greater than 100% of the body, which is obviously not a rational scenario.

It is useful to remember that impairment rating should be an unbiased "medical" determination. Ideally, it should be reproducible among different physicians. The settlement that is made to compensate the worker for the injury is an administrative decision. Although the physician's determination of impairment obviously weighs heavily in the making of this decision, it is not the physician's role to play advocate for the patient by giving a rating that is higher or lower than is justified. Patients sometimes argue for a higher rating, but this is not something that doctors should allow themselves to be manipulated into.

When Applicable, Apportion the Rating

Persons often have a history of previous injury. If, for instance, a person had a back injury in an accident 5 years ago with some residual dysfunction, and now has a new work-related back impairment, then the PPI may not be due entirely to the most recent injury. In this case, the physician should apportion the rating, deciding that, for instance, 25% of the impairment is due to the most recent injury. This apportioning is very subjective, and one must use the best judgment followed by careful explanation of the reasoning behind the apportionment.

Points of Summary

1. The worker's compensation system is a no-fault insurance system for injuries that are work-related.
2. Workers receive compensation for wage replacement as well as medical care.
3. Claims adjustors and case managers work for the insurance company to approve treatments and expedite the care of the injured worker.
4. Patients must achieve maximal medical improvement in order to be discharged from treatment.
5. Workers who suffer permanent loss of function are given a permanent partial impairment rating.
6. The permanent partial impairment rating is a medical decision; the disability determination is an administrative decision.
7. Most practitioners and states use the AMA *Guides for the Evaluation of Permanent Impairment* in rating the worker.
8. Functional capacity evaluations can assist in determining what activities the worker can safely perform.
9. The Waddell scale can be used to objectify behavioral components of the worker's symptoms.

References

1. Rischitelli DG. A worker's compensation primer. Ann Allergy Asthma Immunol 1999;83:614–617.

2. Long AB, Brown RS Jr. Worker's compensation introduction for physicians. Va Med Q 1995;122:108–111.
3. Gerdes DA. Worker's compensation, an overview for physicians. S D J Med 1988;148:341–348.
4. Pye H, Orris P. Worker's compensation in the United States and the role of the primary care physician. Prim Care 2000;27:831–844.
5. Nadler SF, Mulford GJ, Wagner KL, et al. Improving the workers compensation system. Am J Phys Med Rehabil 2000;79:97–99.
6. Cocchiarella L, Andersson GBJ. Guides to the Evaluation of Permanent Partial Impairment (5th ed). Chicago: AMA Press, 2001.
7. Robinson JP, Rondinelli RD, Scheer SJ, Weinstein SM. Industrial rehabilitation medicine. 1. Why is industrial rehabilitation medicine unique? Arch Phys Med Rehabil 1997;78:S3–S9.
8. Rondinelli RD, Robinson JP, Scheer SJ, Weinstein SM. Industrial rehabilitation medicine. 4. Strategies for disability management. Arch Phys Med Rehabil 1997;78:S21–S28.
9. Braddom RL. Industrial Rehabilitation: An Overview. In EW Johnson (ed), Physical Medicine and Rehabilitation Clinics of North America. 1992;3:499–512.
10. Waddell G, McCulloch JA, Kummel E, et al. Nonorganic physical signs in low back pain. Spine 1980;5:117–125.
11. Dictionary of Occupational Titles (4th ed, revised). Washington, D.C.: U.S. Department of Labor, 1991.

Suggested Readings

Cocchiarella L, Andersson GBJ. Guides to the Evaluation of Permanent Partial Impairment (5th ed). Chicago: AMA Press, 2001.

Johnson EW (ed). Physical Medicine and Rehabilitation Clinics of North America: Rehabilitation of the Injured Worker, 1992;3.

Supplement to Arch Phys Med Rehabil 1997;78:No 3S.

15 Complex Regional Pain Syndrome

Randall L. Braddom

Historical Aspects of Complex Regional Pain Syndrome

What we now refer to as *complex regional pain syndrome* (CRPS) was first described by S. Weir Mitchell in 1864.[1] Mitchell noted that approximately 10% of his Civil War patients with a partial nerve injury developed a painful and disabling clinical syndrome. He called this syndrome *causalgia* and defined it as burning pain after peripheral nerve injury. He also described other changes that typically occur, including swelling, smoothness of the skin, temperature changes, and hypersensitivity to stimuli. Studies since the time of Mitchell have shown that causalgia occurs in 2–14% of partial nerve injury cases.[2] Leriche in 1916 was the first to report that sympathectomy relieved causalgia.[3] By World War II it was widely held that sympatholysis relieved causalgic pain.[4]

Sudeck in 1902 was the first to report that this syndrome could also occur in patients who did not have a peripheral nerve injury.[5] A number of triggers were identified, including myocardial infarction, fracture, frostbite, burns, stroke, and soft tissue damage. It was recognized that the syndrome could occur outside the region affected by the triggering event. For example, myocardial infarction and chest pain could lead to the syndrome occurring in the upper limb(s). By the time of World War II it was accepted that this syndrome could occur in the absence of a peripheral nerve injury.[6] It was also commonly held that sympathetic block could relieve the syndrome. Evans eventually named this syndrome *reflex sympathetic dystrophy* (RSD) in 1946.[7]

Diagnosis and Taxonomy

A new taxonomy for this syndrome was suggested by a group of pain experts who met in Orlando, Florida, in 1993. They advocated *complex regional pain syndrome* (CRPS) as the new name for this symptom complex.[8] The name was developed to help clear up some of the diagnostic confusion in RSD, and also to avoid having the name contain a direct reference to the sympathetic ner-

TABLE 15.1 International Association for the Study of Pain diagnostic criteria for complex regional pain syndrome

Presence of an initiating noxious event or a cause of immobilization*

Continuing pain, allodynia, or hyperalgesia in which pain is disproportionate to any inciting event

Evidence (at some time) of edema, changes in skin blood flow, or abnormal sudomotor activity in the region of pain

Note: This diagnosis is excluded by the existence of conditions that would otherwise account for the degree of pain and dysfunction.
*Not required for diagnosis.
SOURCE: *Reprinted with permission from RN Harden. A clinical approach to complex regional pain syndrome. Clin J Pain 2000;16(2 Suppl):S26–S32.*

vous system. They believed this was prudent because it was no longer clear that the pathophysiology of RSD or causalgia actually required the involvement of the sympathetic system.

Patients with classic RSD symptoms brought on by a noxious event other than a peripheral nerve injury are said to have chronic regional pain syndrome type I. Patients with the same syndrome, but with the initiating event being a peripheral nerve injury, are said to have chronic regional pain syndrome type II. In general, the old RSD is now CRPS I, and the old causalgia is now CRPS II. These terms are used interchangeably in this chapter.

The diagnostic criteria coming from the consensus conference in 1993 and then adopted by the International Association for the Study of Pain (IASP) are listed in Table 15.1. Note that the criteria require continuing pain and allodynia or hyperalgesia that is disproportionate to the inciting event. Part of being disproportionate is that the pain is regional, and not limited to the territory of a single nerve. Also required is evidence of current or past edema, skin blood flow abnormalities, or abnormal sudomotor activity in the painful region. Note that osteoporosis (Sudeck's atrophy) is not required to make the diagnosis, as it tends to occur only in severe cases.

The Orlando consensus conference group was also concerned that the diagnosis of RSD was being made too indiscriminately.[8] One result of this was the requirement that the diagnosis of CRPS not be made in a case in which there was another condition that would reasonably account for the symptoms. They cited the example of a patient with diabetic peripheral neuropathy with a stocking and glove distribution of allodynia, skin color changes, and so on. These findings can be explained by diabetic neuropathy, which excludes the diagnosis of CRPS.

The new diagnostic criteria[9] are the latest example of the difficulty clinicians have had since the time of Mitchell[1] in diagnosing, classifying, and treating CRPS. Arguments continue to rage about pathophysiology, best types of treatment, and even whether it is a purely psychiatric diagnosis. Schwartzman reports that this confusion in diagnosis is due to the fact that RSD "has many variations, often follows minor injury, and evolves and spreads over time."[10] There are five main types of symptoms: pain, autonomic dysfunction, edema, movement disorder, dystrophy and atrophy.[10,11] Most patients report that the pain is burning in nature and seems to spread quickly from a dermatomal or limited area to a regional distribution. Hyperalgesia (more pain than would be expected from a painful stimulus) and allodynia (pain from an innocuous stimulus) are common. Hyperpathia (abnormally painful reaction to a stimulus) often occurs. Nails develop changes including ridging, thickening, and brittleness. Hair may become darker and grow more rapidly in an affected area. In the distal portion of the affected extremity, temperature changes may occur, along with hyperhidrosis, livedo reticularis, delayed capillary refill, dusky cyanosis, and diffuse mottling.[10] If treatment is unsuccessful, patients may develop increased burning pain, hyperalgesia, allodynia, disruption of sleep, anxiety, and depression.[10] The later stages often show loss of hair, cyanosis, and mottling of the skin. Radiographs of bones may show cystic and subchondral erosion and osteoporosis (often referred to as *Sudeck's atrophy*).[10]

Schwartzman and Kerrigan[12] have described the movement disorders in RSD as including weakness, tremor, muscle spasms, dystonia, and an inability to initiate movement. These can precede the onset of the pain, and curiously can occur even in the contralateral side of the body. Posturing of a limb can lead to contractures. A typical posture in the upper limb is adduction and internal rotation of the shoulder, and flexion of the elbow. This often resembles the upper limb hemiplegic posture seen in patients with stroke. Patients often hold the ankle and foot in inversion and plantar flexion, also typical of that seen in many patients with stroke.

Some investigators arbitrarily divide the course of CRPS into three stages of severity.[13,14] Stage I is the acute stage, and patients typically complain of severe pain of a burning quality. There is also cyanosis and mottling of the skin (livedo reticularis), as well as edema, which is often out of proportion to the injury. Many also have hypothermia or hyperthermia, hyperhidrosis, and changes in hair and nail growth. Allodynia and hyperalgesia are commonly present. Stage II is the dystrophic stage, and the pain spreads proximally and regionally. Patients often have a cold and cyanotic extremity with brawny edema and mottling of the skin. The joints involved become stiff and begin to develop contractures (Figures 15.1 and 15.2). Integumentary changes include the hair getting darker and growing more rapidly, and the nails thickening and splitting. Stage II usually lasts 3–6 months. Stage III is the atrophic stage (Figure 15.3). The pain spreads proximally in the limb and can migrate to the opposite side as well. The skin becomes shiny and atrophic, and hair loss is common. Joint contractures and shortening of tendons occurs. Radiographs show periarticular and subchondral bony reabsorptive changes (Figure 15.4).

Epidemiology and Triggering Conditions

RSD can affect all ages, from children to the elderly.[8] Many of the descriptive reports of RSD in the older literature involved series of military cases. A series more relevant to civilian practice was recently reported by Allen et al.[15] They examined the epidemiologic factors in a series of 134 consecutive patients with CRPS referred to a large university pain center over a 6-year period. The mean age was 42 years (18–71). There was a 2.3 to 1.0 female to male ratio. The causes were 29% sprain or strain, 24% post-surgical, 16% fractures, 8%

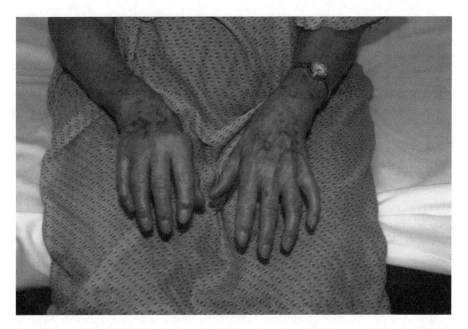

FIGURE 15.1   Sixty-year-old woman who presented with right upper limb complex regional pain syndrome after surgery for right carpal tunnel syndrome. Note the edema of the digits of the right hand.

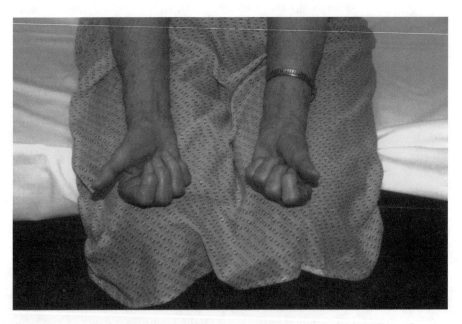

FIGURE 15.2   Same patient as in Figure 15.1. Note the right-hand inability to flex the fingers sufficient to make a full fist.

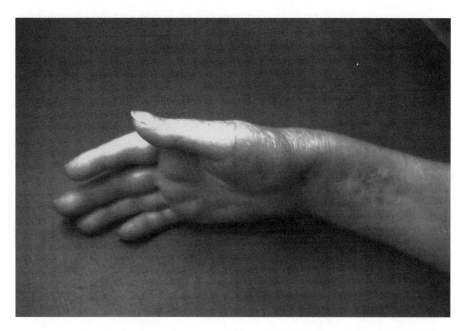

FIGURE 15.3   *Fifty-five-year-old woman with a work-related penetration wound of the wrist, followed by complex regional pain syndrome. The patient has edema, contractures, allodynia, hyperesthesia, and loss of function of the right hand.*

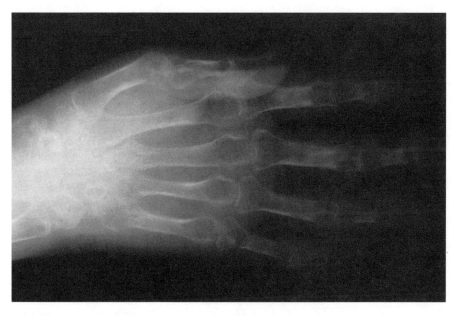

FIGURE 15.4   *Radiograph of the patient in Figure 15.3 showing marked osteoporosis.*

TABLE 15.2   Conditions that can give rise to chronic regional pain syndrome type I

Trauma
   Fracture
   Soft tissue injury
Iatrogenic
   Venipuncture
   Intramuscular injection
   Dental extraction
   Casts
   Medications (anticonvulsants, barbiturates, antituberculous agents)
Ischemic
   Myocardial
   Cerebrovascular
Carcinoma
   Breast
   Esophageal
   Bronchial
Infections
   Osteomyelitis
Neurologic
   Multiple sclerosis
   Spondylosis
   Stroke
   Seizure
   Peripheral neuropathy
Arthritic

SOURCE: *Reprinted with permission from RG Phelps, S Wilentz. Reflex sympathetic dystrophy. Int J Dermatol 2000;39:481–486.*

contusion or crush injury, 6% spontaneous, and 17% other or unknown. The injuries in this series occurred on the job in 56% of the cases. One patient developed symptoms in the jaw region, 7% in multiple extremities, and the remainder in one extremity. The ratio of lower to upper limb cases in this series was 48 to 44.

Table 15.2 lists some of the common conditions that give rise to RSD.[16] Subluxation of the shoulder in patients with hemiplegia has also been implicated as a trigger for RSD. Dursun et al.[17] compared 35 patients with hemiplegia and RSD to 35 patients having hemiplegia without RSD. Patients with hemiplegia having rotator cuff rupture, brachial plexus injury, or spasticity greater than stage II on the Ashworth scale were excluded. All patients were assessed for the presence and grade of subluxation from radiographs, using a 5-point scale. The degree of shoulder pain was assessed on a visual analog scale of 0–10 points. Glenohumeral subluxation was found in 74% of the patients with RSD, but in only 40% of the non-RSD group. One of the implications of the study is that aggressive attempts to prevent and control subluxation of the shoulder after hemiplegia might lessen the incidence and severity of RSD.[17]

Some believe that there is a genetic predisposition to RSD. This relationship was investigated using the human leukocyte antigen (HLA) system in a Dutch study in which 52 unrelated patients with RSD, (according to the IASP criteria for CRPS type I), were studied with serologic HLA typing.[18] Their results were compared to a random control group of 295 unrelated healthy individuals who were believed to be representative of the Dutch population. The frequency of DQ1 was increased from 42% in the normal group to 69% in the patients with RSD. No other major histocompatibility antigens differed in frequency between the two groups. The authors speculated that these HLA antigens possibly relate to factors involved in the repair of damaged neural tissue. They also noted that multiple sclerosis and narcolepsy have also been associated in other studies and with the same HLA antigens.[18]

Pathophysiologic Theories

Clinicians agree that patients have symptoms and signs that we refer to as *CRPS*, but there is no agreement on the etiology and pathophysiology. Schwartzman theorizes that RSD is initiated by trauma in which nociceptive terminals are injured.[10] He cites the animal studies of Bennett showing that "allodynia, thermal hyperalgesia, sympathetic maintenance (in which case sympathetic blockade relieves the pain), dystonia, and altered pain behavior are consistent with lowered pain thresholds."[19] Some believe that the end result of injury to nociceptive terminals is a complicated cascade of events ending in a central sensitization that amplifies pain response in the affected area.[20]

Denervation Hypersensitivity

In CRPS type II (causalgia) it has generally been held that the partial nerve injury causes impairment of sympathetic nerve function and produces a relative state of sympathetic denervation. This leads to decreased local sympathetic activity immediately after the injury, with resulting vasodilation. The affected blood vessels react to this lack of sympathetic innervation by an up-regulation of adrenoceptors, which causes them to be more affected by circulating catecholamines. Studies in rats have shown initial vasodilation (warm limb) after nerve constriction, followed by a cold limb.[21] The vasoconstriction and chronically cold limb is presumed to be due to hypersensitivity of the adrenoceptors and not excessive sympathetic activity.

Centralization Theory

The commonly observed phenomenon of the spreading of symptoms over a wide area of the limb, and even distant from the site of initial injury, has led a number of investigators to suggest a central origin of the sensory changes.[22,23] The autonomic abnormalities such as swelling, skin blood flow and sweating have also been cited as evidence of a central origin.[24] A 1999 Japanese study[25] reported the results of iodine 123–labeled iodoamphetamine single-photon emission computed tomography of 10 patients with CRPS. Uptake was high in the contralateral thalamus in patients with CRPS for up to 7 months. Uptake was lower in the contralateral thalamus in patients with chronic CRPS (24+ months). This is consistent with the finding that acute pain increases thalamic perfusion and activity, while chronic pain reduces it. The authors speculate that the thalamus undergoes adaptive change during the course of CRPS.

Denervation hypersensitivity is a better explanation for causalgia than for RSD, because RSD does not involve nerve injury and sympathetic denervation. Even in causalgia, the patient typically develops these autonomic changes outside the territory of the injured nerve. Hyperhidrosis is a common finding in CRPS, which is curious because sweat glands do not develop denervation hypersensitivity.[26] Baron et al.[24] have speculated that this increased sweat production is due to increased activity in sympathetic sudomotor neurons. This increased activity would require a central origin. During the first 6 months of RSD, patients demonstrate a functional inhibition of cutaneous sympathetic vasoconstrictor activity in the affected limb, causing skin vasodilatation and warming.[24] Measurement of the norepinephrine levels in the venous effluent proximal to the area of pain are consistently reduced in the affected limb.[27] After 6 months, most patients show hyperactive sympathetic reflex patterns in the affected limb,[24] suggesting disturbed sympathetic reflexes.

It is also possible that a combination of central and peripheral mechanisms might be causative in CRPS. Baron et al. suggest that centrally induced inhibition of vasoconstrictor activity could lead to secondary end-organ super-sensitivity (so-called *decentralization super-sensitivity*).[24] This could cause excess sympathetic activity because of the hypersensitivity of end organs.

Goldstein et al.[28] reported a brilliant series of measurements on 30 patients with RSD, 14 of whom had undergone sympathectomy. Their extensive studies on these patients included positron emission tomography scans. They concluded that patients with chronic RSD have "decreased perfusion of the affected limb, symmetrical sympathetic innervation and norepinephrine synthesis, variably decreased release and turnover of norepinephrine in the affected limb, and failure of ganglion blockade to improve the pain in most cases."[28] They went on to state that: "These findings suggest augmented vasoconstriction, intact sympathetic terminal innervation, possibly impaired sympathetic neurotransmission, and pain usually independent of sympathetic neurocirculatory outflows."[28]

Inflammatory Theory

Another theory is that RSD is an inflammatory condition. An inflammatory component for RSD, especially in the acute phase, is suggested by the classic signs of inflammation that occur. These include rubor, dolor, and tumor.[24] It is unclear, however, whether these classic signs are the result or a cause of RSD. A 1998 study[29] compared a number of immune components in patients with RSD and in normal subjects. There was no significant difference in the two groups in terms of their lymphocyte populations (T, B, and NK cells) and activated

T cells. This study casts considerable doubt on the possibility that inflammation is the etiology of RSD.

The term *sympathetically maintained pain* was first suggested in 1986 by Roberts.[4] Sympathetically maintained pain has come to be used synonymously with RSD. Some patients do not respond to sympathetic blockade, and Campbell et al.[30] suggested the term *sympathetically independent pain* for these cases. A number of other authors support the concept of the sympathetic nervous system enhancing or even generating neuropathic pain.[4,11,30,31]

The current confusion about the etiology and pathophysiology of CRPS is exemplified in the separate statements about it for the upper and lower limbs in the American Medical Association's *Guides to the Evaluation of Permanent Impairment*.[32] The upper limb section follows the IASP suggested terminology of CRPS I and II (pages 495–496), whereas the lower limb section lists causalgia as a separate diagnosis and equates CRPS to RSD (page 553).

Could CRPS be purely a psychiatric illness, as some have proposed?[33] Certainly depression and anxiety are frequently seen in these patients.[34] Livingston stated that "The ultimate source of this dysfunction is not known but its organic nature is obvious and no one seems to doubt that these classical pain syndromes are real."[35] A number of studies have suggested that psychiatric disturbances are more likely to be the result, rather than the cause, of CRPS.[36,37]

Ochoa has been particularly blunt in debunking CRPS.[33] Ochoa states:

> "*The shifting paradigm of reflex sympathetic dystrophy-sympathetically maintained pain complex regional pain syndrome is characterized by vestigial truths and understandable errors, but also unjustifiable lies. It is true that patients with organically based neuropathic pain harbor unquestionable and physiologically demonstrable evidence of nerve fiber dysfunction leading to a predictable clinical profile with stereotyped temporal evolution. In turn, patients with psychogenic pseudoneuropathy, sustained by a conversion-somatization-malingering, not only lack physiological evidence of structural nerve fiber disease but display a characteristically, atypical, half-subjective, psychophysical sensory-motor profile.*"[33]

Ochoa reports that the concept of sympathetically maintained pain is based on "embarrassing conceptual errors."[33] These errors "include historical misinterpretation of vasomotor signs and symptomatic body parts, and misconstruing symptomatic relief after 'diagnostic' sympathetic blocks, due to lack of consideration of the possible effect which explains the outcome."[33] He further states: "While conceptual errors are not only forgivable, but natural to inexact medical signs, lies—particularly when entrepreneurially inspired—are condemnable and call for peer intervention."[33]

Ochoa goes on to point out that patients who display a clinical profile such as those with CRPS do not necessarily have a disease with a single etiology. He even objects to the symptoms being called a *syndrome*, having various potential etiologies by a common pathophysiology. He believes that these patients merely have a "symptom complex," with any number of possible physiologic or psychological explanations. He points out that objective autonomic changes do not necessarily indicate sympathetic dysregulation.[33]

He goes on to state: "The conceptual error of invoking the necessary sympathetic cause for the common circulatory changes found in body segments with RSD, as well as for the pain and sensory motor phenomena, was sustained throughout most of the twentieth century. Another reinforcing fallacy: anecdotal, subjective outcomes of sympathetic blocks were taken to offer proof of a sympathetically maintained pain as these blocks often relieve the pain in RSD patients."[33] Kingery[38] reviewed the literature and found only minimal evidence for scientifically proven efficacy of sympathetic blockade in CRPS patients.

Ochoa points out that as early as the work of Verdugo[39] in Chile in 1994, it has been known that the relief obtained after diagnostic-therapeutic sympathetic blocks amounts to nothing more than a placebo. Ochoa points out other authors who have had similar findings, including Jadad et al.,[40] Ramamurthy et al.,[41] and Valentin et al.[42]

Ochoa also debunks the "centralization" phenomenon.[33] Centralization is a hypothetical supposition that the sensory or motor complaints in RSD patients can be explained by central nervous system changes. Ochoa believes that these central changes do not occur in the absence of neural fiber injury and would not occur in the great majority of patients having the diagnosis of RSD.

There is also some evidence that the so-called *objective* signs that occur in RSD (including allodynia, hypothermia, sensory loss, motor loss, and even an abnormal brain positron emission tomography scan), can occur in individuals who experimentally have had a normal limb casted to produce immobilization.[43]

Diagnostic Tests

There is no specific confirmatory test for CRPS. However, a number of laboratory tests are currently being used in the diagnosis of CRPS.

Temperature Measurement

Perhaps the most popular test for CRPS is the temperature measurement of the affected versus the contralateral limb. Frequently used methods include thermometry, infrared, telethermometry, or thermography.[44] Most authors require a side-to-side difference in temperature in the limbs of 1.5°C to represent a significant change.

Blood Flow

Peripheral blood flow has also been used and can be measured by laser Doppler flow meters. Some believe this is an early predictor of sympathetic dysfunction.[45]

Quantitative Sweat Testing

The quantitative sudomotor axon reflex test looks at abnormalities of resting and evoked sweat production. It has been stated that an alteration can reflect pathologic changes of peripheral autonomic function.[46] A common method is to apply 10% acetylcholine with iontophoresis, with the response recorded by a sudorometer. In a prospective series of 102 patients with RSD, quantitative sudomotor axon reflex testing was normal in 38%, increased in 24%, and decreased in 38%.[47]

Sympathetic Skin Response

The sympathetic skin response test studies the conductance of the skin, comparing the affected and nonaffected extremities.[48]

Plain Films

Changes in bone on plain films are typically seen only in severe cases of CRPS. Osteoporosis is the main feature, with periarticular dominance.

Three-Phase Bone Scintigraphy

Three-phase bone scintigraphy can be used to demonstrate an abnormality in blood flow. The bony uptake of a radionuclide tracer is measured at various times, representing the arterial phase, the soft-tissue phase, and the mineral phase. A reduction in blood flow typically occurs in the early phase of CRPS.[6] Increased periarticular uptake occurs in the subacute phase of patients with CRPS. The sensitivity of this scanning procedure has been reported to be 60%, with a specificity of 86%. Others have reported as high as a 30% false-positive or false-negative response rate.[49] In a series of 134 patients described by Allen et al.,[15] 38% had a bone scan, and 53% of these had a radiologist's official reading of being consistent with RSD. Some clinicians actually find the results more confusing than helpful in making the diagnosis.[9]

Ischemia Test

In the ischemia test,[11] the painful limb is wrapped with an Esmarch bandage and a blood pressure cuff is then inflated to reduce the circulation in the extremity. The pain is reduced in 1–2 minutes. Some believe that a positive test indicates that the patient will respond to sympatholytic procedures.[50]

Phentolamine Test

Phentolamine is an alpha-adrenoceptor antagonist that can be injected intravenously into a limb for relief of pain.[51] The rationale is that blockade of alpha-adrenoreceptors prevents the excitation of nociceptive afferent neurons by noradrenaline. Some believe that patients who have a positive response are more likely to have the sympathetic nervous system involved in the generation of their pain.[51]

Guanethidine Test

In the guanethidine test, guanethidine is injected intravenously in a limb distal to a cuff that is suprasystolic.[11] The test is positive if the patient has increased burning pain or paresthesias, and then reduced pain approximately 15 minutes after the cuff is released. The rationale for this is that the guanethidine depletes postganglionic axons (causing an increased excitation of nociceptors), but then prevents further release for 1–2 days.

Treatment

The treatment of CRPS has been as controversial as its etiology and pathophysiology. Harden recently pointed out that, "To date there are no substantial scientific trials of any particular therapy or medication in the specific diagnosis of CRPS."[9] When the clinician is presented with a patient having CRPS, however, he or she doesn't have the luxury of waiting until these controversies are settled to come up with a rational plan of care. A Dahlem-style conference of experts was held in 1998 to try to reach a consensus on a model of treatment.[44] These experts emphasized the importance of functional restoration as the mainstay of therapy (Figure 15.5). Drugs, blocks, and psychotherapy are reserved for those patients who fail to respond to functional restoration techniques. Harden states: "Interdisciplinary pain management techniques emphasizing functional restoration are thought to be the most effective therapy, perhaps by resetting altered central processing and normalizing the distal environment." The term *interdisciplinary* is used rather than *multidisciplinary* because the patient is not just being treated by different types of clinicians. The patient needs to be treated by a team of clinicians who are working together, communicating with the patient and each other, and following a cohesive treatment program whose total impact is greater than the sum of its parts.

The key to a good outcome in CRPS treatment is to begin the treatment as early as possible. This requires a high index of suspicion on the part of the physician. Early treatment of CRPS can typically head off potentially devastating impairment and disability. It is much more difficult to get patients back to a normal level of comfort and function once they have reached the stage of constant pain, edema, contractures, and disuse atrophy.

Reactivation techniques are designed to enhance the patient's functional activity level. They involve gentle active movements that the patient can tolerate, which are gradually increased to more demanding movements. The goal is to reactivate the limb to its normal levels of function and activity. An example of reactivation is gradually increasing the degree of weight bearing on an affected lower limb during gait.

Desensitization is needed because of the hyperalgesia and allodynia. Harden's examples[9] of these include gradually increasing the temperature difference in contrast baths and rubbing the skin with progressively rougher types of cloth. If the patient is unable to tolerate reactivation or desensitization, sympathetic or somatic blocks might present a "window of opportunity"[9] for more aggressive therapy. Contrast baths are an ancient treatment that the author has anecdotally found to be helpful in stopping CRPS in its earliest stages. The author has the patient use contrast baths as part of a home program if there is even a suspicion that CRPS is developing. Another frequent desensitization technique is to use transcutaneous electrical nerve stimulation (TENS). In addition to helping to relieve pain, the stimulation from the TENS electrodes is a form of afferent input that aids in desensitization.

Reactivation

Contrast baths

Desensitization

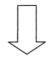

Flexibility

Edema control

Peripheral electrical stimulation

Isometric strengthening

Diagnosis and treatment of secondary myofascial pain

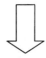

Range of motion (gentle)

Stress loading

Isotonic strengthening

General aerobic conditioning

Postural normalization and balanced use

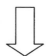

Ergonomics

Movement therapies

Normalization of use

Vocational/functional rehabilitation

FIGURE 15.5   *Compound diagram of the physical and occupational therapy modalities that are used in a stepwise fashion to achieve functional restoration. The listing of each modality does not absolutely imply a specific order or priority. (Reprinted with permission from RN Harden. A clinical approach to complex regional pain syndrome. Clin J Pain 2000;16[2 Suppl]:S26–S32.)*

Control of edema is needed at every stage of treatment (see Figure 15.5). Getting the patient to move the extremity, rather than holding it immobile, is often all that is needed to mobilize the edema. Active muscle activity causes the "muscle pump" to move fluid out of the limb toward the heart. Elevation, elastic wraps, compression stockings, or gloves are sometimes necessary.[52] The wraps, stockings, and gloves can also assist in desensitization. Patients with allodynia often can't tolerate more than a few minutes of the use of these devices. This time can be gradually extended until the patient is wearing them for several hours at a time.

Maintaining flexibility is critical in the care of patients with CRPS. Simple active range-of-motion (ROM) exercise is often all that is needed to maintain normal ROM in the affected limb. The patient can be shown how to do these as part of a home exercise program. If the patient has considerable pain, or already has lost some ROM, "active-assisted" ROM exercise can be added. Active-assisted ROM techniques involve having the patient perform as much active ROM as much as possible, and then having the therapist apply gentle external force toward normal ROM. Passive ROM techniques involve having the therapist provide the ROM force toward normal ROM. Passive ROM is used to maintain or enhance joint ROM only until the patient can begin actively participating in the exercise.[53] Dynamic splinting can be used if patients have contractures that are resistant to ROM exercise. For example, a hand splint with rubber bands can be used to put gentle tension on contracted finger joints. This also provides sensory input that assists the desensitization process.

Heating an extremity during the stretching or ROM exercise process has a number of benefits. It makes soft tissues more extensible and increases the likelihood that flexibility and ROM will improve. It also relieves pain (unless the patient has severe heat allodynia) and helps in the desensitization process. Typical kinds of heating (depending on the limb involved and the available equipment) include whirlpool, paraffin dip and wrap, fluidotherapy, hot silicon gel packs, infrared bulbs, and Kenny packs.[54]

Maintaining or regaining strength is an important aspect of the therapy program, especially to combat disuse atrophy. Isotonic exercise that takes the joints through a full ROM is usually the best technique, as it improves strength and flexibility and is relatively inexpensive.[55] It can be done with ordinary barbells, weight machines, or even with homemade weights. For example, the patient can place a small can of soup in each of two socks, tie the socks together, and drape them across the wrist for wrist flexion and wrist extension strengthening exercises. Isokinetic exercise can also be used, but this requires expensive equipment and isn't practical outside the physical therapy gymnasium. Isokinetic exercise involves exerting muscle force against a preset, rate-limiting device.[55] Isokinetic exercise does not exist in nature, but is often helpful in motivating patients because it can be computerized. Patients can get the "biofeedback" of observing their progress on a computer screen or on hard copies of charts and graphs. Isometric strengthening techniques can be used to begin a strengthening exercise in situations in which isotonic or isokinetic exercise is too painful.[55] Isometric exercise is usually done by tensing a muscle for 10 seconds and repeating this 10 times. Isometric exercise is relatively painless, because there is no joint movement. As soon as the patient can tolerate it, the isometric exercise should be changed to isotonic or isokinetic exercise.

Harden[9] believes that patients often have an associated myofascial pain syndrome. He advocates aggressive treatment of myofascial pain syndrome to help relieve the pain and get the patient moving toward more functionality.

Medications are often used in CRPS, despite the fact that few double-blind, randomized, controlled trials have been done.[56] The use of various medicines in the treatment of CRPS is clearly more a part of the "art," rather than the science, of medicine. Tricyclic antidepressants are frequently used to treat depression, anxiety, pain, and insomnia. Harden anecdotally reported disappointing results with serotonin reuptake inhibitor antidepressants in his patients.[9] Anti-epileptic drugs such as gabapentin, carbamazepine, phenytoin, and lamotrigine are frequently prescribed because of their successful use in treating patients with neuropathic pain. They have not been studied in randomized, controlled trials in patients with CRPS. Nonsteroidal anti-inflammatory drugs are often used, but have not been formally studied in CRPS.[38] Although a short course of oral steroids has some theoretical rationale, there is little or no rationale for a chronic course of steroids.

The use of opioids in patients with CRPS is controversial. Opioids are probably best reserved for crisis management situations or to assist in therapy when progress is slow or nonexistent. Skin preparations such as lidocaine patches, eutectic blend of local anesthetics (EMLA) cream, and capsaicin are often used, but there are no formal studies on their efficacy in CRPS. Some use nifedipine to control vasoconstriction, but again, no formal studies exist for its use in patients with CRPS.

Schwartzman[10] suggests that the first line of treatment of RSD should include early diagnosis, treatment of the underlying cause (if identifiable), treatment with sympathetic blockade when appropriate, and intensive physical therapy. In a series of 134 patients reported by Allen et al.,[15] the treatments used (in order of frequency) were physical therapy (88%), nerve blocks (82%), tricyclic antidepressants (78%), opiates (70%), anticonvulsants (60%), psychological (50%), immobilization (47%), occupational therapy (45%), serotonin reuptake inhibitors (38%), and spinal cord stimulation (6%). The author believes that immobilization should rarely be used. In the author's experience immobilization fosters disuse atrophy, contractures, and osteoporosis, and can even lead to an "alienation phenomenon" in which the brain seemingly forgets how to use the muscles in the immobilized area, even though they are not technically denervated.

Sympatholytic treatments abound in the treatment of CRPS.[57,58] The three basic types include surgical sympathectomy, sympathetic ganglion blocks, and regional intravenous use of medicines that deplete norepinephrine in the postganglionic axon (such as guanethidine, bretylium, and reserpine). Systemic intravenous phentolamine has also been used.

Sympathetic ganglion blockade can have false-negative results due to a number of factors. Baron et al.[24] report that these include failure to get adequate concentration of drug at the site of action, anatomic variability of the sympathetic chain, and the fact that neurons down to T2 can contribute to the upper limb innervation and escape blockade. Another potential cause of failure is that CRPS is often over-diagnosed, and patients are believed to have CRPS when actually they have vague symptoms of some other diagnosis, and would not be expected to respond to sympathetic blockade. Baron et al.[24] noted that up to 85% of CRPS patients respond acutely to sympathectomy or sympathetic block, but critics have pointed out many other reasons why patients might have relief from these procedures. Ochoa[33] reports that the major factor is a placebo effect. Others point out that these results have not been as impressive in controlled studies of blocks. It is also possible that many other types of nerves are being blocked along with the sympathetics, and the effect has little or nothing to do with the sympathetics.

Surgical and chemical sympathectomy techniques can be used to get a permanent sympathectomy, but patients having these procedures are known to have a disappointingly high rate of pain recurrence.[59]

Subcutaneous lidocaine has also been used for CRPS, going back as far as the work of Leriche in 1938.[60] Linchitz and Raheb[61] treated nine patients with 4–8 weeks of subcutaneous infusion of 10% lidocaine in an uncontrolled manner. Their chronic CRPS patients had already had extensive failed treatments, including epidural blocks, stellate ganglion blocks, lumbar sympathetic blocks, axillary blocks, trigger point injections, bier blocks, physical therapy, TENS, spinal cord stimulator, nonsteroidal anti-inflammatory drugs, tricyclic antidepressants, serotonin reuptake inhibitor antidepressants, sedatives and hypnotics, mexiletine, gabapentin and carbamazepine, beta blockers, clonidine, lidocaine skin cream, intravenous albuterol sulfate (Ventolin), subcutaneous morphine infusion, and intrathecal morphine pump. All of these patients had CRPS ranging from 30 months to 96 months in duration. Five of the nine patients were able to complete the infusion treatment. They reported significant improvement in their pain and other symptoms, and improvements were maintained after discontinuation of treatment.

A Dutch study compared the use of spinal cord stimulation alone with spinal cord stimulation plus physical therapy in patients with CRPS type I (RSD).[62] The patients were carefully selected to meet the IASP criteria for CRPS type I (see Table 15.1). Conventional pain medicines, sympathetic blocks, TENS, and physical therapy had been used on these patients without favorable results. The 36 study subjects received implanted spinal cord stimulators, a treatment introduced as far back as 1967.[63] The control group of 18 patients did not get spinal cord stimulation, but both groups received physical therapy. Test stimulation was done using a temporarily implanted spinal cord stimulator. The spinal cord stimulator was permanently implanted only if the test stimulation was successful. A permanent stimulator was implanted in 24 of the 36 patients who reported improvement in their symptoms with the temporary spinal cord stimulation. Patients were assessed with a visual analog pain scale, functional status measure, and a health-related quality of life assessment. The patients having spinal cord stimulation and physical therapy had a mean reduction of 2.4 cm in the intensity of their pain on a 10-cm visual analog scale. The control group receiving only physical therapy reported a mean increase of 0.21 cm in their visual analog pain assessment. Six patients receiving the permanent stimulator had complications and one patient had to have the device removed. The authors stated that the success of spinal cord stimulation depended on the use of strict criteria for the selection of patients. This was particularly true with the exclusion of patients having psychiatric disorders. Also listed as a critical success factor was having the temporary stimulation cause full coverage of the painful area by paresthesias. The paresthesias that occur on spinal cord stimulation created a problem in blinding this study. In spite of this limitation, the outcome was supported by the 1-month and 6-month results being similar, the fact that pain relief was not achieved unless the entire painful area was covered by paresthesias, and the fact that the pain recurred when the electrode was moved. Functional status did not improve in either group of patients.

Intravenous clodronate was used to treat CRPS type I in a 2000 randomized, double-blind, controlled study of 32 patients with RSD who were randomized into two groups.[64] The treatment group received i.v. clodronate at a rate of 300 mg daily for 10 consecutive days. The control group received a placebo. Forty days later the patients receiving the clodronate showed significant decreases in pain on a visual analog scale and improvement on a clinical global assessment device.

Korpan et al.[65] used acupuncture to treat 14 patients who had a history of CRPS for 1–6 months. They were randomly assigned to get either classical or "sham" acupuncture. The patients were than evaluated with a visual analog scale and clinical examination. The clinical parameters and the visual analog scale improved in both groups to almost normal levels within 6 months. There was no significant difference in outcome of the classical acupuncture or sham acupuncture treatment groups.

Perhaps the most bizarre and unintentional treatment for CRPS was reported by Shibata et al.[66] This case report involved a 51-year-old architect with chronic, right upper limb CRPS type I who had received stellate ganglion blocks, regional i.v. guanethidine, cervical epidural block, dorsal column stimulation at the cervical level, and various medications. All treatments were unsuccessful and he had been unable to return to work. He used a glove on his right hand and held his hand against his chest, refusing to allow anyone to touch it. The right upper limb showed hyperhydrosis and radiographs showed osteoporosis. Ten years after the onset of CRPS, the patient fell and accidentally struck his head. He lost consciousness for approximately an hour, and cerebral scans showed a cerebral contusion in the left temporal lobe with a 3-cm hematoma. He was transiently confused and in a post-traumatic delirium. After the accident he stopped complaining of the pain in the right upper limb and began to spontaneously use it to write and shake hands. He lost all symptoms including allodynia, coloration changes, and temperature changes. He had only a mild residual loss of ROM in the finger joints. The authors noted that the patient's recovery occurred after a temporal lobe injury, but could offer no clear explanation of his sudden recovery.

Vitamin C has been used to attempt to reduce the incidence of RSD after wrist fractures.[67] A Dutch study took 123 patients with wrist fracture and acceptable reduction by conservative means and treated half with 500 mg of vitamin C daily and the other half with placebo. The treatment began on the day of the fracture and continued for 50 days. The diagnosis of RSD was standardized by requiring at least four of the following six findings: unexplained diffuse pain, skin temperature different from opposite limb, skin color different from opposite limb, diffuse edema, loss of active ROM, or occurrence of increase in these signs and symptoms after activity. RSD occurred in 8% of patients in the vitamin C–treated group and 22% in the placebo group, which represented a significant difference. The authors were unable to draw a direct line between vitamin C and the pathophysiology of RSD, except for the possible presence of "toxic oxygen radicals" and the vitamin's antioxidant effect.

Points of Summary

1. Chronic regional pain syndrome (CRPS) is a potentially disabling condition that comes on after trauma (even minor trauma) and typically affects a limb. It spreads beyond the area of injury to involve the entire limb, and can even involve the contralateral limb.
2. Pain is the most common presenting symptom, particularly allodynia and hyperalgesia; the pain usually has a burning quality. Later in the course of the syndrome, the affected limb develops edema, loss of flexibility and contractures, changes in skin color and temperature, dystrophic changes of the integument, weakness due to disuse atrophy, osteoporosis, and even abnormal movements.
3. The etiology and pathophysiology of CRPS are still in question, especially in regard to the involvement of the sympathetic nervous system.
4. The current mainstay of treatment is to use functional restoration techniques.
5. The current trend in treatment is to reserve the use of a full interdisciplinary team and sympathetic and somatic blocks for the more difficult cases.

References

1. Mitchell SW, Morehouse G, Keen WW. Gunshot Wounds and Other Injuries of the Nerves. Philadelphia: JB Lippincott, 1864.
2. Richards RL. Causalgia. A centennial review. Arch Neurol 1967;16:339–350.
3. Leriche R. De la causalgie envisagee comme une nevrite dusympathique et de son traitement par la denudation et l'excision des plexus nerveux peri-arteriels. Presse Med 1916;24:178–180.
4. Roberts SJ. A hypothesis on the physiological basis for causalgia and related pains. Pain 1986;124:297–311.
5. Sudeck P. Uber die acute (trophoneurotische) knochenatrophie nach entzundungen und traumen der extremitaten. Dtsh Med Wocheschr 1902;28:336–342.
6. Baron R, Levine JD, Fields HL. Causalgia and reflex sympathetic dystrophy: Does the sympathetic nervous system contribute to the generation of pain? Muscle Nerve 22:678–695, 1999.
7. Evans JA. Reflex sympathetic dystrophy. Surg Clin North Am 1946;26:435–448.
8. Stanton-Hicks M, Janig W, Hassenbusch S, et al. Reflex sympathetic dystrophy: changing concepts and taxonomy. Pain 1995;63:127–133.
9. Harden RN. A clinical approach to complex regional pain syndrome. Clin J Pain 2000;16(2 Suppl):S26–S32.
10. Schwartzman RJ. New treatments for reflex sympathetic dystrophy (Editorial). N Engl J Med 2000;343(9):654–656.

11. Blumberg H, Janig W. Clinical Manifestations Reflex Sympathetic Dystrophy and Sympathetically Maintained Pain. In PD Wall, PD Melzack (eds), Textbook of Pain (3rd ed). Edinburgh: Churchill Livingstone, 1994;685–697.
12. Schwartzman RJ, Kerrigan J. The movement disorder of reflex sympathetic dystrophy. Neurology 1990;40:57–61.
13. Schwartzman RJ, Maleki J. Postinjury Neuropathic Pain Syndromes. In JH Cullen (ed), Med Clin North Am 1999;83(3):597–626.
14. Bonica JJ. Causalgia and Other Reflex Sympathetic Dystrophies. In JJ Bonica (ed), The Management of Pain (2nd ed). Philadelphia: Lea & Febiger, 1990;200–243.
15. Allen G, Galer BS, Schwartz L. Epidemiology of complex regional pain syndrome: a retrospective chart review of 134 patients. Pain 1990;80:539–544.
16. Phelps RG, Wilentz S. Reflex sympathetic dystrophy. Int J Dermatol 2000;39:481–486.
17. Dursun E, Dursun N, Ural CE, Cakci A. Glenohumeral joint subluxation and reflex sympathetic dystrophy in hemiplegic patients. Arch Phys Med Rehabil 2000;81:944–946.
18. Kemler MA, van de Vusse AC, van den Berg-Loonen EM, et al. HLA-DQ1 associated with reflex sympathetic dystrophy. Neurology 1999;53:1350–1351.
19. Bennett GJ. Animal Models of Neuropathic Pain. In GF Behhart, DL Hammond, T Jensen (eds), Proceedings of the 7th World Congress of Pain. Progress in Pain Research and Management. Vol. 2. Seattle: IASP Press, 1994;495–510.
20. Woolf CJ, Salter MW. Neuronal plasticity: increasing the gain in pain. Science 2000;288:1765–1769.
21. Kurvers HA, Tangelder GJ, De Mey JG, et al. Skin blood flow abnormalities in a rat model of neuropathic pain: result of decreased sympathetic vasoconstrictor outflow? J Auton Nerv Syst 1997;63:19–29.
22. Gracely RH, Lynch SA, Bennett GJ. Painful neuropathy: altered central processing maintained dynamically by peripheral input. Pain 1992;51:175–194.
23. Wasner G, Backonja MM, Baron R. Traumatic neuralgias: complex regional pain syndromes (reflex sympathetic dystrophy and causalgia): clinical characteristics, pathophysiological mechanisms and therapy. Neurol Clin 1998;16:851–868.
24. Baron R, Blumberg H, Janig W. Clinical Characteristics of Patients with Complex Regional Pain Syndromes in Germany with Special Emphasis on Vasomotor Function. In M Stanton-Hicks, W Janig (eds), Progress in Pain Research and Management: Reflex Sympathetic Dystrophy—a Reappraisal (vol 6). Seattle: IASP Press, 1996;22–36.
25. Fukumoto M, Ushida T, Zinchuk VS, et al. Contralateral thalamic perfusion in patients with reflex sympathetic dystrophy syndrome. Lancet 1999;354:1790–1791.
26. Fleming WW, Westfall DP. Adaptive Supersensitivity. In U Trendelenburg, N Weiner (eds), Handbook of Experimental Pharmacology (vol 90/I). New York: Springer, 1988;509–559.

27. Drummond PD, Finch PM, Smythe GA. Reflex sympathetic dystrophy: the significance of differing plasma catecholamine concentrations in affected and unaffected limbs. Brain 1991;114:2025–2036.
28. Goldstein DS, Tack C, Li S. Sympathetic innervation and function in reflex sympathetic dystrophy. Ann Neurol 2000;48:49–59.
29. Ribbers GM, Oosterhuis WP, van Limbeek J, de Metz M. Reflex sympathetic dystrophy: is the immune system involved? Arch Phys Med Rehabil 1998;79:1549–1552.
30. Campbell JN, Meyer RA, Raja SN. Is nociceptor activation by alpha-1-adrenoreceptors the culprit in sympathetically maintained pain? APSJ 1992;1:3–11.
31. Janig W, McLachlan E. The Role of Modifications in Noradrenergic Peripheral Pathways after Nerve Lesions in the Generation of Pain. In HL Fields, JC Liebeskind (eds), Pharmacological Approaches to the Treatment of Chronic Pain: New Concepts and Critical Issues. Progress in Pain Research and Management (vol 1). Seattle: IASP Press, 1994;101–129.
32. Cocchiarella L, Andersson GBJ (eds). Guides to the Evaluation of Permanent Impairment (5th ed). Chicago: AMA Press, 2001;495–496,553.
33. Ochoa JL. Truths, errors, and lies around "Reflex Sympathetic Dystrophy" and "Complex Regional Pain Syndrome." J Neurol 1999;246:875–879.
34. Lynch ME. Psychological aspects of reflex sympathetic dystrophy: a review of the adult and pediatric literature. Pain 1992;49:337–347.
35. Livingston WK. In HL Fields (ed), Pain and Suffering. Seattle: IASP Press, 1998:87–91.
36. Ciccone DS, Bandilla EB, Wu W. Psychological dysfunction in patients with reflex sympathetic dystrophy. Pain 1997;71:323–333.
37. Covington EC. Psychological Issues in Reflex Sympathetic Dystrophy. In M Stanton-Hicks, W Janig (eds), Progress in Pain Research and Management: Reflex Sympathetic Dystrophy—A Reappraisal (vol 6). Seattle: IASP Press, 1996;192–196.
38. Kingery WS. A critical review of controlled clinical trials for peripheral neuropathic pain and complex regional pain syndromes. Pain 1997;73:123–139.
39. Verdugo R, Campero M, Ochoa J. Phentolamine sympathetic block in painful polyneuropathies. II. Further questioning of the concept of "sympathetically maintained pain." Neurology 1994;44:1010–1014.
40. Jadad AR, Carroll D, Glynn CJ, McQuay HJ. Intravenous regional sympathetic blockade for pain relief in reflex sympathetic dystrophy: a systematic review and a randomized double-blind cross over study. J Pain Symptom Manage 1995;10(1):13–20.
41. Ramamurthy S, Hoffman J, Abadir A, et al. Intravenous regional guanethidine in the treatment of reflex sympathetic dystrophy/causalgia: a randomized, double-blind study. Anesth Analog 1995;81:718–723.
42. Valentin N. Reflex sympathetic dystrophy treated with guanethidine. Time for a change of name and strategy. Acta Anaesthesiol Scand 1996;401:171–172.
43. Butler S, et al. Abstracts 165 & 166. Vienna: World Congress on Pain, 1999.

44. Stanton-Hicks M, Baron R, Boas R, et al. Consensus report: complex regional pain syndromes: guidelines for therapy. Clin J Pain 1998;14:155–166.
45. Schurmann M, Grad LG, Andress HJ, et al. Assessment of peripheral sympathetic nervous function for diagnosing early post-traumatic complex regional pain syndrome Type I. Pain 1999;88:149–159.
46. Low PA, Amadio PC, Wilson PR, et al. Laboratory findings in reflex sympathetic dystrophy: a preliminary report. Clin J Pain 1994;10:235–239.
47. Sandroni P, Low PA, Ferrer T, et al. Complex regional pain syndrome I (CRPS I): prospective study and laboratory evaluation. Clin J Pain 1998;14:282–289.
48. Knezevic W, Bajada S. Peripheral autonomic surface potential: quantitative technique for recording autonomic neural function in man. Clin Exp Neurol 1985;21:201–210.
49. Kozin F, Genant HK, Bekerman C, et al. The reflex sympathetic dystrophy syndrome. II. Roetgenographic and scintigraphic evidence of bilaterality and of periarticular accentuation. Am J Med 1976;60:332–338.
50. Blumberg H, Hoffmann U. Der ischamie-test-ein neues verfahren in der klinischen diagnostic der sympathetichen reflexdystrophia (Kausalgie, M Sudeck). Der Schmerz 1992;7:196–198.
51. Arner S. Intravenous phentolamine test: diagnostic and prognostic use in reflex sympathetic dystrophy. Pain 1991;46:17–22.
52. Strakowski JA, Wiand JW, Johnson EW. Upper Limb Musculoskeletal Pain Syndromes. In RL Braddom (ed), Physical Medicine & Rehabilitation (2nd ed). Philadelphia: Saunders, 2000;815–816.
53. Buschbacher RM, Porter CD. Deconditioning, Conditioning and the Benefits of Exercise. In RL Braddom (ed), Physical Medicine & Rehabilitation (2nd ed). Philadelphia: Saunders, 2000;707–708.
54. Weber DC, Brown AW. Physical Agent Modalities. In RL Braddom (ed), Physical Medicine & Rehabilitation (2nd ed). Philadelphia: Saunders, 2000;440–455.
55. deLateur BJ. Therapeutic Exercise. In RL Braddom (ed), Physical Medicine & Rehabilitation (2nd ed). Philadelphia: Saunders, 2000;392–411.
56. Haddox JD, Van Alstine D. Pharmacologic therapy for reflex sympathetic dystrophy. Phys Med Rehabil 1996;10:297–307.
57. Stanton-Hicks M, Raj PP, Racz GB. Use of Regional Anesthetics for Diagnosis of Reflex Sympathetic Dystrophy and Sympathetically Maintained Pain: A Critical Evaluation. In W Jannig, M Stanton-Hicks (eds), Reflex Sympathetic Dystrophy: A Reappraisal: Progress and Pain Research and Management (vol 6). Seattle: IASP Press, 1996;217–237.
58. Stanton-Hicks M, Janig W. Progress in Pain Research and Management: Reflex Sympathetic Dystrophy—A Reappraisal. Seattle: IASP Press;1996.
59. Schwartzman RJ, Liu JE, Smullens SN, et al. Long-term outcome following sympathectomy for complex regional pain syndrome type 1 (RSD). J Neurol Sci 1997;150:149–152.
60. Leriche R. Intra-arterial therapy of infectious and other diseases. Mem Acad Chir 1938;64:220.
61. Linchitz RM, Raheb JC. Subcutaneous infusion of lidocaine provides effective pain relief for CRPS patients. Clin J Pain 1999;15:67 72.

62. Kemler MA, Bariendse GAM, Van Kleef M, et al. Spinal cord stimulation in patients with chronic reflex sympathetic dystrophy. N Engl J Med 2000;343(9):618–624.
63. Shealy CN, Mortimer JT, Reswick JB. Electrical inhibition of pain by stimulation of the dorsal columns: a preliminary clinical report. Anesth Analg 1967;46:489–491.
64. Varenna M, Zucchi F, Ghiringhelli D, et al. Intravenous clodronate in the treatment of reflex sympathetic dystrophy syndrome. A randomized, double blind, placebo controlled study. J Rheumatol 2000;27(6):1477–1483.
65. Korpan MI, Dezu Y, Schneider B, et al. Acupuncture in the treatment of posttraumatic pain syndrome. Acta Orthop Belg 1999;85(2):197–201.
66. Shibata M, Kazuhisa N, Galer BS, et al. A case of reflex sympathetic dystrophy (complex regional pain syndrome-type I) resolved by cerebral contusion. Pain 1999;79:313–315.
67. Zollinger PE, Tuinebreijer WE, Kreis RW, Breederveld RS. Effect of vitamin C on frequency of reflex sympathetic dystrophy in wrist fractures: a randomized trial. Lancet 1999;354:2025–2028.

Suggested Readings

Bonica JJ. Causalgia and Other Reflex Sympathetic Dystrophies. In JJ Bonica (ed), The Management of Pain (2nd ed). Philadelphia: Lea & Febiger, 1990;200–243.

Gupta MA, Haddox JD, Raja SN. Complex Regional Pain Syndromes and Sympathetically Maintained Pain. In SE Abram, JD Haddox (eds), The Pain Clinic Manual (2nd ed). Philadelphia: Lippincott, Williams & Wilkins, 1999;177–184.

Janig W. The Sympathetic Nervous System in Pain: Physiology and Pathophysiology. In M Stanton-Hicks (ed), Pain and the Sympathetic Nervous System. Boston: Kluwer, 1990.

Ochoa JL. Truths, errors, and lies around "Reflex Sympathetic Dystrophy" and "Complex Regional Pain Syndrome." J Neurol 1999;246:875–879.

16   Muscle Pain Syndromes: Fibromyalgia and Myofascial Pain Syndrome

Rina M. Bloch

Muscle pain syndromes have been recognized for years, both as components of other diseases and as distinct entities in themselves. They may be somewhat elusive, both because they are often a diagnosis of exclusion and because there are no tests to serve as a "gold standard" to prove the diagnosis. The literature is confusing because a number of different terms have been used over the years to describe these problems—terms such as *fibrositis*, *nonarticular rheumatism*, *tension rheumatism*, *myofasciitis*, and *fibromyositis*, among others. Also, it is still being argued as to what these entities are—collections of symptoms, syndromes—or if indeed they exist at all. Today it is generally accepted that there are two distinct clinical entities of muscular pain: fibromyalgia (FM) and myofascial pain syndrome (MPS).

Fibromyalgia

Fibromyalgia is a systemic disorder characterized by chronic, diffuse musculoskeletal pain, aching, stiffness, fatigue, and disturbed sleep. It is also associated with exaggerated tenderness at specific, reproducible locations. These are known as *tender points* (Figure 16.1). Associated complaints include anxiety, headache, urinary urgency, history of dysmenorrhea, and Raynaud's phenomenon.[1] Symptoms of FM are typically aggravated by cold, humid weather, tension, fatigue, inactivity, and overactivity, and are decreased by heat, moderate physical activity, stretching, massage, and restful sleep. Fibromyalgia is much more common in women than in men, and its prevalence appears to increase with age.[1,2]

Etiology

The exact etiology of fibromyalgia is unclear. Biopsy studies to detect muscle abnormality have been equivocal, and in general do not support the concept

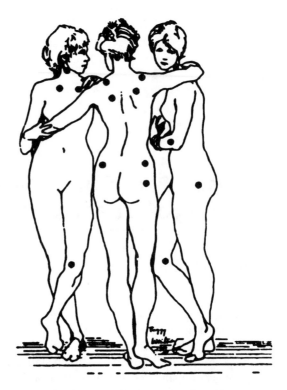

FIGURE 16.1   *Tender point locations for the 1990 classification criteria for fibromyalgia (The Three Graces, after Baron Jean-Baptiste Regnault, 1793, Louvre Museum Paris). (Reprinted with permission from F Wolfe, et al. The American College of Rheumatology 1990 criteria for the classification of fibromyalgia. Arth Rheum 1990;33[2]:160–172. Wiley-Liss, Inc., a subsidiary of John Wiley and Sons, Inc.)*

of intrinsic muscle pathology as the cause.[3,4] Studies investigating possible abnormal muscle metabolism in FM patients have shown no consistent abnormalities.[5] Abnormal electromyographic (EMG) activity has not been found in most studies, although one study did find small areas of spontaneous activity.[6] FM does not appear to be caused by "muscle spasm."[3]

Psychological factors appear to play a role in the development of FM. Compared with a control group of women with other rheumatologic disorders, women with FM reported a significantly higher incidence of sexual and physical abuse.[7] FM patients report a higher prevalence of depression, "severe" allergies, stomach problems, and hypertension than do rheumatoid arthritis patients.[7] FM is also associated with the presence of irritable bowel syndrome.[8] It is difficult to know whether these patients are self-reporting more problems, have a different interpretation of symptoms, or have a truly higher incidence of these other problems.[9] They may have a different threshold for perceiving pain and a different central processing of pain.[2,10,11] FM is associated with failure to complete high school and a lower household income.[2] However, although there is research support for a relationship between psychological factors and FM, it is not a factor in all cases, and the strength of the relationship varies widely among individual patients.

FM symptoms can present after Lyme disease, after coxsackievirus and parvovirus infections, and in conjunction with the human immunodeficiency virus.[12] Infection may not be a direct cause, but may lead to a behavior pattern which then leads to FM.

Sleep disturbance is a common complaint among persons with FM, and may in fact be linked to causation of the clinical syndrome. Normally, alpha rhythm is present during quiet wakefulness and disappears with the onset of stage 1 sleep.[13] Patients with FM appear to have an alpha wave abnormality during non-rapid eye movement sleep. It has been demonstrated that patients with FM have a lack of stage IV non-rapid eye movement sleep. Disrupting the sleep of normal sedentary people may induce symptoms similar to FM.[14]

Diagnosis

Criteria for diagnosing FM were established by the American College of Rheumatology for clinical and epidemiologic use.[1] These are listed in Table 16.1. Although tender points are related to the presence of FM, a complete tender point count is not absolutely necessary to make the clinical diagnosis. Some FM patients may have more diffuse tenderness. Others may have the disorder but not meet the strict tender point count. It is important to not get caught up in the tender point count to the exclusion of evaluating the person as a whole. It should also be noted that the points over the trapezius, occiput, and epicondyle might be tender in normal subjects.

Laboratory, x-ray, and EMG studies are normal in FM, and other conditions that cause similar symptoms, such as hypothyroidism and connective tissue diseases, must be ruled out before the diagnosis can be made.

Treatment

The foundation for a treatment plan in FM is patient education. This includes a realistic discussion of diagnosis and prognosis. Patients should be aware that FM is a relatively common syndrome and that there are no specific laboratory findings to suggest the disease. Patients should also be made aware that FM is neither life-threatening nor degenerative, nor does it cause structural deformities.

Because FM is a systemic disorder, it requires systemic treatment. Because sleep disturbances are a common complaint, and particularly in light of the evidence that suggests that sleep disturbance by itself can produce muscle aches, one should try to normalize the patient's sleep patterns. This includes discouraging the use of caffeinated beverages and alcohol.

An aerobic exercise program of moderate intensity, which gradually improves cardiovascular fitness, flexibility, muscle tone, and posture, has been shown to significantly decrease pain symptoms in FM patients.[15] The exercise should be instituted gradually and should not be overly vigorous. Too much exercise can worsen symptoms.

Stress and a resultant lack of sleep have been shown to aggravate FM; therefore, attention should be paid to obvious stress factors. Relaxation training, possibly through biofeedback, is useful. Patients should be encouraged to plan

TABLE 16.1   The American College of Rheumatology 1990 criteria for the classification of fibromyalgia*

History of widespread pain.

Definition—Pain is considered widespread when all of the following are present: pain in the left side of the body, pain in the right side of the body, pain above the waist, and pain below the waist. In addition, axial skeletal pain (cervical spine or anterior chest or thoracic spine or low back) must be present. In this definition, shoulder and buttock pain is considered as pain for each involved side. "Low back" pain is considered lower segment pain.

Pain in 11 of 18 tender point sites on digital palpation.

Definition—Pain, on digital palpation, must be present in at least 11 of the following 18 tender point sites:

Occiput: bilateral, at the suboccipital muscle insertions.

Low cervical: bilateral, at the anterior aspects of the intertransverse spaces at C5–C7.

Trapezius: bilateral, at the midpoint of the upper border.

Supraspinatus: bilateral, at origins, above the scapula spine near the medial border.

Second rib: bilateral, at the second costochondral junctions, just lateral to the junctions on upper surfaces.

Lateral epicondyle: bilateral, 2 cm distal to the epicondyles.

Gluteal: bilateral, in upper outer quadrants of buttocks in anterior fold of muscle.

Greater trochanter: bilateral, posterior to the trochanteric prominence.

Knee: bilateral, at the medial fat pad proximal to the joint line.

Digital palpation should be performed with an approximate force of 4 kg. For a tender point to be considered "positive," the subject must state that the palpation was painful. "Tender" is not to be considered "painful."

For classification purposes, patients will be said to have fibromyalgia if both criteria are satisfied. Widespread pain must have been present for at least 3 months. The presence of a second clinical disorder does not exclude the diagnosis of fibromyalgia. SOURCE: Reprinted with permission from F Wolfe, et al. The American College of Rheumatology 1990 criteria for the classification of fibromyalgia. Arth Rheum 1990;33(2):160–172. Wiley-Liss, Inc, a subsidiary of John Wiley and Sons Inc.

activities, alternate work with rest periods, and find avocational activities that ease tension. Attention to sleep and to proper posture at work and home are also important.

Physical modalities such as massage, ice, acupuncture, ultrasound, and transcutaneous electrical nerve stimulation may be beneficial in individual patients, but the results are usually temporary.

Medications

Medications that have been found to benefit patients with FM in placebo-controlled studies include amitriptyline (Elavil) and cyclobenzaprine (Flexeril),[16–18] and a fluoxetine-amitriptyline combination.[19] These medications can be beneficial if given in low doses before bedtime. For example, amitriptyline can be used at a dosage of 10–50 mg per day.[20]

The anxiolytic alprazolam has also been studied in the treatment of FM, and data supports its effectiveness.[20,21] Analgesics and nonsteroidal anti-inflammatory medications have limited benefit in the treatment of FM, and narcotics should be avoided, as in most chronic pain states.[21] Growth hormone has shown promise in the treatment of FM, but it has not yet been proven to have long-term benefits and is very expensive.[22]

Counseling
Because psychological issues are of great importance in FM, patients may require psychological counseling or psychiatric intervention, sometimes with antidepressant medication.

Other
Acupuncture has not been proven to be beneficial in the treatment of FM.[23] Hypnotherapy may help, possibly because of improved sleep[24]; biofeedback also seems to be beneficial.[25]

Fibromyalgia and Disability
FM patients often come to the doctor seeking disability statements. In general, this runs counter to the goal of maintaining function. Although many forms of activities, including hobbies and work, may increase the subjective symptoms, FM is not considered to be caused by work. Patients should be counseled that they need to learn to live with their pain. Although patients with FM may be unable to engage in physically strenuous jobs without significant aggravation of their symptoms, some work is helpful from a pain management perspective for lessening deconditioning and illness behavior.

Myofascial Pain Syndrome

MPS is a syndrome of regional pain complaints, often accompanied by "trigger points" and, less commonly, by autonomic symptoms. The regional complaints are of an aching, sore, and stiff muscle or group of muscles. The patient sometimes reports that pain, numbness, or tingling radiates distally or to the head. Autonomic symptoms such as vasoconstriction, sweating, pilomotor response (gooseflesh), or a feeling of coldness may be noted. However, these complaints are rare.

MPS is extremely common, and an element of the syndrome is found accompanying a wide variety of other problems, ranging from cervical strain to postoperative pain.

All patients with MPS have regional pain. It is usually present as an acute or subacute problem, although it can become chronic. Both sexes are affected equally, and it is not associated with sleep disturbance (except that pain by itself may make sleep troublesome), generalized fatigue, or other disease.

Trigger Points

A *trigger point* is a hyperirritable spot found in skeletal muscle that is associated with a hypersensitive palpable nodule in a taut band. The spot is painful on compression, and palpation can give rise to characteristic referred pain, motor dysfunction, and autonomic phenomena. A *latent trigger point* is tender to palpation, but does not cause spontaneous pain. A *taut band* is composed of tight muscle fibers extending from a trigger point to the muscle attachments.

Sometimes a local *twitch response* is noted with palpation. This is a transient contraction of a group of muscle fibers that traverse a trigger point. The fibers may contract due to stimulation such as "snapping" palpation or insertion of a needle.[26]

Trigger points are the subject of controversy in MPS. Some argue that the condition can only be diagnosed if such points are present. Others deny that they exist. The truth probably lies somewhere between these extremes. When present, the trigger points refer symptoms in a pattern characteristic to the muscle in which they are located. The spontaneous pain of which the patient complains does not always occur at this same spot. Many patients with MPS have such trigger points, and palpating them causes a referred pain pattern that is highly suggestive of this syndrome. Other patients have only local tenderness at these spots. Only rarely does palpation of a trigger point cause autonomic symptoms.

Trigger points in the neck and shoulder often refer pain to the head and are potential causes of headache. They can also refer pain into the arm, and may mimic the symptoms of radiculopathy. They can be differentiated from radiculopathy because pressing on the muscle, rather than compressing the nerve (such as with a Spurling maneuver), reproduces the distal symptoms. Back and pelvic trigger points may refer symptoms to the legs.

Etiology

MPS can be caused by overwork fatigue of a muscle, by trauma, or by overstretching of the muscle. It may develop after the initiation of a new activity or exercise, such as carrying around a new infant and baby equipment. It can also be caused by structural factors such as leg length discrepancy, poor posture, or after injury or surgery when body kinematics have changed. Underlying diseases that cause muscle splinting, such as herniated disk, may also aggravate MPS. Increased muscle tension from anxiety can worsen symptoms.

As in FM, laboratory, EMG, and x-ray studies are normal in MPS (except, of course, when other concomitant conditions aggravate or cause MPS).

Treatment

As in FM, patient education plays an important role in the treatment of MPS. Each patient must take responsibility for complying with the treatment regimen. Structural and postural modifications can be made, if needed, to avoid muscle overwork. Any underlying medical problems must be addressed.

MPS is treated as a regional pain problem. Having said that, it is still important to normalize sleep patterns, which are often disrupted just by virtue of being in pain. Any underlying biomechanical or musculoskeletal abnormalities (e.g., leg length discrepancy, poorly designed workplace) should be corrected.

A reconditioning program, beginning with stretching, aerobic exercise, and then progressive resistance exercises aimed at the affected muscles, should be instituted. This reinforces an active role for the patient in treating the condition.

Ice massage and hot packs are often useful to facilitate relaxation and stretching. The spray and stretch technique is also often used. A vapocoolant spray is directed over the trigger points parallel to the course of the muscle fibers to cool the muscle. This is followed by stretching.[26]

Ischemic compression is a technique of applying local pressure to the trigger point. This causes an initial ischemia and subsequent reactive hyperemia, and can be taught to patients to treat their trigger points at home. The beneficial mechanisms of the procedure are unknown; it may be that the reactive hyperemia relaxes the tight muscle and reduces symptoms. In any case, the compression can be applied multiple times daily. It can be performed by hand, by leaning against or lying on a tennis ball, by leaning against doorframes, or with special cane-like devices to reach the back. It should involve firm, even pressure. Excessive rubbing or massage should be avoided, as they may actually worsen the pain.

Trigger points or tender spots can also be injected. Although no one knows exactly how such injections work, they are done in an attempt to deactivate the particular area of muscle that is felt to be affected. Efficacy has been demonstrated with the injection of sterile saline, lidocaine, bupivicaine, diclofenac, and prednisolone, as well as with "dry needling."[27] The best clinical response is seen if injection causes a local twitch response. Dry needling causes more postinjection soreness.[28]

Points of Summary

1. Fibromyalgia (FM) is a syndrome of generalized pain complaints accompanied by sleep disturbance and fatigue, and is more common in women.
2. Myofascial pain syndrome (MPS) involves local or regional pain complaints, and shows no preference for either sex.
3. FM is associated with tender points; MPS is associated with trigger points (and sometimes with other tender spots).
4. FM tends to become chronic; MPS usually resolves.
5. FM is treated with moderate aerobic exercise and medication to help normalize the sleep cycle.
6. MPS is treated with physical modalities, stretching, injections, and strengthening.
7. MPS is often related to repetitive activities, and can also be brought on by structural abnormalities. The triggers of fibromyalgia are less clear.

References

1. Wolfe F, Smythe HA, Yunus MB, et al. The American College of Rheumatology 1990 criteria for classification of fibromyalgia: report of the multicenter criteria committee. Arthritis Rheum 1990;33:160–172.
2. Wolfe F, Ross, K, Anderson J, et al. The prevalence and characteristics of fibromyalgia in the general population. Arthritis Rheum 1995;38:19–28.
3. Simms R. Is there muscle pathology in fibromyalgia syndrome? Rheum Dis Clin North Am 1996;22:245–266.
4. Bengtsson A, Henriksson KG, Larsson J. Muscle biopsy in primary fibromyalgia: light microscopical and histochemical findings. Scand J Rheumatol 1986;15:1–6.

5. Simms RW. Fibromyalgia is not a muscle disorder. Am J Med Sci 1998;315:346–350.
6. Hubbard D, Berkoff G. Myofascial trigger points show spontaneous needle EMG activity. Spine 1993;18:1803–1807.
7. Boisset-Pioro MH, Esdaile JM, Fitzcharles, M. Sexual and physical abuse in women with fibromyalgia syndrome. Arthritis Rheum 1995;38:235–241.
8. Yunus M, Masi AT, Calabro JJ, et al. Primary fibromyalgia (fibrositis): clinical study of 50 patients with matched normal controls. Semin Arthritis Rheum 1981;11(1):151–171.
9. Wolfe F, Anderson J, Harkness D, et al. A prospective, longitudinal, multicenter study of service utilization and costs in fibromyalgia. Arthritis Rheum 1997;40:1560–1570.
10. Bennett RM. Emerging concepts in the neurobiology of chronic pain: evidence of abnormal sensory processing in fibromyalgia. Mayo Clin Proc 1999;74:385–398.
11. Mikkelsson M, Latikka P, Kautiainen H, et al. Muscle and bone pain threshold and pain tolerance in fibromyalgia patients and controls. Arch Phys Med Rehabil 1992;73:814–818.
12. Goldenberg DL. Do infections trigger fibromyalgia? Arthritis Rheum 1993;36:1489–1492.
13. Moldofsky H. Sleep and fibrositis syndrome. Rheum Dis Clin North Am 1989;15:91–103.
14. Moldofsky H, Scarisbrick P, England R, Smythe H. Musculoskeletal symptoms and non-REM sleep disturbance in patients with "fibrositis syndrome" and healthy subjects. Psychosom Med 1975;37:341–351.
15. McCain GA. Role of physical fitness training in the fibrositis/fibromyalgia syndrome. Am J Med 1986;81(Suppl 3A):73–77.
16. Campbell SM, Galter RA, Clark S, et al. A double blind study of cyclobenzaprine versus placebo in patients with fibrositis. Arthritis Rheum (Suppl) 1984;27:576.
17. Carette S, Bell M J, Reynolds WJ, et al. Comparison of amitriptyline, cyclobenzaprine, and placebo in the treatment of fibromyalgia. Arthritis Rheum 1994;37:32–40.
18. Goldenberg DL, Felson DT, Dinerman H. A randomized, controlled trial of amitriptyline and naproxen in the treatment of patients with fibromyalgia. Arthritis Rheum 1986;29:1371–1377.
19. Goldenberg D, Mayskiy M, Mossey C, et al. A randomized double-blind crossover trial of fluoxetine and amitriptyline in the treatment of fibromyalgia. Arthritis Rheum 1996;39:1852–1859.
20. McCain G. A cost-effective approach to the diagnosis and treatment of fibromyalgia. Rheum Dis Clin North Am 1996;22:323–349.
21. Alarcon G, Bradley L. Advances in the treatment of fibromyalgia: current status and future directions. Am J Med Sciences 1998;315:397–404.
22. Bennett R, Clark SC, Walczyk J. A randomized double-blind placebo controlled study of growth hormone in the treatment of fibromyalgia. Am J Med 1998;104:227–231.
23. Berman BM, Ezzo J, Hadhazy, V, Swyers JP. Is acupuncture effective in the treatment of fibromyalgia? J Fam Pract 1999;48:213–218.

24. Haanen HC, Hoenderdos HW, van Romunde LJ, et al. Controlled trial of hypnotherapy in the treatment of refractory fibromyalgia. J Rheumatol 1991;18:72–75.
25. Ferraccioli G, Ghirelli L, Scita F, et al. EMG-biofeedback training in fibromyalgia syndrome. J Rheumatol 1987;14:820–825.
26. Simmons DG, Travell JG, Simons LS. Travell and Simons' Myofascial Pain and Dysfunction: The Trigger Point Manual (vol 1, 2nd ed). Baltimore: Williams & Wilkins, 1999.
27. Borg-Stein J, Stein, J. Trigger points and tender points: one and the same? Does injection treatment help? Rheum Dis Clin North Am 1996;22:305–322.
28. Hong C. Lidocaine injection versus dry needling to myofascial trigger point: the importance of the local twitch response. Am J Phys Med Rehab 1994;73:256–263.

Suggested Readings

Goldenberg, Don L. Fibromyalgia Syndrome a Decade Later: What Have We Learned? Arch Int Med 1999;159:777–785.

Leventhal, LJ. Management of fibromyalgia. Ann Intern Med 1999;131:850–858.

Yunus MB, Kalyan-Raman UP, Kalyan-Raman K. Primary fibromyalgia syndrome and myofascial pain syndrome: clinical features and muscle pathology. Arch Phys Med Rehabil 1988;69:451–454.

Musculoskeletal Problems in the Pediatric Population

Denise L. Carpenter and Binduben A. Patel

Musculoskeletal problems in children generally present differently than in adults. Immaturity and active growth of the musculoskeletal system lead to injuries and disorders specific to the pediatric patient. From birth through adolescence the skeleton is changing. Therefore, the frequency and types of diseases and injuries change as the child ages. Some conditions improve and others worsen with age.

Traumatic injury in children often affects the cartilaginous growth sites of the long bones or the tendon insertion sites. The child's immature bones are softer than mature adult bones, whereas the periosteum is thicker. Traumatic forces applied to young bones, therefore, result in bone bending with incomplete buckle or greenstick fractures rather than complete fractures. When children reach adolescence and bone has begun to strengthen, the growth plate remains immature and becomes the weak link. Therefore, in adolescence, fractures of the growth plate become more common. The occurrence of Osgood-Schlatter disease and other types of overuse injuries also increase in adolescence.

A complete overview of musculoskeletal problems in children is far beyond the scope of this chapter. What follows are descriptions of some of the more common disorders, as well as a general treatment approach. Systemic disorders such as juvenile rheumatoid arthritis and seronegative spondyloarthropathis should also be kept in the differential, but are not covered here.

Shoulder Girdle

Shoulder Instability

Glenohumeral dislocations and subluxations are the most common sports injuries of the shoulder. Most occur anteriorly, and when seen in children they often recur.[1,2] An aggressive rehabilitation program may reduce the incidence of recurrence.[2–4]

Sprengel's Deformity

Sprengel's deformity is due to failure of the scapula to descend during development. It may be unilateral or bilateral. Patients complain of limited range of motion of the scapulothoracic joint. Radiographs and physical examination reveal an elevated scapula. The deformity can be associated with Klippel-Feil syndrome or scoliosis. Surgical treatment may provide increased range of motion (ROM) at the neck and shoulder.

Elbow

A common elbow injury seen in young children, usually toddlers, is a subluxation of the radial head, known as *nursemaid's elbow*. This occurs when the arm is pulled, and can occur with seemingly minor trauma. It is usually easily reduced by flexing and supinating the elbow. Radiographs may be necessary to rule out associated fracture.

Throwing Injuries

Throwing athletes experience repetitive valgus stress at the elbow, which may affect the medial or lateral condyles. Although this type of injury ultimately results in elbow pain and dysfunction, three different presentations can be outlined.

Little league elbow is the result of apophysitis of the medial humeral epicondyle. It is gradual in onset, and the clinical complaint is of activity-related aching pain and tenderness over the affected area. Mild swelling and decreased ROM may be present. X-ray may be normal or demonstrate avulsion fragments or excess calcium deposition at the medial epicondyle.

In the 9- to 12-year-old age group, a sudden forceful pitch may result in avulsion of the medial epicondyle. This results in significant acute swelling and pain. If the avulsion fracture is complete, surgery is indicated.

Panner's disease and *osteochondritis dissecans* of the capitellum generally occur in children younger than 10 years of age and older than 13 years of age, respectively. Both injuries involve the lateral elbow, with osteonecrosis of the capitellum. In younger children, Panner's disease resembles Legg-Calvé-Perthes pathology and has a good prognosis; loose bodies within the joint are generally not encountered. In adolescents, osteochondritis dissecans is often associated with loose joint bodies and prognosis is guarded. In addition to the presentation of activity-related elbow pain with tenderness over the lateral condyle, complaints of the elbow locking may be present if an osteochondral loose body is present.

X-rays may show irregular or delayed development of the capitellum in Panner's disease and osteochondritis dissecans. In older children with osteochondritis, small osteochondral fragments in the joint space may be visualized. There may also be a lucency of the capitellum due to compromise of growth of the subchondral bone from traumatic vascular compromise.

Treatment of these elbow injuries includes rest of the affected elbow with no throwing for up to 6 weeks, followed by a rehabilitation program of generalized arm strengthening and progressive stretching of the anterior elbow capsule. Residual symptoms are more likely to occur in the adolescent with osteochondritis dissecans of the elbow. Those injuries involving complete avulsion of the medial epicondyle or pathology of the capitellum with loose fragments require surgical repair.

Hip

The hip is a relatively common area of problems in children. Newborns may present with developmental dysplasia of the hip. This is often detected shortly after delivery or during well-baby checkups. Other serious hip problems are described in the following sections.

Legg-Calvé-Perthes Disease

Legg-Calvé-Perthes disease is an idiopathic osteonecrosis of the hip that primarily affects young males between 4 and 10 years of age. There is a 4 to 1 ratio of males to females, and the peak incidence occurs at 5–7 years of age. It is rare in blacks and American Indians.[5] Although the cause is unknown, it involves an avascular necrosis of the femoral head. There is ischemic necrosis, followed by collapse and then repair of the femoral head. Ten to twenty percent of cases are bilateral.[5,6] The disease process itself is generally self-limiting, lasting 2–4 years; however, patients suffer from early onset degenerative changes and are often significantly impaired.

Presentation most often includes an antalgic, limping gait, with mild groin pain that may radiate to the thigh and knee. Hip internal rotation is limited early in the disease process; later, general hip motions become decreased, with loss of abduction being the most significant.

Evaluation includes x-rays of the hips, which may be normal early in the disease process. Bone scan or magnetic resonance imaging may reveal abnormalities before they are detected by radiographs. Treatment goals include reduction of synovitis, pain control with the use of nonsteroidal anti-inflammatory drugs, and preservation of the shape of the femoral head. The femoral head is positioned so that it is completely contained within the acetabulum; this is achieved by bracing the leg in abduction or, if necessary, by surgery. Containment is effective only if carried out before the healing phase. Surgical intervention is often indicated in older children or in those with severe disease.[7,8] These children should be evaluated by an orthopedic surgeon.

Prognosis is better for those children who present with the disease before 8 years of age and with less than 50% involvement of the femoral head.

Slipped Capital Femoral Epiphysis

Slipped capital femoral epiphysis is a developmental problem seen in adolescents, usually overweight males. It most commonly involves a posteroinferior displacement of the epiphysis on the proximal femoral metaphysis (the head of the femur slips off of the neck of the femur).[6] This condition affects boys twice as often as girls, with peak ages at 13 years and 11 years, respectively. Blacks are disproportionately affected,[5] and bilateral involvement occurs in 20–40% of cases. The etiology appears to be a decrease in the mechanical integrity of the proximal physis of the femur, which is associated with endocrine disorders and with pubertal children.

The evolution of slipped capital femoral epiphysis depends on the severity. Mild slips can lead to deformities that increase the risk for arthritis. Severe slips may cause the femoral head to become totally displaced from the neck, causing hip stiffness and abductor weakness. Osteonecrosis of the femoral head may also occur.

Clinical presentation is with a painful limp and external rotation of the affected leg. Onset of pain may or may not be associated with a recent injury. Pain typically occurs in the hip and groin or may be referred to the medial knee (sometimes without hip pain), complicating or delaying diagnosis. Pain is worsened with walking, high-impact activity, and internal rotation. Physical examination reveals loss of internal rotation of the hip and shortening of the affected leg by 1–3 cm.

X-rays are diagnostic; the lateral view of the hip joint reveals the posterior slip of the femoral head and the anteroposterior view shows widening of the growth plate.

Treatment involves immediate cessation of weight bearing and surgical evaluation for stabilization of the growth plate. Screw or pin fixation is generally indicated for mild to moderate slips, whereas osteotomy is occasionally required for severe slips.

Transient Synovitis

Transient synovitis is actually a sterile effusion and inflammatory synovitis of the hip joint. The etiology is unknown but the condition often presents after a viral illness (upper respiratory infection) or mild trauma. Boys are affected approximately two times more often than girls. Children between 2 and 5 years of age are most commonly affected, with an age range of 2–15 years.[9] The effusion usually resolves without complication. Septic arthritis must be ruled out and should not be overlooked in the differential diagnosis.

Clinically, the child presents with a history of acute onset of a limp or refusal to bear weight on the affected side; the thigh may be spontaneously held in abduction. If the child is old enough, there may be complaints of hip or groin pain. ROM is mildly restricted.

Evaluation must be thorough enough to distinguish transient synovitis from septic arthritis. Hip x-ray of transient synovitis is usually normal or may show a mild effusion; septic arthritic joints are more likely to demonstrate a widened joint. White blood cell counts in transient synovitis are normal but may be elevated with a septic joint. Sedimentation rate should be normal to less than 25 mm per hour with transient synovitis, but is often greater than 25 mm per hour with septic arthritis. Fever may be absent or low grade with transient synovitis and moderate to high with a septic hip. The child with transient synovitis may display mild irritability, but a good appetite persists and there are no signs of systemic toxicity. The child with arthritis generally appears more "toxic," with fever and worsening of hip pain over time.

The course of transient synovitis is improvement over an average of 3–10 days. The child is often improved by the time medical attention is sought. Hip ROM restrictions remain minimal during the process. Treatment with rest and nonsteroidal anti-inflammatory drugs is generally effective in managing symptoms. If the child is afebrile and improving within 3 days of onset, observation may be continued. If symptoms persist, further evaluation is warranted.[9]

Prognosis is excellent with no associated sequelae, but the condition can recur. Legg-Calvé-Perthes may subsequently develop in up to 3% of cases, but it is unclear if there is a direct correlation.

Knee

Osgood-Schlatter Disease

Osgood-Schlatter disease is a traction apophysitis of the tibial tubercle. It is associated with micro-avulsion injuries at the insertion of the infrapatellar tendon on the tibial tubercle. It is a repetitive injury that is seen in adolescence. Athletic males present more frequently than athletic females, with a ratio of 4 to 1. It is most common in the 10 to 15-year-old age group and is bilateral 25% of the time.

Clinical complaints include anterior knee pain with running and jumping, along with "knobby knees." The affected tibial tubercles are swollen or enlarged and tender to palpation. X-rays may be normal or reveal fragmentation of the tibial tubercle, although many children who are asymptomatic may also have this x-ray finding. X-rays should be obtained to rule out tumor.

This is generally a self-limiting disorder that resolves over the course of 12–18 months. Treatment includes rest (especially from sports), icing, activity modification, and analgesics for pain control. Quadriceps, hamstring, and iliotibial band stretches may be helpful in maintaining knee mobility. A knee guard or immobilizer may help relieve pain, but if no improvement is seen after 3 weeks of conservative treatment, an orthopedic referral is indicated for evaluation for a cylinder cast. When symptoms subside, tubercle enlargement persists.

Sinding-Larsen-Johansson Syndrome

A similar problem can occur at the inferior pole of the patella. It is called *Sinding-Larsen-Johansson syndrome* ("jumper's knee"). It is treated similarly to Osgood-Schlatter disease, and generally resolves within 3–12 months.[10]

Genu Valgum and Genu Varum

Knock-knees and bowlegs, or *genu valgum* and *varum*, are two common parental concerns in young children. At birth, infants have a bowlegged posture or a normal genu varum of 10–15 degrees. It nearly always straightens to 0 degrees by 12–18 months of age. Physiologic bowing, involving the tibia and the distal femur, often occurs during the second year of life. It is more common in blacks. In most children, the condition spontaneously resolves by the age of 3. Bracing does not change the course of the process and it is not recommended.[6]

As the child grows, a knock-kneed type of posture develops. This is also known as genu valgum, and angulation of 12–15 degrees at 3–4 years of age is not unusual. Valgus posturing is more obvious in the obese child. Fortunately, it too decreases with age. By adolescence, the genu valgum approaches the normal alignment of 5–10 degrees.

Evaluation beyond history and physical examination is indicated only when pathology is suspected. If the child is less than the twenty-fifth percentile for height, if there is a severe or increasing deformity, or if there is excessive tibial torsion, radiographs are indicated. If bone dysplasia or physeal arrest is suspected, a skeletal survey or tomogram, respectively, should be ordered.

The differential diagnosis for genu varum should include hypophosphatemic rickets, infantile tibia vara (infantile Blount disease), and metaphyseal chondrodysplasia. The differential diagnosis for genu valgum should also include hypophosphatemic rickets, epiphyseal dysplasia, and pseudoachondroplasia.

Not all cases resolve spontaneously. One should always carefully document measurements from the initial patient visit and continue with close follow-up. The progression of a valgus deformity can be documented by measuring the intermalleolar distance. If the distance is less than 10 cm, observation is the treatment of choice. Should the condition persist into puberty, surgery is recommended. Both osteotomy and hemiepiphysiodesis have been shown to be effective.[11]

Neck

Congenital Muscular Torticollis

Congenital muscular torticollis is a deformity of the head and neck due to unilateral contracture of the sternocleidomastoid (SCM) muscle. It may occur at birth or within the first 2 months of life. The etiology was originally thought to be secondary to birth trauma, which was thought to cause a hematoma and, later, the formation of scar tissue, which then shortened the muscle and pulled the head into a tilted and rotated position.

Currently, two other theories have been proposed. First, an intrauterine vascular insult may result in scarring and shortening of the SCM. Second, intrauterine head position may cause the fibrosis and shortening.

Congenital muscular torticollis is painless and usually affects the right SCM. Often, a small olive-sized mass is palpable within the muscle. This mass spontaneously resolves after approximately 3 months. If the torticollis is not corrected within the first year, facial asymmetry, along with skull deformities, may develop.

Radiographs must be completed to rule out other causes of torticollis, such as bony anomalies, tumors, fractures, dislocations, or rheumatoid arthritis.

Hip dysplasia exists in 20% of the cases; therefore, ultrasound or x-ray of the hip should be performed to rule out this possibility.

The majority of cases resolve by 12 months of age. Treatment consists of stretching the contracted muscle multiple times a day. For a child older than 1 year of age, a custom-molded brace with a helmet may be prescribed. If the condition persists, surgery should be performed before the age of 3 years.[7,12]

Klippel-Feil Syndrome

Patients with Klippel-Feil syndrome have a congenital abnormality of the cervical spine due to incomplete segmentation of the vertebrae. Cases vary from fusion of two vertebrae to complete fusion of the entire cervical region. The etiology is unknown.

Children with this syndrome are often asymptomatic. The classic patient is described as having a short neck, low posterior hairline, and limited neck motion. However, all three of these characteristics are found in fewer than 50% of the cases. Klippel-Feil syndrome is associated with Sprengel's deformity, scoliosis, congenital heart disease, nervous system and genitourinary defects, along with hearing impairments.[7]

Radiographs confirm the anomalies, and the patient should be referred to an orthopedic surgeon.

Cervical Instability

Children with Down's syndrome relatively frequently have occipitocervical or atlantooccipital instability. This can present with gait abnormality, neck pain, mild weakness, and decreased exercise tolerance. Periodic cervical x-ray evaluations in children with Down's syndrome are probably reasonable.[13]

Back

Scoliosis

Scoliosis is a non-painful lateral curvature of the spine. It is present in 2% of the population, and occurs equally in both genders until 10 years of age. After this age, the condition predominates in females. In general, the deformity most commonly observed is a right thoracic curve.

Scoliosis can be classified into three major types: congenital, idiopathic, and neuromuscular. The idiopathic type accounts for 80% of the cases.

Idiopathic scoliosis occurs more often in females than males and the peak age of incidence is from 9 to 12 years. The exact etiology is unknown. Some believe it is an autosomal dominant trait, whereas others consider it to be multifactorial. A thorough physical examination reveals asymmetric shoulder height, pelvic obliquity, and exaggerated flank creases and rib fullness. Radiographs display the lateral curve associated with rotation of the vertebrae. For curves less than 20 degrees, observation is recommended. Curves between 20 and 40 degrees require bracing for approximately 23 hours a day. Curves greater than 40 degrees require surgery.

Congenital scoliosis is due to partial or complete failure of formation or segmentation of the vertebrae. Children with thoracic deformities have an increased incidence of cardiac abnormalities, whereas those with a lumbar defect often have gastrointestinal or renal anomalies. Fifty percent of the cases progress and require surgery. With rapid progression, magnetic resonance imaging should be obtained to rule out a tethered cord, syrinx, or intraspinal anomaly.[14]

Neuromuscular scoliosis is frequently seen in cerebral palsy, Friedreich's ataxia, spinal muscular atrophy, and muscular dystrophy. The curve is usually long and sweeping, and the cervical spine may be involved. It is due to abnormal muscular force (or lack of force) on the spine. Treatment consists of strengthening exercises along with bracing. Progression of the deformity requires surgical fusion.

Scheuermann's Disease

Scheuermann's disease is a common spine disorder affecting 0.5–8.0% of the adolescent population. It involves a familial osteochondrosis of the thoracic spine that causes vertebral wedging and kyphosis. It occurs more often in males, and peaks at 14–17 years of age. The etiology is unknown. Physical examination reveals a child with a rounded shoulder appearance, a thoracic kyphosis (which is not flexible), and a compensatory lumbar hyperlordosis. Tight hamstring muscles are also common, and neurologic examination is usually normal. The patient may complain of pain that is located over the apex of the kyphosis.

Radiographs help confirm the diagnosis. Common findings include (1) anterior wedging of three or more adjacent vertebrae (greater than 5 degrees, with an overall curve greater than 45 degrees from T5 to T12); (2) irregular vertebral end plates; and (3) Schmorl's nodes.[9]

Initial treatment consists of postural exercises and a gentle flexibility program, along with a Milwaukee brace. After 1 year, if the deformity has been corrected, the patient may be weaned from the brace. However, if the skeletally mature curve is greater than 70 degrees, surgery is recommended.[15]

Spondylolisthesis

Spondylolysis can be seen in the young athlete whose sport requires repetitive hyperextension of the lumbar spine. Gymnastics, football, high diving, and weight lifting are all activities that impart repetitive mechanical stress to the pars interarticularis, which fractures in this condition. As in adults, forward slippage of the involved vertebrae, usually L5, can occur, resulting in spondylolisthesis.

Clinical history and symptoms may include a recent growth spurt in addition to complaints of back pain over the lumbosacral level. On physical examination there may be flattening of the normal lumbar lordosis; loss of the ability to bend forward to touch the toes, with tight hamstring muscles;

and rarely, symptoms of nerve compression. There may be a palpable stepoff at the level of the slipped vertebra. X-ray findings are the same as those seen in adults.

Treatment varies according to the degree of displacement of the fracture and clinical symptoms. Acute injury may be treated with immobilization in a body jacket. For mild to moderate slippages, aggravating activity should be avoided and a brace may be considered. For severe slippage, orthopedic evaluation and possible surgical treatment is indicated.[10]

Foot

Calcaneal Apophysitis

Calcaneal apophysitis, or Sever's disease, results from the repeated pull of the Achilles tendon on the calcaneal apophysis. Repetitive microtrauma occurs at the tendon-bone junction leading to apophysitis of the heel. This condition is unique to prepubertal athletes who are skeletally immature. When the apophysis matures and fuses to the calcaneus, this condition generally resolves. Apophyseal fusion is usually complete by 9 years of age in girls and 11 years of age in boys.

Clinically, children complain of heel pain and may walk with a limp. On physical examination, compression of the posterior heel at the Achilles tendon insertion causes discomfort.

X-rays may reveal fragmentation of the apophysis or sclerosis of the secondary ossification centers (a normal finding). Therefore, x-rays may be non-diagnostic. If, however, there is pain at only one heel, x-rays may demonstrate a tumor or bone cyst on that side.

Treatment is with activity modification, a heel pad, and Achilles tendon stretching. If symptoms persist, casting may be considered. This is a self-limiting condition and usually lasts 6–12 months.[10]

Points of Summary

1. Bones in children may break as "greenstick" rather than complete fractures.
2. Traumatic adolescent bone injuries occur commonly at the epiphyseal plate.
3. Overuse syndromes in children commonly affect the apophyses, such as with Osgood-Schlatter disease, Sinding-Larsen-Johansson syndrome, and Sever's disease.
4. Shoulder dislocation in adolescents or young adults often recurs. An aggressive rehabilitation program may reduce the incidence of recurrence.
5. Nursemaid's elbow is a subluxation of the radial head, usually seen in toddlers and caused by pulling on the arm. It is easily reduced by flexion and supination of the forearm.

6. Limping in children can be a sign of serious problems such as Legg-Calvé-Perthes disease or slipped capital femoral epiphysis, or a benign problem such as transient synovitis.
7. Throwing injuries in children often affect the medial elbow.
8. A variety of congenital or developmental abnormalities may be detected in children.
9. Congenital torticollis should be treated with an aggressive stretching program.
10. Children with Down's syndrome should be observed for cervical instability.
11. Back pain in adolescents who participate in hyperextension during sports activity may be a sign of spondylolysis/spondylolisthesis.

References

1. Rowe CR, Sakellarides HT. Factors related to recurrences of anterior dislocations of the shoulder. Clin Orthop 1961;20:40–47.
2. Sanders JO, Song KM. Fractures, Dislocations, and Acquired Problems of the Shoulder in Children. In CA Rockwood Jr, FA Matsen III (eds), The Shoulder (2nd ed). Philadelphia: Saunders, 1999;1239–1295.
3. Aronen JG, Regan K. Decreasing the incidence of recurrence of first time anterior shoulder dislocations with rehabilitation. Am J Sports Med 1984;12(4):283–291.
4. Burkhead WZ Jr, Rockwood CA Jr. Treatment of instability of the shoulder with an exercise program. J Bone Joint Surg 1992;74A:890–896.
5. Mier RJ, Brower TD. Pediatric Orthopedics: A Guide for the Primary Care Physician. New York: Plenum, 1994.
6. Molnar, G, Alexander, M. Pediatric Rehabilitation. Philadelphia: Hanley & Belfus, 1999.
7. Richard, B. Orthopaedic Knowledge Update Pediatrics. Rosemont, IL: American Academy of Orthopaedic Surgeons, 1996.
8. Poussa M, Yrjonen T, Hoikka V, et al. Prognosis after conservative and operative treatment in Perthes' disease. Clin Orthop 1993;297:82–86.
9. Snider, R. Essentials of Musculoskeletal Care. Rosemont, IL: American Academy of Orthopaedic Surgeons, 1997.
10. Staheli LT. Fundamentals of Pediatric Orthopedics (2nd ed). Philadelphia: Lippincott–Raven, 1998.
11. Morrissy R, Weinstin S. Lovell and Winter's Pediatric Orthopaedics. Philadelphia: Williams & Wilkins, 2001.
12. Wirth CJ, Hagena FW, Wueklker N, et al. Biterminal tenotomy for the treatment of congenital muscular torticollis: long-term results. J Bone Joint Surg 1992;74A:427–434.
13. Herman MJ, Pizzutillo PD. Cervical spine disorders in children. Orthop Clin North Am 1999;30:457–466.
14. McMaster MJ, Ohtsuka K. The natural history of congenital scoliosis: a study of two hundred and fifty-one patients. J Bone Joint Surg 1982;64A:1128–1147.

15. Sachs B, Bradford D, Winter R, et al. Scheuermann kyphosis: follow-up of Milwaukee-brace treatment. J Bone Joint Surg 1987;69A:50–57.

Suggested Readings

Mier RJ, Brower TD. Pediatric Orthopedics: A Guide for the Primary Care Physician. New York: Plenum, 1994.

Snider, R. Essentials of Musculoskeletal Care. Rosemont, IL: American Academy of Orthopaedic Surgeons, 1997.

Staheli LT. Fundamentals of Pediatric Orthopedics (2nd ed). Philadelphia: Lippincott–Raven, 1998.

18   Geriatrics

Angela T. Carbone and Ralph M. Buschbacher

Musculoskeletal disorders are the most common cause of pain among the elderly. Although these disorders are not unique in this population, they are certainly more prevalent and may lead to a higher degree of disability. Treatment in this group of patients has its own set of unique challenges due to the natural aging process and the higher prevalence of comorbidities. The American population is aging, with the 65-and-older group making up the fastest growing segment.[1] This chapter explains the effects of aging on the musculoskeletal system and addresses a few special issues that arise more often in the elderly.

Aging, Disuse, and Effects on the Body

Muscular System

It is often difficult to distinguish between primary (or "natural") aging and secondary aging from disease and environmental factors. The aging process is a complex set of events that are influenced by genetics and environmental factors. Regardless of a person's level of activity, there is an overall decline in all systems of the body. The rate of this decline is strongly influenced by the person's physical activity level, life stresses, and environmental exposures, such as smoking, sun damage, and diseases.

The muscular system undergoes significant changes throughout life. There is a loss in lean muscle mass, with an increase in the type I– to type II–fiber area ratio and a reduction in fiber number and size. Decrements in strength, but not overall endurance, have also been observed.[2,3,4] The elderly tend to be less active than their younger counterparts. Therefore, many of the changes seen in the muscular system are not only related to advancing age but can also be explained by disuse.

A person who is active throughout life maintains more muscle mass, strength, and coordination than one who is sedentary. However, the sedentary elderly individual can regain some muscle strength and endurance through a regular and consistent training program, even if the program is begun late in life.[5,6,7] Despite maintaining a continuous and somewhat strenuous exercise program, however, declines in overall strength are still observed. This is largely due to the reduction in the number of functional motor units with age.[8]

Relative endurance does not seem to be affected by age. Brown[4] noted that as long as an older individual worked at the same relative intensity (same percentage of maximum strength) as someone younger, there was no difference in the length of time a task could be performed.

Skeletal System

The skeletal system goes through a variety of changes throughout life. There appears to be a rapid increase in bone metabolism during adolescence. This process begins to slow during the third decade. Before this time, bone density is increasing because deposition is occurring at a faster rate than resorption. Sometime during the fourth decade the rate of resorption exceeds the rate of deposition and bone density begins to decline. The rate of bone loss differs among men and women and is strongly influenced by hormones, diet, and activity. As with the muscular system, an increase of physical activity (mainly weight-bearing exercises) can reduce the rate of bone loss so that osteoporosis and its complications will not become a serious risk until extremely late in life.

Tendons, ligaments, and joint capsules lose elasticity with age. This leads to a loss of flexibility. Inflexibility may increase the risk of soft tissue injury and falls. Gait pattern changes in the elderly population are mainly due to inflexible joints, tendons, and ligaments.

Nervous System

There is a loss of brain mass over time. This is largely due to an increase in neuronal death and glial cell proliferation. There is also a reduction in the number of peripheral motor and sensory neurons, and a change in motor unit recruitment patterns as we age. There is an increase in variability in the discharge rate of motor units as well as an increase in coactivation of the antagonist muscle group, leading to a decline in steadiness of low-force isometric and anisometric muscle contractions.[9] These changes in the nervous system can lead to poor coordination, a prolongation of reaction time, a reduction in fine motor skills, and a loss of balance and proprioception.

Other Changes

Other body organ systems also change with age. Changes include a rise in systolic blood pressure, a decrease in cardiac output, a decrease in pulmonary vital capacity, an increase in body fat, and a decrease in renal, hepatic, and immune system functions. There is a decline in the ability to recover from injury or disease, which has a strong impact on the individual's ability to age successfully.

Diagnosis and Treatment of Specific Disorders

Degenerative Joint Disease

Degenerative joint disease (DJD) is one of the most common causes of pain and disability in middle-aged and older people. It is also commonly referred to as *osteoarthritis, degenerative arthritis, osteoarthrosis,* or *hypertrophic arthritis*. DJD is characterized by pain, stiffness, and decreased range of motion (ROM). There is a progressive loss of articular cartilage, remodeling of subchondral bone, and, in many instances, the formation of osteophytes. The most common joints affected are the knees, hips, hands, feet, and spine.

DJD is not necessarily an inevitable consequence of aging. In fact, there is no evidence that a normal joint, used normally, will break down over time. The main risk factor for the development of DJD is repetitive overload to the joint. This is usually in the form of heavy lifting, obesity, abnormal work positions, vibration, and continuously repeated motions. Regular moderate or even strenuous exercise does not appear to cause or accelerate the onset of DJD (this does not include contact sport–type activities). In fact, activity stimulates connective tissue matrix synthesis, whereas immobility causes its degradation and can eventually lead to degenerative changes.[10]

On physical examination there may be joint tenderness to palpation and crepitus with active or passive ROM. Joint effusions may or may not be present. In advanced DJD there are joint deformities, limited joint ROM, bony hypertrophy, and joint instability. Radiographic findings include joint-space narrowing, subchondral sclerosis, marginal bone spurs, and subchrondral cysts. There is often a great discrepancy between the severity of patient symptoms and the severity of radiographic findings. Patients who complain of minimal pain may have severe degenerative changes on x-ray and vice versa. Other studies that can help to evaluate DJD include bone scan, computed tomography (CT), and magnetic resonance imaging (MRI).

The treatment of DJD is directed toward controlling pain and maintaining adequate function. Pain is controlled with the use of pharmacologic and non-pharmacologic therapies. This includes the judicious use of nonsteroidal anti-inflammatory drugs (NSAIDs) and other analgesics, as well as intra-articular steroid or hyaluronic acid injections. As a rule, medications are used on an as-needed basis. This decreases the risk of untoward effects such as gastrointestinal bleeding. There is a subset of patients that use NSAIDs continually and do well without any long-term deleterious effects. These patients need close monitoring.

Intra-articular steroid injection in combination with an anesthetic can be extremely helpful, especially in the presence of joint inflammation. In general, steroid injections are given sparingly; most clinicians inject a particular joint 3–4 times a year, or once every 3–4 months, to reduce the possibility of hastening joint deterioration.

The non-pharmacologic treatments of DJD include physical and occupational therapy to provide energy conservation techniques that are applicable to daily activities; proper joint protection; ROM and strengthening exercises; and, when applicable, gait retaining to help promote proper joint loading.

Typically, a therapist is instructed to use modalities before and after treatment sessions to help minimize pain and promote joint movement. Modalities that can be used include ultrasound, ice, and heat. Assistive devices such as canes and walkers can also help diminish pain associated with activity as well as facilitate continued independence. These devices decrease the force that is applied to the joint during weight bearing. Shoe orthotics may also help change the kinetics of the lower extremity and decrease the stress on the legs and the back. Splints for the upper and lower extremities can offer protection to joints through immobilization during a phase of acute inflammation.

A recent randomized study of patients with DJD of the knee found that manual physical therapy was beneficial. The treatment group received passive ROM, muscle stretching, and soft-tissue mobilization, primarily to the knee. The hip, ankle, and lumbar spine were given the same treatment if these areas also showed limited ROM, were symptomatic, or were contributing to overall lower limb dysfunction. The treatment group also performed closed kinetic chain strengthening exercises and received instructions for a home exercise program. The results showed that the patients benefited in regard to ROM. They had decreased pain with activity and improved quality of life. The percentage that required surgery at 1-year follow-up was significantly reduced.[11] Other studies have shown exercise to be extremely beneficial in decreasing pain, decreasing analgesic and physician use, improving quality of life, and reducing functional impairments. Cardiopulmonary parameters also improve.[12–14]

In severe cases of DJD, with intractable pain and considerable impairments, joint arthrodesis (fusion), osteotomy (changing the angle of the bone), or arthroplasty (joint replacement) may be necessary. Arthrodesis is currently preferred in the ankle, whereas joint replacement gives better results in the hips and knees. Younger patients tend to wear out their joint replacements within their longer remaining life spans; elderly patients generally do well with such replacements.

Neck and Back

Neck and back pain occur in all age ranges; however, the causes of pain do vary with age. Young adults may suffer from connective tissue disease such as Reiter's syndrome or ankylosing spondylitis, which mainly cause low back and sacroiliac pain. In middle age, common causes of neck pain include myofascial pain syndrome and post-traumatic pain. Back pain is commonly caused by mechanical low back disorder. Herniated disks occur most commonly in this age group. Older individuals may suffer from DJD, osteoporotic fractures, or spinal stenosis.

Degenerative Joint Disease
DJD commonly affects the facet joints. These joints are equipped to provide a weight-bearing surface, yet in a lifetime of improper spinal mechanics they may be injured and begin to degenerate. If facet arthropathy develops, extension or rotation of the spine may exacerbate pain. Flexion may relieve the symptoms. Treatment consists of instruction in proper back mechanics,

strengthening of the back muscles, and NSAIDs. Facet joint injections may be necessary in some cases. When degeneration allows the vertebrae to slip on each other (a condition known as *spondylolisthesis*), treatment may consist of an isometric flexion strengthening program and possibly lumbosacral orthoses. Such degenerative spondylolisthesis is different from isthmic spondylolisthesis, which involves a fracture of the pars interarticularis (spondylolysis) and is found in younger patients.

Osteoporosis

Osteoporotic fractures are the dreaded end result of osteoporosis. In the spine they often occur as wedge-shaped compression fractures of the thoracic or lumbar vertebrae. Pain from such fractures generally resolves as the bone heals, usually in a few months. The fracture leaves a deformity that leads to kyphosis. If no neurologic deficit occurs, the acute compression fracture is treated with a short period of rest, analgesics, and return to activity as soon as tolerated. Positions of flexion are avoided. Back braces, which are useful in younger patients with traumatic compression fractures, are usually not tolerated in the elderly.

Spinal Stenosis

Spinal stenosis is a narrowing of the vertebral canal due to a buildup of bone. It can occur in the cervical and lumbar spine. It can also involve the intervertebral foramina where the spinal nerves exit the vertebral canal. It is more likely in those with a relatively small spinal canal.

When stenosis affects the cervical spine, it can cause myelopathy, or damage to the spinal cord. This may produce lower motor neuron signs of damage at the involved level and upper motor neuron signs below the injury. The patient may complain of numbness, weakness, and tingling of the limbs, mainly in the arms and hands. In more advanced cases there may be spasticity, lower extremity hyperreflexia, and the presence of pathologic reflexes (especially in the lower extremities). Diagnosis can be suggested electromyographically and confirmed with MRI, CT, or myelogram. Treatment can be conservative, with a cervical collar, NSAIDs, and physical therapy, to maximize function. If symptoms become significant enough to interfere with activities of daily living, a surgical decompression of the spinal cord may be indicated.

In stenosis of the lumbar spine there may be symptoms of neurogenic claudication, or pseudoclaudication. In true claudication, poor arterial blood flow to the legs causes leg pain after a predictable interval of exercise. In neurogenic claudication, the lumbar stenosis causes similar symptoms due to compression of the lumbar spinal contents. Symptoms of pseudoclaudication are more variable than in true claudication. They occur with back extension and during standing (not just walking). The symptoms do not occur during exercise if the spine is flexed, as when riding a bicycle or walking in a stooped position. This helps differentiate this condition from true vascular claudication, which occurs with any lower extremity activity and is relieved by rest, no matter what position the spine is in.

Lumbar spinal stenosis can often be treated with a program of lumbar flexion exercise, a lumbosacral corset, and shock-absorbing shoe inserts. Surgical decompression may be necessary in some cases.

When spinal stenosis causes a narrowing of the intervertebral foramina (lateral stenosis), it pinches the corresponding spinal nerves and may lead to radiculopathy. Diagnosis of such nerve damage can be made by electromyography. Oblique spine x-ray films, MRI, or CT can be used to image the narrowing. Conservative care with NSAIDs; epidural, oral, or nerve root sleeve corticosteroid injection; and physical therapy may be successful. Surgical decompression may be necessary in some cases.[15] In cases of herniated nucleus pulposus concomitant with such lateral stenosis, surgery is more likely to be necessary.[16]

Other

In addition to the conditions already discussed, which are relatively more common in the elderly than in young patients, the older patient is also at higher risk of developing neck or back pain from cancer metastases, neck pain from rheumatoid arthritis involvement, and post-traumatic pain. The ligamentum flavum in the posterior of the spinal canal is flexible and elastic in the younger population. As a person ages, it becomes less elastic. Thus in a hyperextension injury, such as a flexion-extension (whiplash) motion in motor vehicle accident, the less elastic ligamentum flavum may pinch the spinal cord, leading to neck pain or, in severe cases, a partial spinal cord injury.

Shoulder

Almost all disorders of the shoulder described in Chapter 8 can be found in the elderly. The older individual is, however, more likely to suffer specifically from a few of them. Chronic rotator cuff tears are more common, as is impingement syndrome. Treatment is similar to that for younger patients; however, in these more chronic conditions, conservative care is typically more useful than surgery. If surgery is performed, care must be taken to avoid prolonged immobilization. Such immobilization is more likely to cause adhesive capsulitis in the elderly than in the young. Adhesive capsulitis can also be triggered by anything from trauma to myocardial infarction. Often, the cause is unknown.

Another condition that may be more common in the older population is rupture of the biceps tendon. This produces a bulge in the anterior arm due to a retraction of the muscle belly. This reduces the strength of the biceps, although most patients do not complain of weakness. Surgery is helpful in a patient who requires full biceps strength.

DJD of the shoulder can cause severe symptoms, which can be incapacitating in the elderly. The humeral head may migrate superiorly and become virtually locked onto the acromion. Surgical care with arthrodesis or, more commonly, total joint replacement, usually provides relief of pain and dysfunction.

The shoulder can also be a site of referred pain in the elderly. The primary pathology may lie in the heart, cervical spine, paraspinal and neck muscles, in the brachial plexus, or in apical lung tumors (Pancoast's tumor). Avascular necrosis of the humeral head may occur in patients treated with oral steroid medication.

Hip

The hip is a constrained joint that can withstand great compressive loads. Consequently, any degeneration and inflammation can lead to symptoms. Pain can be severe and may be present even when the hip is not bearing weight.

Degenerative disease of the hip can often be treated conservatively with NSAIDs, a cane, and gentle exercises. Hip replacement surgery is a generally well-tolerated treatment for more severe cases of DJD.

Fractures of the hip, often due to osteoporosis in the elderly, require assessment and treatment by an orthopedic surgeon and are not discussed further here.

Other causes of hip pain may be trochanteric bursitis, peripheral vascular disease, abdominal or pelvic tumors, or pseudogout (chondrocalcinosis). Avascular necrosis is also a diagnosis to consider in patients who have been treated with corticosteroids.

Knee and Leg

Knee disorders are probably more common in younger patients than in the elderly. Meniscal tears, cruciate ligament tears, and chondromalacia are common disorders usually seen in a sports medicine setting. The elderly develop a different set of knee disorders, mainly degenerative meniscal tears and DJD.

Treatment of degenerative meniscal tears is usually conservative, with NSAIDs and gentle strengthening exercises. Sometimes joint injections, arthoscopic débridement, and even meniscectomy are necessary. DJD of the knee is similarly often treated conservatively with NSAIDs, a cane, joint injections, and exercises. In severe cases, total knee replacement surgery offers a generally effective way to reduce pain and increase function.

Other causes of knee pain in the elderly may include a Baker's cyst, referred hip pain, and pseudogout. Baker's cyst is a posterior outpouching of the synovial membrane of the knee. If it ruptures it may mimic deep venous thrombosis.

Leg pain can be due to any number of causes in the elderly. One of the most common is intermittent claudication. Although not truly a musculoskeletal disorder, it belongs in this book because it mimics musculoskeletal disorders. Claudication is due to arterial disease, which causes symptoms of ischemic leg pain after performing a certain amount of muscular activity. Typically the patient reports that pain starts after walking a set distance. The distance remains remarkably constant from day to day. Symptoms are relieved by rest, although not necessarily by sitting down (differentiating this from pseudoclaudication). Symptoms may be reduced with a progressive exercise program. Surgery is required if the vascular disease progresses to the point of threatening limb viability.

Foot

The foot is an anatomically complex part of the body that serves as a lever for ambulation and as a platform for standing. Foot problems in the elderly are due to several classes of etiology. One is the anatomic changes in the foot that are a part of normal aging. In addition, there are problems that occur from a lifetime of wearing improper footwear. Other causes include overuse and disease states.

With aging, the fat pads on the plantar surface of the foot become atrophic. These pads act as shock absorbers, and their atrophy places increased stress on the rest of the foot. Elderly patients also have more osteoarthritis of the joints of the foot. Medical conditions such as peripheral vascular disease, peripheral neuropathy, and connective tissue diseases take their toll on the foot as well.

Achilles tendonitis is an overuse condition, and can usually be successfully treated with conservative care. Achilles bursitis is an inflammation of the retrocalcaneal bursa, and is often caused by mechanical irritation from shoes. Again, treatment should be conservative in most cases.

Painful heel pads probably occur due to heel pad atrophy and are worsened by obesity. The pain in this condition is felt on the major weight-bearing portion of the calcaneus. Plantar fasciitis is a common condition in young and old patients. It causes pain to be felt at the anterior border of the calcaneus, where the plantar fascia inserts into this bone. It can usually be treated with warm soaks (or ice), NSAIDs, stretching, and shoe orthotics.

Acquired pes planus in the geriatric population is often due to posterior tibial tendon rupture. Pes cavus and associated claw toes can be due to a progressive neurologic disease. Treatment should include stretching and strengthening exercises as well as shoe modification.

Hallux valgus is common in the elderly. It is seen more frequently in women than in men and is felt to be due to high-heeled shoes and narrow toe boxes. Hallux rigidus is usually due to DJD.

Metatarsalgia is commonly seen in those older than age 40, especially in women, and is thought to be caused by atrophy of the fat pads of the foot as well as by wearing high-heeled shoes. It can also be caused by trauma in those who stress their feet with poor footwear.

Falls

Falls are a common and feared problem in the elderly. They can result in fractures that cause morbidity and even mortality. Subsequent deconditioning, fear of further falling, and medical complications such as deep venous thrombosis often start the patient on a gradual decline in activity and quality of life. Falls in the elderly are more likely than in the younger population because of decreased strength, balance, coordination, reaction time, vision, and flexibility. They are also sometimes the first presenting signs of medical conditions such as orthostatic hypotension, syncope, or Parkinson's disease.

Falls in the elderly must be taken seriously. After dangerous medical reasons for the falls are ruled out, the patient often benefits from a strengthening and conditioning program, as well as the possible use of a cane or other adaptive equipment.

Medications

There are a number of bodily changes that occur with aging that affect the pharmacology and side effects of medications used in musculoskeletal medicine.

With age come changes in the gastrointestinal (GI) system that decrease the absorption of drugs. This effect is usually fairly minor and in general does not require higher doses of a prescribed drug. There are also changes in body composition in the elderly, as described earlier. A higher body fat content means that fat-soluble drugs are more likely to be stored in body fat. This increases the time required for these drugs to show clinical effects and retards their complete elimination from the body when they are discontinued. A lower body water content makes the serum levels of water-soluble drugs higher in the elderly, and lower serum albumin increases the serum concentration of drugs that normally bind to this protein. The elderly have a reduced capacity to eliminate medications by the two usual methods, hepatic metabolism and renal clearance. In general they are also more susceptible to drug side effects and adverse reactions. Because older patients are often on numerous medications for various illnesses and diseases, they are also more likely to suffer from adverse drug interactions.

Nonsteroidal Anti-Inflammatory Drugs

NSAIDs are probably the most frequently prescribed medications in any age group. In the elderly, they are especially likely to cause problems of GI ulcers and bleeding and acute renal failure. The salicylates cause more metabolic acidosis in the elderly. Sulindac may be less harmful to the kidneys. The new Cox-2–specific NSAIDs are promising. They have the same efficacy as the non-specific NSAIDs, but clinical trials indicate that the incidence of GI upset and GI bleeding are significantly less.[17,18] However, current data indicate that Cox-2–specific NSAIDs do not have particularly favorable effects on renal function. These renal effects appear to be similar to those of the nonspecific NSAIDs.[19,20]

Acetaminophen

Acetaminophen is a very safe medication; however, in the elderly it may have an increased serum half-life, and in patients with impaired liver function it may cause further liver damage if ingested in high doses.

Narcotic Analgesics

The elderly have no special problems with this class of drugs except that they may be more likely to experience side effects such as central nervous system depression, respiratory depression, and constipation.

Corticosteroids

Corticosteroids are powerful medications that can suppress the adrenal glands. In older patients, as well as in younger ones, this can create problems in times of bodily stress, such as during surgery. Patients who have been on chronic systemic corticosteroid medication within a year of such stress may need steroid supplementation to avoid complications such as shock. Corticosteroids also worsen diabetes and, when used chronically, can cause or worsen osteoporosis. These are special concerns in the elderly.

Tricyclic Antidepressants

Older individuals are more susceptible to the anticholinergic side effects of tricyclic antidepressants. This includes problems of orthostatic hypotension, confusion, dry mouth, urinary retention, and blurred vision.

Other Medications

Virtually any drug can have adverse effects, especially in the elderly. Phenytoin may exhibit a higher serum level, and thus a higher level of side effects, in the elderly. Diazepam has an increased half-life and is stored in body fat. Beta-blockers reduce the rise in heart rate with exercise. These effects, along with many others, must be watched for when dealing with the elderly population. To maximize safety it is best to use the lowest dose of medication possible, and to increase the dose only slowly, as needed. If possible, drugs should be avoided altogether.

Points of Summary

1. Virtually every body system deteriorates with age to some extent; this may be due to the primary effects of aging, as well as disuse.
2. The elderly suffer from different musculoskeletal problems compared with younger individuals.
3. Falls are common in the elderly. They may be due to less of a physical margin of safety or may be signs of medical disease.
4. Medication side effects are generally amplified in the elderly; the lowest doses possible should be used.
5. Successful aging can be achieved with a healthy lifestyle, which includes a well-balanced diet and regular exercises. Smoking and excessive alcohol intake should be avoided.

References

1. Spencer G. Projections of the Population by Age, Sex, and Race: 1988–2080. Current Population Reports, Series P-25, No 1018. Washington, DC: United States Census, Government Printing Office, 1989.
2. Anniasonn A, Hedberg M, Henning G, et al. Muscle morphology, enzymatic activity and muscle strength in elderly men: a follow up study. Muscle Nerve 1986;9:585–591.
3. Lexell J. Aging and human muscle: observations from Sweden. Can J Appl Physiol 1993;18:2–18.
4. Brown M. Selected physical performance changes with ageing. Top Geriatr Rehabil 1987;2:68–76.
5. Frontera WR, Meredith CN, O'Reilly KP, et al. Strength conditioning in older men: skeletal muscle hypertrophy and improved function. J Appl Physiol 1988;64:1038–1044.
6. Chandler JM, Hadley EC. Exercise to improve physiologic and functional performance in old age. Clin Geriatr Med 1996;12:761–784.

7. Rogers MA, Evans WJ. Changes in skeletal muscle with aging: effects of exercise training. Exerc Sport Sci Rev 1993;21:65–102.
8. Campbell M, McComas A, Petito F. Physiological changes in aging muscle. J Neurol Neurosurg Psychiatry 1973;36:174–182.
9. Laidlaw DH, Bilodeau M, Enoka RM. Steadiness is reduced and motor unit discharge is more variable in older adults. Muscle Nerve 2000;23:600–612.
10. Buckwalter JA, Martin J. Degenerative joint disease. Clin Symp Ciba-Geigy 1995;47(2):1–32.
11. Deyle GD, Henderson NE, Matekel RL, et al. Effectiveness of manual physical therapy and exercise in osteoarthritis of the knee, a randomized controlled trial. Ann Intern Med 2000;132:173–181.
12. Ettinger WH Jr, Burns R, Messier SP, et al. A randomized trial comparing aerobic exercise and resistance exercise with a health education program in older adults with knee osteoarthritis: the Fitness Arthritis and Seniors Trial (FAST). JAMA 1997;277:25–31.
13. Ries MD, Philibin EF, Groff GD. Relationship between severity of gonarthrosis and cardiovascular fitness. Clin Orthop 1995;313:169–176.
14. Van Baar ME, Dekker J, Oostendorp RAB, et al. The effectiveness of exercise therapy in patients with osteoarthritis of the hip or knee: a randomized clinical trial. J Rheumatol 1998;25:2432–2439.
15. Turner JA, Ersek M, Herron L, et al. Surgery for lumbar spinal stenosis—attempted meta-analysis of the literature. Spine 1992;17:1–8.
16. Saal JA, Saal JS. Nonoperative treatment of herniated lumbar intervetebral disc with radiculopathy: an outcome study. Spine 1989;14:431–437.
17. Silverstein FE, Faich G, Goldstein JL, Simon LS, et al. Gastrointestinal toxicity with celecoxib vs nonsteroidal anti-inflammatory drugs for osteoarthritis and rheumatoid arthritis. The CLASS study: a randomized controlled trial. JAMA 2000;284(10):1247–1255.
18. Lipsky, et al. Analysis of the effects of COX-2 specific inhibitors and the recommendations for their use in clinical practice. J Rheumatol 2000;27:1338–1340.
19. Whelton A, Schulman G, Wallermark C, et al. Effects of celecoxib and naproxen on renal function in the elderly. Arch Intern Med 2000;160:1465–1470.
20. Perazella MA, Eras J. Are selective COX-2 inhibitors nephrotoxic? Am J Kidney Dis 2000;35(5):937–940.

Suggested Readings

Alonso JA, Cote LJ. Biology of Aging in Humans. In JD Dowey, SJ Myers, et al. (eds), The Physiological Basis of Rehabilitation Medicine (2nd ed). Boston: Butterworth–Heinemann, 1994;689–704.

American College of Rheumatology Subcommittee on Osteoarthritis Guidelines. Recommendations for the medical management of osteoarthritis of the hip and knee, 2000 update. Arthritis Rheum 2000;43:1905–1915.

Elward K, Larson EB. Benefits of exercise for older adults. Clin Geriatr Med 1992;8:35–50.

19 Musculoskeletal Issues and Related Medical Concerns in Women

Joanne B. (Anne) Allen and Katherine L. Dec

Musculoskeletal conditions in the United States are the number one cause of visits to physicians' offices and are estimated to cost the United States more than $215 billion yearly.[1] Approximately one in seven Americans has a musculoskeletal impairment, and these impairments rank number one for men and women of all major racial groups.[2] As an increasing number of women are exercising and participating in sports as well as in the workforce, the number of musculoskeletal issues in women is likely to continue an upward trend.[3,4]

General Anatomic and Physiologic Issues

Anatomy

The average woman typically weighs less, has less bone mass, and has a larger surface area to mass than the average man.[5] The average body fat of the female is approximately 18–22% of her body weight, and women average approximately 10% more body fat than men.[5] Women also tend to have bones that are thinner and lighter than men do and experience a rapid loss of bone after menopause, contributing to an increased risk of osteoporosis.

A woman's pelvis differs in shape from that of a man, with a wider pelvic inlet to accommodate childbearing. Actual absolute width of the female pelvis can vary and appears wider when measured relative to height.

Anatomic alignment of the lower limbs in the female has been associated with a higher incidence of patellofemoral problems. The alignment is due to the relatively wider pelvis and a higher prevalence of increased femoral anteversion.[5,6] This is also known as the *miserable malalignment syndrome*—the knee is in slight valgus (knock-kneed), the femur is anteverted, the tibia is externally rotated, and there is resultant excessive pronation at the feet. The angle at which the quadriceps pulls on the patella is greater in women than in men. This can play a significant role in patients who present with knee pain. Women also tend to have smaller Achilles tendons and narrower heels than men do, which can impact footwear issues.

In the upper extremity, the elbow-carrying angle is increased in women, with a greater valgus position noted at rest. This may contribute to medial elbow strain and ulnar nerve symptoms. It has been noted that women suffer more than 60% of all repetitive motion injuries, many of which result in carpal tunnel syndrome and tendonitis.

The relative proportion of fast-twitch and slow-twitch fibers is similar in men and women.[5] The difference in muscle strength between men and women appears to be due to muscle size. Men and women have similar numbers and patterns of muscle fibers, but the fibers in women are smaller.

Physiology

Most of the research in exercise physiology in women has been done for endurance training. $\dot{V}O_2max$, the maximum rate of oxygen uptake, is a general measure of cardiovascular endurance. When measuring $\dot{V}O_2max$ and comparing it in athletes with similar lean body mass and training regime, women have 5% less aerobic capacity compared to men.[7] This is due, in part, to a proportionately greater amount of body fat, a lower muscle mass, and a lower hemoglobin concentration, compared to men. It has been reported that women have smaller hearts, smaller thoracic cages, and lower blood volumes than men. This is said to reduce their maximum oxygen carrying capacity, but it is unclear from the literature whether these differences are absolute or simply related to women's smaller physical size.

Musculoskeletal Injuries in Women

Musculoskeletal disorders affect a large segment of the population in the United States, with more than 21 million acute musculoskeletal injuries occurring per year and more than 40 million people with chronic conditions. Some of these diseases occur frequently in women, including arthritis, osteoporosis, low back pain, shoulder impingement, myofascial pain syndrome, carpal tunnel syndrome, and specific sports injuries such as anterior cruciate ligament (ACL) tears and patellofemoral dysfunction. Much of the research addressing such disorders has been conducted either in the workplace or in the athletic arena. Women suffer 63% of all repetitive motion injuries, accounting for 69% of lost work time cases from carpal tunnel syndrome and 61% of lost work time cases from tendonitis.[3,8]

In athletic venues, injury patterns generally have been shown to be sport-specific rather than gender-specific. However, there are exceptions to this finding, as epidemiologic studies have revealed that the ACL injury rate is much higher in women than in men, especially in the jumping and pivoting sports.[9,10] Griffen[11] reported that shoulder impingement, low back pain, ACL injuries, patellofemoral dysfunction, shin splints, stress fractures, Achilles tendonitis, and foot problems are common in women due to either gender-related anatomic differences or participation in specific sports.

Knee Injuries

Knee problems, including ACL injuries, are a serious concern among female athletes. The incidence of ACL injuries among women may be affected by a combination of anatomic, physiologic, and training issues; this is especially true in young women.[9] Multiple theories have been voiced as to why the incidence may be higher in women, including smaller intercondylar notch size, increased ligament laxity, greater angle of limb alignment, less muscle strength, less coordination, hormonal and endocrine influences, and specific sport-related skills. Research, however, has been inconclusive as to the cause of a gender difference.

Patellofemoral disorders are also more common in women than in men.[9,12] These syndromes are caused by problems in the knee extensor mechanism and surrounding soft tissue attachments. Patellar instability usually occurs secondary to instability due to traumatic forces, although chronic laxity and malalignment may be contributing factors as well. Patellar dislocation has been thought to recur more frequently in women, but further research is needed to determine if gender-specific anatomic differences such as increased quadriceps angle and a hypoplastic vastus medialis obliquus play a role in injury mechanisms and thus influence treatment.

Patellofemoral dysfunction without instability is poorly understood, but is frequently thought to be associated with the miserable malalignment syndrome often seen in women. Radiographic evaluations may be helpful, but often do not necessarily confirm alignment changes, making patellofemoral dysfunction difficult to treat. Recommendations for treatment include a closed-chained strengthening program that focuses on the quadriceps and extensor mechanism but includes the entire lower limb; posture modifications; possible orthotics for overpronation control; and McConnell taping or braces as needed as an adjunct to rehabilitation.[9]

Foot Injuries

Foot problems are also common in women, whether due to heredity or footwear. Bunions are caused by bursal inflammation over the prominence of the first metatarsal, and with enough pressure can contribute to the formation of a hallux valgus deformity. Further pressure on the second phalanx can cause hammertoes and plantar calluses. High-heeled shoes with a narrow toe box, along with an overpronated foot, can aggravate such deformities, and also contribute to Achilles tendonitis. Proper shoe-fitting advice includes sizing shoes to fit the larger foot, choosing a shoe that allows enough room in the toe box, and avoiding high heels. Careful selection of athletic shoes, paying special attention to motion and shock absorption, may also help prevent injury.

Carpal Tunnel Syndrome

Carpal tunnel syndrome is more common in women than men. This may be due to the types of jobs that women typically have or due to activities at home. Pregnant women are particularly predisposed to developing a transient carpal tunnel syndrome. Diagnosis should be with electrodiagnostic studies correlated with clinical findings. Treatment includes wrist splints to maintain a neutral position, nonsteroidal anti-inflammatory drugs, and avoidance of aggravating activity. In refractory or severe cases, surgical release may be necessary. Addressing proper ergonomics in the workplace and at home may help to prevent this condition.

Low Back Pain

Low back pain is common in men and women, but it is a particular problem in pregnant women. This is due to the altered biomechanics of carrying a child but also may be related to hormonal changes. The incidence appears to increase with age, repeat pregnancy, abdominal muscle weakness, and natural changes in posture and body habitus that accompany pregnancy. In addition, it has been suggested that the effects of relaxin on connective tissue may predispose the pregnant woman to sacroiliac pain.

Fibromyalgia

Fibromyalgia is more common in women than in men. It is covered in Chapter 16.

Training Issues

Women respond similarly to men to a strength training regimen, with an increase in the cross sectional area of their muscles. Because they have less testosterone, however, they do not experience the same increase in muscle mass. They do benefit from improved neural control of strength and synchronization of muscle firing and can therefore increase functional strength.[13] They also benefit from the bone-building aspects of activity.

Women's response to endurance training is comparable to that of men. When women and men train at similar levels of effort for similar tasks they have nearly identical rates of increases in $\dot{V}O_2max$, at least for up to 7 weeks of training.[14] At submaximal exercise loads, their heart rates decrease similarly. Endurance training increases slow-twitch (fatigue-resistant) muscle fiber area to a similar extent in women and men.[15] Of note, endurance training in pregnant women is influenced by the physiologic effects of pregnancy, which include the thermoregulatory and the cardiovascular systems.

Females are more flexible than males regardless of activity level or body weight.

Exercise in Pregnancy

Exercise is encouraged throughout pregnancy in those without medical conditions that otherwise limit activity.[16] Women with abnormal vaginal bleeding, hypertension, previous high-risk pregnancy, or cardiopulmonary disease should not exercise vigorously. General guidelines for exercise were modified in 1994 by the American College of Obstetrics and Gynecology[17] and are worth reviewing.

Pregnant women should avoid multijoint exercises after the first trimester, and in general should limit intensity and volume of strength training, with no prolonged supine lifting exercises late in pregnancy. Elite athletes who are not experiencing a high-risk pregnancy can continue an intense level of training if they are closely monitored by their medical team, and if training changes are individualized to their symptoms. Most women choose moderate activities such as swimming or walking. Activities that predispose pregnant women to either heat stress or abdominal trauma should be avoided. Women carrying twins may also be cautioned that the extra oxygen required by two fetuses might be compromised by overly vigorous exercise.

There is no clear-cut safe limit for maximum heart rate during pregnancy. The cardiovascular and metabolic effects of pregnancy limit the ability to use heart rate as a training gauge. Some prefer the Borg scale of perceived exertion and generally recommend that fatigue be the rate/intensity limiting factor. Activity should be in the "mild to moderate exertion" phase and should be carried out approximately three times per week as a general guideline.

Postpartum Training

The type of delivery may dictate the kind of activity and the time frame in which one can return to regular exercise postpartum. Vaginal delivery often results in a quicker return to previous training or exercise programs than does a Caesarian section. Caesarian section, as an abdominal surgery, causes trauma to the muscle layers that must be given time to heal before strenuous exercise is resumed. Most women undergoing Caesarian sections for childbirth will need to wait at least 6 weeks before return to their training or exercise programs; and a gradual progression of such a program is highly recommended. Dr. Shangold has noted some *minimum* waiting periods for resumption of activities, but very few women can return this quickly[18]:

> Following a vaginal delivery or a second-trimester abortion, weight training may be resumed the same day; aerobic exercise, except water sports, may be resumed in 2 days; water sports may be resumed when bleeding has ceased. . . . Following a cesarean delivery or other abdominal surgery (requiring an incision), light aerobic exercise outside of water and light weight training may be resumed in 7 days; intense aerobic exercise (speed work), submaximal weight training and water sports should be postponed at least 21 days.

Related Medical Concerns

Menstruation

Despite the fact that many women feel that menstruation impairs their athletic performance, there is no evidence of a consistent change in athletic performance at different parts of the menstrual cycle.[19] Occasionally, women may perform better during the follicular phase of their cycles, and if they are elite athletes, manipulation of their cycle with birth control pills to coincide with major athletic competition is an option.[18] However, performance benefits are small with this practice. No changes in training regimes are necessary during the menstrual bleeding phase of the cycle; however, women with anemia and profuse bleeding may become fatigued during this phase. Exercise, overall, does not cause any adverse effects on the menstrual cycle. However, vigorous exercise, especially in long-term training regimes, may lead to amenorrhea or oligomenorrhea. This is usually reversible and should be evaluated medically. Prolonged amenorrhea can impair bone density.

Because of menstrual losses, women obviously require adequate intake of iron.

Female Athlete Triad

The etiology of the female athlete triad (disordered eating, menstrual cycle irregularities, and osteoporosis) has not been conclusively defined in scientific research. However, it involves an intricate interaction between the hormonal, physiologic, and psychological systems in the female body. The triad is estimated to affect 25–30% of collegiate athletes. In addition, there is a disconcerting prevalence of young females with body image issues. Although the triad can be present in all types of sports, there appears to be a higher incidence in sports with weight class requirements or that stress body appearance. As young women begin to age, body weight and size are often seen as a driving force that encourages them to begin exercising, even if they have not previously been athletic. With the second decade being the peak bone density acquisition years, this may be a particularly bad time to develop these problems. Premature loss of bone density or lesser bone growth in this age group can lead to potentially irreversible bone weakening.

Treatment of the female athlete triad is aimed at prevention. Education includes teaching proper nutrition, training parameters, and recognition of physical symptoms that may signal physiologic energy imbalance. When physical symptoms are present, testing is aimed at the presenting issue (i.e., oligomenorrhea, stress fracture, fatigue).

Breast

Breast issues have received significant media attention regarding the rising rates of breast cancer and legal issues surrounding the risk of breast implants. Traumatic injuries to the breast can occur, although not commonly, especially in women who participate in contact sports; for this reason, implants are not recommended in some elite athletes. Implants also reduce the proportion of lean body mass and thus slightly reduce athletic performance. Prevention of breast injuries of any type—contusions, hematomas, abrasions, or otherwise—is especially recommended in athletic women through proper bra selection. Supportive bras may also decrease postexercise breast pain. Suggestions include a firm, nonelastic bra, in women with a cup size of at least a B, to reduce excessive breast movement during running or bouncing activities.

Osteoporosis

Osteoporosis is a major public health problem in the United States, affecting 20 million people per year and accounting for more than a million fractures annually. Women lose up to 4–6% of bone mass in the first 4–5 years after menopause. Weight-bearing exercise, adequate calcium intake, avoidance of amenorrhea, and, possibly, hormone replacement or other drug therapy may help to reduce the problems associated with this condition.

Points of Summary

1. Women have less muscle mass than men, and are limited in building muscle mass because they have less testosterone.
2. Women have a lower $\dot{V}O_2$max than do men. This is due to many reasons, including greater body fat proportion and lower hemoglobin.
3. Women are predisposed to certain musculoskeletal problems, including anterior cruciate ligament (ACL) tears, patellofemoral dysfunction, carpal tunnel syndrome (CTS), and foot problems.
4. Heat stress and abdominal trauma should be avoided during pregnancy.
5. Mild to moderate exercise should be encouraged in pregnant women in whom exercise is not contraindicated.
6. Menstruation has minimal, if any, effects on athletic performance.
7. The female athletic triad can result in permanent bone weakening.

References

1. Praemer A, Furner S, Rice DP. Musculoskeletal Conditions in the U.S. Rosemont, IL: American Academy of Orthopaedic Surgeons, 1999.
2. Ehrilich, M. Statement to the House Labor/Health and Human Services/ Education Subcommittee on Appropriations. American Academy of Orthopaedic Surgeons. February 4, 1998.
3. Rosenstock L, Lee L. Women, work, and health. J Am Med Women's Assoc 1999;55.
4. Fullerton H. Labor force projections to 2008: steady growth and changing composition. Monthly Labor Review 1999;11:19–32.
5. Sanborn C, Jankowski C. Gender-Specific Physiology. In R Agostini (ed), Medical and Orthopedic Issues of Active and Athletic Women. Philadelphia: Hanley & Belfus, 1994.
6. Staheli LT. Rotational problems of the lower extremities. Orthop Clin North Am 1987;18:503–512.
7. Sparling PB. A metaanalysis of studies comparing maximal oxygen uptake in men and women. Res Q Exerc Sport 1980;51:542.
8. Survey of Occupational Injuries and Illnesses, 1998. Washington, DC: US Department of Labor, Bureau of Labor Statistics, 1999.
9. Arendt EA. Common musculoskeletal injuries in women. Phys Sports Med 1996;24:7.

10. Arendt E, Dick R. Knee injury patterns among men and women in collegiate basketball and soccer: NCAA data and review of literature. Am J Sports Med 1995;23:694–701.
11. Griffen LY. Orthopedic Concerns. In M Shangold, G Mirkin (eds), Women and Exercise: Physiology and Sports Medicine (2nd ed). Philadelphia: FA Davis, 1994;235.
12. Whiteside PA. Men's and women's injuries in comparable sports. Phys Sports Med 1980;8:130–140.
13. Pauls J. Soft tissue disorders: the female athlete. Orthop Phys Ther Clin North Am 1996;5:137–167.
14. Eddy DO, Sparks KL, Adelizi DA. The effects of continuous and interval training in women and men. Eur J Appl Physiol 1977;37:83–92.
15. Drinkwater BL. Women and exercise: physiological aspects. Exerc Sport Sci Rev 1984;12:21–51.
16. Williams KR, Cavanaugh PR, Qiff JL. Biomechanical studies of elite female distance runners. Int J Sports Med 1987;8(S2):107–118.
17. American College of Obstetrics and Gynecology. Exercise during pregnancy and the postpartum period. Technical Bulletin No. 189, Feb 1994.
18. Shangold MM, Mirkin G (eds). Women and Exercise: Physiology and Sports Medicine. Philadelphia: FA Davis, 1988.
19. Brooks-Gunn J, Gargiulo J, Warren MP. Menstrual Cycle and Athletic Performance. In JL Puhl, CH Brown (eds), The Menstrual Cycle and Physical Activity. Champaign, IL: Human Kinetics Publishers, 1986;13–28.

Suggested Readings

Agostini R (ed). Medical and Orthopedic Issues of Active and Athletic Women. Philadelphia: Hanley & Belfus, Inc., 1994.

American College of Obstetrics and Gynecology. Exercise during pregnancy and the postpartum period. Technical Bulletin No. 189, Feb 1994.

Shangold M, Mirkin G (eds). Women and Exercise: Physiology and Sports Medicine (2nd ed). Philadelphia: FA Davis, 1994.

20 Musculoskeletal Issues in Persons with Disabilities

Joanne B. (Anne) Allen and Rayden C. Cody

The modern era has witnessed, for the first time, a large group of aging persons with significant physical disabilities. This group is remaining active through sports and independent activity. It is recognized that people with disabilities can enhance their cardiovascular health, flexibility, mobility, and coordination by participating in regular exercise.[1] However, this is resulting in a significant number of persons with disability who are developing primary or secondary musculoskeletal problems.

The impact of musculoskeletal dysfunction on a physically disabled individual can have far-reaching implications that may further limit the capacity for independent activity. A secondary musculoskeletal injury in a disabled person can increase physical demands on support structures that are otherwise required for normal activities, thus severely limiting independence. This type of difficulty is the primary focus of this chapter.

Musculoskeletal Injuries in the Disabled

Epidemiology

There have been numerous investigations describing injury profiles in the disabled.[2-7] A large number of these have involved retrospective questionnaires given to paralympic wheelchair athletes; many may have been subject to recall bias and inadequate injury definitions, resulting in over-reporting. Nevertheless, the sports medicine model functions well as an approach to addressing musuloskeletal injuries in the disabled.

A 1990 review concluded that injury patterns in disabled athletes are similar to those seen in able-bodied athletes.[2] The majority of these injuries involve soft tissues (sprains, strains, and overuse syndromes). It has also been noted that within the disabled athletic population, injury location is disability- and sport-dependent. In a cross-disability, retrospective study of 426 disabled athletes, 57% of wheelchair athlete injuries involved the shoulder, whereas athletes with cerebral palsy have a 21% incidence of knee injury.[3]

The Athletes with Disabilities Injury Registry[8] has reported an injury rate of 9.3 per 1,000 athlete exposures, which is similar to what has been reported for college football and soccer but higher than that observed in men's and women's basketball. It is obvious from this registry that musculoskeletal injuries are commonly seen in the athletic disabled population, as they are in the able-bodied.

Overuse Injuries

The disabled population experiences a large number of overuse injuries. The location of these injuries varies with the type of disability and the activity or sport. Individuals in wheelchairs are more likely to sustain upper extremity overuse injuries, whereas lower extremity injuries are more commonly encountered in the ambulatory disabled—that is, those with amputations and cerebral palsy.[3,7,9] Because of these differences, this chapter addresses upper and lower extremity problems separately. Because of the limits of space, only the more common conditions, and those with special features related to disability, are covered. Disabled persons can obviously also have any of the numerous other problems covered in this book.

Upper Extremity Injuries

Shoulder

Prolonged, repetitive, and forceful overhead activities predispose to shoulder problems, especially impingement. It is little wonder then that wheelchair users, who are lower to the ground than standing individuals, are particularly susceptible to shoulder problems. These individuals also have to transfer and propel themselves, which further stresses the shoulder.

Stroke patients often have shoulder problems due to inferior subluxation of the humeral head. This is due to a loss of scapular stabilization, which causes the shoulder to tilt downward, resulting in loss of ligamentous restraint to this subluxation. Proper positioning is essential early on.

Impingement Syndrome or Rotator Cuff Tendinosis

Wheelchair users are often diagnosed with impingement syndrome or rotator cuff tendinosis. These are related overuse conditions that involve the repetitive entrapment of the subacromial bursa and the tendon of the supraspinatus between the humeral head below and the coracoacromial arch above. Repeated shoulder external rotation, internal rotation, and overhead activities predispose persons to these conditions. With continued insult, the bursa becomes inflamed and the tendon shows signs of degeneration, resulting in pain and decreased function.

During wheelchair propulsion, the shoulder is maintained at approximately 70 degrees of abduction.[10] At the beginning of the propulsive phase of motion, the shoulder is extended and internally rotated. At the end of this motion, the shoulder is flexed and externally rotated. It is these repetitive motions that often cause wheelchair users to have well-developed shoulder flexors, internal rotators, and abductors. However, these individuals often have poorly developed external rotators and scapular stabilizers. The repetitive nature of the wheelchair push, coupled with these muscular imbalances and poor wheelchair posture, predispose wheelchair users to rotator cuff impingement and, later, tendinosis. Transfers place more significant loads on the shoulder and can cause acute injury in a joint weakened by overuse.

The proper treatment of rotator cuff impingement or tendinosis involves a period of rest to control pain and inflammation. This is often difficult in the wheelchair-dependent, as they rely exclusively on their upper limbs for mobility and weight-bearing tasks. Once the pain and inflammation has been controlled, a flexibility and graduated functional strengthening program is initiated, targeting the muscle imbalances and identified inadequacies described above. In severe cases in which degeneration has resulted in a rotator cuff tear, a motorized wheelchair or surgery may be warranted. A motorized chair, however, alters the patient's self-image of independence and leads to reduced physical activity and deconditioning.

Bicipital Tendinosis
Bicipital tendinosis and full or partial tearing of the long head of the biceps tendon should always be considered in the differential diagnosis of shoulder pain in manual wheelchair users. A study by Gellman et al. found it to be the most common shoulder injury in his group of wheelchair athletes.[11] It is often associated with impingement and can be a particular problem during transfers.

The treatment of bicipital tendinosis is similar to rotator cuff problems and involves an initial period of rest, followed by a graduated, functional strengthening program with emphasis on eccentric strengthening exercises.

Elbow and Wrist

Like the shoulder, the elbow is predisposed to overuse injuries in the wheelchair-dependent population.[5–7] The most common diagnosis reported is wrist extensor tendinosis (lateral epicondylitis).

Ulnar neuropathy at the elbow and carpal tunnel syndrome (CTS) have also been described in the wheelchair population. This association is due to a variety of predisposing factors, including repetitive elbow and wrist flexion and extension and direct compression (especially of the median nerve).

Wrist Extensor Tendinosis
Wrist extensor tendinosis is an overuse injury involving the extensor carpi radialis brevis. Histologic studies demonstrate a degenerative process in the tendon 1–3 cm from its origin on the lateral epicondyle. During wheelchair propulsion, the elbow is forcefully extended and the wrist goes from flexion-supination to extension-pronation.[12] Repetition of this motion can lead to overuse syndromes of the wrist extensor-supinator and flexor-pronator complexes. Wheelchair tennis players may be further predisposed to this injury if they have poor form (leading elbow on a backhand stroke) or improper equipment (tennis racquet too heavy or grip too small).

Like any tendinosis, the mainstay of early treatment for wrist extensor tendinosis is unloading the affected tendon. This is accomplished with counter-force bracing and use within the limits of pain. Once the pain is controlled, a flexibility and graduated functional strengthening program is begun, with the emphasis on eccentric exercises, as tolerated.

Ulnar Neuropathy at the Elbow

The ulnar nerve is susceptible to chronic repetitive irritation at the elbow. In the non-disabled sport population, ulnar neuropathy at the elbow is the most common upper limb entrapment neuropathy, whereas in the wheelchair athlete it is second only to CTS.[13] It should be diagnosed by electrodiagnostic study (electromyography [EMG]) correlated with clinical findings. Burnham et al.[13] demonstrated that 19.4% of the 28 wheelchair athletes in their series had EMG evidence of ulnar neuropathy at the elbow. Possible etiologies include entrapment of the nerve between the two heads of the flexor carpi ulnaris during use and prolonged pressure on the elbow and proximal forearm when resting against a wheelchair armrest.

The ulnar nerve is particularly vulnerable to injury in wheelchair racquet sports. Valgus extension overload at the elbow with repeated forehand serve strokes may lead to ulnar collateral ligament insufficiency, in turn leading to increased traction of the ulnar nerve.

Treatment involves protection of the ulnar nerve from further compression with elbow pads, in addition to avoidance of prolonged elbow flexion (nighttime extension splint). Direct pressure on the nerve is avoided, and predisposing activities and poor biomechanics must be corrected. If patients fail such conservative care, surgical decompression or transposition of the nerve may be necessary. Surgery should be avoided if at all possible, as it carries significant risks and may not resolve the symptoms.

Carpal Tunnel Syndrome

CTS is commonly seen in the manual wheelchair–dependent population. Possible etiologies include direct repeated compression and frequent wrist extension, both of which occur during wheelchair propulsion. Wrist tendonitis may also be a cause. Carpal tunnel pressures are increased during wrist extension in wheelchair users as compared to ambulatory individuals.[14] A 46% incidence of CTS was found in a series of wheelchair athletes. Few had clinical evidence of carpal tunnel syndrome.[13] Diagnosis should be confirmed by EMG.

Treatment is similar to CTS in the able-bodied population, and includes wrist splints to maintain a neutral position, nonsteroidal anti-inflammatory drugs, and avoidance of aggravating activities (obviously difficult in the wheelchair user). If symptoms do not improve, especially in persons with severe symptoms or in the face of significant nerve damage detected by EMG, surgical release should be considered.

Lower Extremity and Spine Injuries

Lower extremity injuries are seen frequently in individuals with amputations, as well as in those with cerebral palsy.[8,15] In amputees, an ill-fitting or worn-out prosthesis is often to blame, and special attention must be paid to the length and composition of the stump and any weakness, contractures, or muscle imbalances that may be present.

In cerebral palsy, injuries are frequently caused by the stressors of inefficient ambulation, compounded by spasticity. Falls are also more common than in the general population.

Lower extremity injuries can also be seen in other disability groups, including those with stroke, brain injury, and spinal cord injury, but in the current sports-based research, they appear less frequently.

Data collected in the Athletes with Disabilities Registry[8] reveal that the lower extremity is involved in injury at least 21% of the time. Athletes with cerebral palsy appear to sustain injuries to the knee more commonly than injuries to the leg or ankle.[15] In amputees playing soccer, the majority of the injures are to the knee and ankle.[16]

Knee

In below-knee amputees, the knee can have an excessive valgus or varus stress placed on it if the prosthetic foot is situated too medially or laterally. If the foot is too far forward or is plantarflexed, it can cause a back-bending force on the knee, leading to genu recurvatum. If the foot is too far backwards, the socket too flexed, or the ankle too dorsiflexed, it can cause the knee to lurch forward during heel strike, which can lead to loss of balance as well as excessive stress on the quadriceps, extensor mechanism, and patellofemoral joint. All of these things must be considered in evaluating knee problems in a below-knee amputee. Because foot and ankle devices determine the position of the knee, special attention must be given to these areas.

Persons with cerebral palsy, stroke, or other causes of spasticity can have excessive plantiflexion posturing of the foot. This also leads to genu recurvatum, and may need correction with an ankle-foot orthosis. External rotation of the leg during ambulation can cause increased stress on the medial knee structures.

Patellofemoral Dysfunction

Malalignment between the patella and the trochlear groove can cause pain by transmitting abnormal forces to the patellofemoral joint. Most patellofemoral dysfunction occurs because of a muscular imbalance in the extensor mechanism of the quadriceps and its surrounding soft tissue attachments. Patellofemoral pain syndrome can have an insidious onset, with complaints of pain after sitting for a long time or going up and down stairs. These patients often have tenderness of the medial patella and on patellar compression. They often have a relative weakness of the vastus medialis. Treatment in both able-bodied and disabled persons is conservative, emphasizing quadriceps strengthening and proper biomechanics.

Low Back Pain

A frequent complaint of lower extremity amputees is low back pain, which is often related to a limb-length discrepancy or an imbalanced prosthesis. This can often be easily corrected with proper alignment of components. In addition, a lumbar and abdominal strengthening program can be of benefit as the center of gravity can change in amputees, especially in bilateral lower extremity amputees.

Skin Breakdown

A lower extremity that is insensate or has a neuropathic component is also susceptible to skin problems. Proper skin care and adequate self-examination are essential to avoid such complications. This is important in many types of disability, including spinal cord injuries (SCI) and in patients who have sensory loss in the lower limbs. It is particularly a problem in wheelchair athletes, who sometimes spend long periods of time in a streamlined racing position without proper pressure release. In amputees, poor prosthetic fit or inadequate skin care can also lead to skin breakdown.

Other

Myofascial pain syndrome is frequently diagnosed in wheelchair users. Proper sitting posture and wheelchair fitting is required, as is counseling in proper biomechanics and rest.

Osteoporotic fractures are a common complication in SCI. Loss of bone mineral content causes these individuals to have significant predisposition to pathologic lower extremity fractures.[17] The lower extremity fracture incidence has been reported to be between 4% and 6% in the SCI population,[18] which is probably an underestimate. SCI patients who ambulate with braces or other adaptive devices should be made aware of these statistics and cautioned appropriately.

Persons with SCIs can have abnormal thermoregulation. If they engage in athletic pursuits, they can be susceptible to such problems, and care must be taken to avoid complications such as hyperthermia. Bowel and bladder care must also be maintained, especially avoiding overfilling of the bladder or dehydration and urinary tract infections.

Points of Summary

1. The impact of musculoskeletal problems on the disabled can be much greater than similar problems in others.
2. Musculoskeletal problems are common in the disabled due to abnormal biomechanics and compensatory movements.
3. Wheelchair users are particularly susceptible to upper extremity problems.
4. Persons with amputations or cerebral palsy are particularly susceptible to lower extremity problems.
5. Amputee musculoskeletal problems are often due to improper prosthetic fitting.

References

1. Glaser RM, Janssen TW, Suryaprasad AG, et al. The Physiology of Exercise. In DF Apple (ed), Rehabilitation Research and Development Service;

Physical Fitness: A Guide for Individuals with Spinal Cord Injury. Baltimore, MD: Scientific and Technical Publications Section, 1997:3–23.

2. Ferrara MS, Davis RW. Injuries to elite wheelchair athletes. Paraplegia 1990;28:335–341.
3. Ferrara MS, Buckley WE, McCann BC, et al. The injury experience of the competitive athlete with a disability: prevention implications. Med Sci Sports Exerc 1992;24:184–188.
4. Ferrara MS, Peterson CL. Injuries to athletes with disabilities: identifying injury patterns. Sports Med 2000;30(2):137–143.
5. Curtis KA, Dillon DA. Survey of wheelchair athletic injuries: common patterns and prevention. Paraplegia 1985;23:170–175.
6. Hoeberigs JH, Debets-Eggen HB, Debets PM. Sports medical experience from the international flower marathon for disabled wheelers. Am J Sports Med 1990;18(4):418–421.
7. Taylor D, Williams T. Sports injuries in athletes with disabilities: wheelchair racing. Paraplegia 1995;33:296–299.
8. Ferrara MS, Buckley WE. Athletes with disabilities injury registry. Adaptive Physical Activity Quarterly 1996;13:50–60.
9. Burnham R, May L, Nelson E, et al. Shoulder pain in wheelchair athletes: the role of muscle imbalance. Am J Sports Med 1993;21:238–242.
10. Harburn KL, Spaulding SJ. Muscle activity in the spinal cord injured during wheelchair ambulation. Am J Occup Ther 1983;40:629–636.
11. Gellman H, Sie I, Waters RL. Late complications of the weight-bearing upper extremity in the paraplegic patient. Clin Orthop 1988;233:132–135
12. Boninger ML, et al. Wrist biomechanics during two speeds of wheelchair propulsion: an analysis using a local coordinate system. Arch Phys Med Rehab 1997;78:364–372.
13. Burnham RS, Steadward RD. Upper extremity peripheral nerve entrapments among wheelchair athletes: prevalence, location and risk factors. Arch Phys Med Rehabil 1994;75:519–524
14. Aljure J, Eltorai I, Bradley WE, et al. Carpal tunnel syndrome in paraplegic patients. Paraplegia 1985;23:182–186.
15. Stopka C. An overview of common injuries to individuals with disabilities: Part I. Palaestra 1996;12(1):44–51.
16. Kegel B, Malchow D. Incidence of injury in amputees playing soccer. Palaestra 1994;10(2):50–54.
17. Biering-Sorenson F, Bohr H, Schaadt O. Bone mineral content of the lumbar spine and lower extremities years after spinal cord lesion. Paraplegia 1988;26:293–301.
18. Ingram RR, Suman RK, Freeman PA. Lower limb fractures in the chronic spinal cord injured patient. Paraplegia 1989;27:133–139.

Suggested Readings

Bloomquist LE. Injuries to athletes with physical disabilities: prevention implications. Phys Sports Med 1986;14(9):97–105.

Cooper RA. Wheelchair Selection and Configuration. New York: Demos, 1998.

Ferrara MS, et al. The injury experience of the competitive athlete with a disability: prevention implications. Med Sci Sports Exerc 1992;24:184–188.

Stopka C. An overview of common injuries to individuals with disabilities: Part I. Palaestra 1996;12(1):44–51.

Taylor D, Williams T. Sports injuries in athletes with disabilities: wheelchair racing. Paraplegia 1995;33:296–299.

21   Chronic Pain

Angela T. Carbone and Mark S. Randall

Chronic Pain and Chronic Pain Syndrome

Chronic pain is defined as pain present for more than 6 months or present long after the expected time of healing, regardless of whether ongoing tissue injury is present. Pain is more than a physiologic response to injury; there is a large emotional component that may elicit a flight or fight response and can evoke past painful memories. Many studies have established the importance of the psychological state in affecting pain perception.[1] The biomedical model holds that nociception, the transmission and modulation of pain signals, and the feeling of pain are a biologically predetermined course of action. This explanation is rooted in dualistic Cartesian (the mind and body are separate) thinking.[2] The biopsychosocial model advocates a more comprehensive and inclusionary awareness of musculoskeletal pain and psychological factors. Therefore, the biopsychosocial model moves away from the view that organic pain can be explained purely through physiologic mechanisms.

There is a distinction between chronic pain and chronic pain syndrome. Patients who suffer from chronic pain usually have an ongoing chronically painful condition, such as degenerative arthritis, which causes intermittent pain or constant but variable pain intensities throughout the course of the disease. These patients have appropriate behaviors and function in relation to the degree of tissue injury. Chronic pain syndrome is characterized by diffuse pain that is not related to ongoing tissue injury, as well as behavioral changes, sleep disturbance, functional impairments, disruptive personal life, depression, and possible misuse of drugs, braces, and assistive devices.

The treatment of chronic pain syndrome requires a comprehensive, multidisciplinary approach with traditional, behavioral, and complementary medicine. The team includes the patient, family, primary care physician, physician consultants, pain psychologist, physical or occupational therapist, and nurse. Some centers also include a hypnotist, biofeedback specialist, or acupuncturist. Physician consultants who specialize in the management of pain include physiatrists, neurologists, neurosurgeons, anesthesiologists, and orthopedic surgeons. It is important that the appropriate members of the team be identified and that an individualized care plan be closely coordinated. This helps to ensure that ineffective treatments are not repeated and that treatments that may be effective are done in a timely manner. The major goals of a multidisciplinary program are typically focused on returning the patient to work, maximizing function, teaching the patient self-management skills, reducing or eliminating future medical use, avoiding recurrence of injury, and avoiding medication abuse or dependence.[3]

Epidemiology

One of the most common reasons for a patient to seek medical attention is pain. In fact, approximately 75–80% of patient visits are due to a painful condition.[4] It is also estimated that one-third of all Americans have a chronically painful condition and that 17.0–50.4 million Americans are debilitated to some extent by their pain.[5]

Pain Pathways

Nociceptors are pain-sensitive neurons. These small fiber neurons are divided into the thin, myelinated A-δ fibers and the unmyelinated C fibers. Both fibers end in laminae I, II, and X of the dorsal horn. Interneurons in lamina I and III appear to play a role in inhibition of nociceptive afferents by releasing a neurotransmitter known as *γ-aminobutyric acid* or *enkephalin*. These interneurons are stimulated by the inhibitory descending pathway and by large fiber afferent neurons. When these inhibitory mechanisms are compromised (e.g., in nerve damage), the threshold for pain is reduced. Under these conditions, innocuous stimuli can provoke a poorly localized burning pain, hyperalgesia, allodynia, or enlargement of the painful area. This is largely due to structural changes that occur in the central nervous system known as *central plasticity*. Phantom limb pain is the classic example of this mechanism.

There are several neurotransmitters responsible for pain inhibition. First, endogenous opioids, enkephalins, endorphins, and dynorphins act at the same receptor sites in the brain and spinal cord as morphine to produce a significant reduction in pain intensity. Serotonin and norepinephrine in the midbrain activate the descending inhibitory pathway. This pathway then activates the interneurons at the spinal level to release enkephalins and γ-aminobutyric acid, thus producing a decreased pain response.

In 1965, Melzack and Wall[6] proposed the gate control theory. This stated that non-painful stimuli (vibration and light touch via large A-β fibers) could inhibit nociceptive activity. The theory was modified in 1991 based on more recent findings on pain mechanisms.[7] The original theory is supported by evidence that direct stimulation to the nociceptive afferent nerve fibers results in some pain inhibition. This helps explain the pain relieving effect of counterirritants such as heat, cold, and rubbing.

The etiology of chronically painful conditions can be divided into at least four separate categories: somatic, visceral, neuropathic, and psychological. Somatic etiologies include musculoskeletal problems such as degenerative arthritis, vertebral facet arthropathy, rheumatoid arthritis, and fibromyalgia. Visceral pain is pain originating from the soft tissues of the thorax, abdomen, and pelvis. It is poorly localized and poorly defined. Patients complain of diffuse, dull, sharp, throbbing or burning pain. Some common chronic visceral pain syndromes include endometriosis, colitis, interstitial cystitis, and chronic pelvic pain. Neuropathic etiologies include phantom limb pain, reflex sympathetic dystrophy (complex regional pain syndrome), post-stroke central pain syndrome, peripheral neuropathies, and so forth. This type of pain responds poorly to opioid treatment. Psychological etiologies are usually due to life stresses that manifest as pain.

Emotions and Musculoskeletal Pain

Pain is a multidimensional occurrence that includes sensory and affective components.[8] A complete understanding of an individual's pain requires a full understanding of the emotional interaction of anxiety, depression, and anger with reported physical pain.

Depression

The incidence of depression in persons with chronic pain is higher than in the general population. Estimated depression rates of 30–54% among chronic pain syndrome patients indicate that depression is a significant issue among these individuals.[9] Depression acts in synergy with other psychological factors to worsen symptoms. These include somatization (tendency to magnify physiologic sensations), catastrophizing (negative expectations about the future), social/interpersonal impairments, poor life control (decreased perceived control), and interference (intrusion in life activities).[10]

Anxiety

Anxiety has also been found to be more common in chronic pain patients than in the general population. Asmundson et al.[11] found that 17.8% of their study sample of chronic musculoskeletal pain patients met the criteria for a current anxiety disorder. McCracken et al.[12] found that anxiety accounted for 16–54% of the statistical variance in pain report, disability, and pain-related behavior.

Interesting developments in the study of anxiety have also suggested a construct termed *fear/avoidance*.[13] This idea proposes that the avoidance of painful activity results in various chronic pain syndromes characterized by a sequence of decreased activity, fear, loss of self-efficacy, negative affect, and deconditioning that leads to greater avoidance of pain-related behavior.[13]

Anger

In comparison to depression and anxiety, anger has received much less consideration with respect to chronic pain. In a review of the literature by Fernandez and Turk concerning anger and chronic pain conditions, results indicated that many researchers have noted the co-occurrence of anger and hostility among patients with pain conditions.[14] Although the role of anger in causing or perpetuating pain is difficult to study, the end result of anger among patients with pain appears to be noteworthy to treatment dynamics.

Clinical Assessment

An extensive pain history should be taken to prevent repeating unnecessary tests or use of ineffective therapies. The history should include the character of pain (e.g., dull, sharp, burning, numbing, achy), anatomic location, onset (sudden, gradual, inciting event), duration (constant, intermittent), chronicity, intensity, aggravating and alleviating activities or modalities, and associated disturbances (e.g., sleep, depression, libido). A pain diagram is a helpful tool for pain location and character assessment. The visual analog scale can be used to measure pain intensity. The history should also include past medications (and why the medications were discontinued), a complete list of previous physicians, a list of treatment modalities (physical therapy, chiropractic care, injections, and surgeries), and a list of diagnostic tests and results.

The initial psychological workup of a pain patient typically includes an informative pain history, essentially an assessment of the individual's current mental status and pain condition. This information is gathered through various sources, including the patient interview, interviews of significant others (if required), review of medical records, review of past psychological and psychiatric records, and administration of psychological and pain assessment instruments.[15] Psychometric instruments for evaluating pain impairment, disability, pain beliefs, coping strategies, depression, anxiety, and personality are also integral to a comprehensive assessment of the pain patient.[15] Physical examination is performed, focusing on the musculoskeletal and neurologic systems, to identify any treatable causes of the pain. The examination also can help identify any nonorganic components to the patient's pain complaint, and in some cases can lead to performing further diagnostic tests.

Waddell et al. reported five major physical examination findings that are helpful in the assessment of nonorganic low back pain[16]: tenderness (superficial, nonanatomic); overreaction; simulation (axial loading and rotation); distraction; and regional weakness/sensory loss. For example, a patient who has muscle weakness in toe extension, dorsiflexion, and plantarflexion on manual muscle testing but can walk on his heels with his toes extended strongly suggests a nonorganic component to his or her pain complaint. The classic distraction test is the sitting straight leg test versus the supine straight leg test. The clinician gives the patient the impression that the pulses in each foot are being checked as opposed to performing a neural stretch on the sciatic nerve. Most patients complain of pain when supine rather than while sitting. Patients may also demonstrate a ratcheting movement on manual muscle testing. This is non-physiologic and can make it difficult to assess true strength. To get a better sense of a patient's true strength, bilateral muscle groups should be tested simultaneously when possible.

Treatment

The goals of treatment are the "4 A's": Maximize *analgesia* and *activities* of daily living while minimizing *adverse* reactions and *aberrant* behaviors. Based on the history and various assessments, an individualized treatment program is initiated. Patient education includes lifestyle changes (smoking, caffeine intake, inactivity, poor sleep hygiene, and excessive alcohol), coping skills, medication facts, pacing activities, and realistic goal setting. Sleep hygiene and relaxation techniques are also part of patient education. Smoking cessation classes (with or without hypnosis) and dietary consultation for weight reduction can also be helpful in the management of pain.

Treatment for chronic pain syndrome requires various physical and psychotherapeutic strategies to match the patient's particular symptoms. Physical and occupational therapy may be used, but the emphasis should be on teaching the patient to manage the pain, rather than relying on modalities or others to do so. The therapist is a key educator for the patient and family to learn self-massage, ice massage, and distraction techniques to reduce pain non-pharmacologically. Psychological intervention is one of the keys to successful management of chronic pain syndrome and includes techniques such as operant conditioning, cognitive-behavioral therapy, psychodynamic therapy, biofeedback and relaxation therapy, hypnosis and imagery, group therapy, and family therapy. As a broad focus, the psychological treatment should emphasize that the individual has the ability to exert control over his or her responses to pain.

Medications

Medications are almost always used in the treatment of chronic pain and chronic pain syndrome. The World Health Organization promotes a stepladder approach to the treatment of cancer pain. In this approach, mild to moderate pain is treated with acetaminophen or a nonsteroidal anti-inflammatory drug with or without adjuvant therapy, such as physical modalities, ice, heat, and nonopioid medications. If this does not improve the patient's pain, then a combination of opioid and nonsteroidal anti-inflammatory drugs or acetaminophen is tried along with adjuvant treatment. The same principles can apply to chronic pain management; however, there is controversy with regard to the use of opioids in the treatment of chronic pain syndromes. The American Academy of Pain Medicine and the American Pain Society published a consensus statement in support of the prudent use of opioids in a well-controlled environment with frequent re-evaluation of drug efficacy in the management of chronic pain.[17] However, the clinician must keep in mind the mechanisms that are causing the persistence of pain, and use the drugs that have specifically been proven to be effective in the treatment of specific pain syndromes. Some of the more commonly used medications, along with mechanism of action, clinical usefulness, and side effects, are listed in Table 21.1.

Injections

There are several types of injection procedures that are typically part of the armamentarium in the management of pain. These include joint injections, trigger point injections, nerve blocks, and epidural injections. Generally these have short-term benefits, but when used in conjunction with oral medications and physical therapy, activity levels may be increased more rapidly than with oral medications alone. Injections should not be overused in chronic pain states.

TABLE 21.1 Medications commonly used in the treatment of chronic pain

Medications	Mechanism of action	Clinical use	Side effects
Acetaminophen	Weak inhibitor of inflammmation, inhibits prostaglandin production and release	Mild to moderate pain such as headache, myalgias, and arthralgias	Allergic rash, thrombocytopenia, hepatic damage in high doses
Nonsteroidal anti-inflammatories	Strong anti-inflammatory, inhibits prostaglandin production and release	Mild to moderate pain such as headache, myalgias, and arthralgias	Allergic rash, peptic ulcer disease, renal insufficiency, acute renal failure
Capsaicin cream	Stimulates the release of substance P and inhibits the reuptake in the periphery	Osteoarthritis, phantom limb pain, post-herpetic neuralgia	Local irritation, which usually improves with each application
Tricyclic antidepressants	Not well understood; inhibits the reuptake of norepinephrine and serotonin	Neuropathic pain, fibromyalgia, chronic pain syndromes, help with sleep and depression	Dry mouth, headache, AM drowsiness, weight gain, dizziness
Antiseizure	Stabilizes cell membranes to increase the depolarization threshold	Neuropathic pain, trigeminal neuralgia	Sedation, dizziness, confusion, nystagmus, ataxia, gingival hypertrophy, osteomalacia
Benzodiazepines	Inhibit spinal reflexes via the suppression of the brain stem reticular system	Use is limited secondary to side effects; may be used short term as a muscle relaxant or sleep aid	Highly addictive, sedation, confusion, ataxia, vivid dreams, nausea, headache, impaired sexual function
Baclofen	γ-Aminobutric acid derivative inhibiting the pain pathway at the spinal cord level	Myalgias, neuropathic pain, pain associated with muscle spasticity	Drowsiness, weakness, confusion, seizures, dizziness, ataxia
Tizanidine	Central β_2-adrenergic agonist, reduces substance P release	Neuropathic pain, pain associated with muscle spasticity	Hypotension, dizziness, sedation
Opioids	Bind to the mu, kappa, and delta receptors inhibiting the release of excitatory neurotransmitters	Most types of pain, poor response in fibromyalgia and neuropathic pain	Nausea, vomiting, constipation, sedation, pruritis

Invasive Procedures

The use of invasive procedures is considered a last resort. Spinal cord stimulation has shown to be very promising in the treatment of neuropathic, sympathetically mediated and ischemic pain syndromes.[18,19] Neurosurgical techniques such as nerve decompression, laminectomies and carpal tunnel release, intrathecal pumps for baclofen or morphine, and ablation procedures, such as dorsal root rhizotomies, radiofrequency facet denervation, intradiskal electrotherapy, and symphectomy have also been employed in the management of pain.[20]

Acupuncture

Acupuncture is becoming the most popular complementary therapy for the relief of pain. It is currently being used by approximately 1 million Americans annually.[21] There have been several studies in the use of acupuncture and chronic pain syndromes, but the results are inconsistent with regard to its efficacy. There may be a role for acupuncture in the treatment of pain, but further studies and better treatment designs need to be developed to better assess the usefulness of this modality.

Points of Summary

1. The biopsychosocial approach is a comprehensive and inclusionary model that offers the practitioner the ability to consider physiologic, psychological, and social factors in treating the pain patient.
2. A multidisciplinary approach that views pain as a complex, multifactorial phenomenon involving sensory, cognitive, affective, and behavioral components is the best approach to treatment.
3. Depression, anxiety, and anger have been the main emotions researched and studied with respect to musculoskeletal pain.
4. Treatment strategies are multiple and offer specific advantages for various pain syndromes from both a physiologic and psychological perspective.
5. Chronic pain is rarely completely eliminated, but a reduction in the intensity, frequency, and duration of pain, along with increased activity, is the major goal of treatment.

References

1. Baum A, Gatchel RJ, Krantz D. An Introduction to Health Psychology. New York: McGraw-Hill, 1997.
2. Block A, Kremer E, Fernandez E (eds). Handbook of Pain Syndromes. New Jersey: Lawrence Erlbaum Associates, 1999.
3. Gatchel RJ, Turk DC. Interdisciplinary Treatment of Chronic Pain Patients. In RJ Gatchel, DC Turk (eds), Psychosocial Factors in Pain: Critical Perspectives. New York/London: The Guilford Press, 1999;435–444.

4. Turk DC. Clinicians' attitudes about prolonged use of opioids and the issue of patient heterogeneity. J Pain Symptom Manage 1996;11(4):218–230.
5. Bonica JJ. General Considerations of Chronic Pain. In JJ Bonica (ed), The Management of Pain (vol 1). Philadelphia: Lea & Febiger, 1990.
6. Melzack R, Wall PD. Pain mechanisms: a new theory. Science 1965; 150:971–979.
7. Melzack R. The Gate Control Theory 25 Years Later: New Perspectives in Phantom Limb Pain. In MR Bond, JE Charlton, CJ Woolf (eds), Proceedings of the VI World Congress on Pain. Amsterdam: Elsevier, 1991;9–21.
8. International Association for the Study of Pain. Pain terms: a list with definitions and notes on usage. Pain 1979;6:249–252.
9. Banks SM, Kerns RD. Explaining high rates of depression in chronic pain: a diathesis-stress framework. Psychol Bull 1996;119:95–110.
10. Robinson ME, Riley JL. The Role of Emotion in Pain. In RJ Gatchel, DC Turk (eds), Psychosocial Factors in Pain. Critical Perspectives. New York: The Guilford Press, 1999;74–88.
11. Asmundson GJ, Jacobson SJ, Allerdings MD, et al. Social phobia in disabled workers with chronic musculoskeletal pain. Behav Res Ther 1996;34:939–949.
12. McCracken LM, Gross RT, Aikens J, et al. The assessment of anxiety and fear in persons with chronic pain: a comparison of instruments. Behav Res Ther 1996;34:927–933.
13. Vlaeyen JWS, Linton SJ. Fear avoidance and its consequences in chronic musculoskeletal pain: a state of art. Pain 2000;85:317–332.
14. Fernandez E, Turk DC. The scope and significance of anger in the experience of chronic pain. Pain 1995;61:165–175.
15. Eimer BN, Freeman A. Pain Management Psychotherapy: A Practical Guide. New York: Wiley, 1998;31–65.
16. Waddell G, McCulloch JA, Kummel E, Venner RM. Nonorganic physical signs in low back pain. Spine 1980;5:117–125.
17. Consensus statement from the American Academy of Pain Medicine and the American Pain Society. The use of opioids for the treatment of chronic pain. Clin J Pain 1997;13:6–8.
18. ten Vaarwerk IA, Staal MJ. Spinal cord stimulation in chronic pain syndromes. Spinal Cord 1998;36:671–682.
19. Kemler MA, Barendse GAM, van Kleef M, et al. Spinal cord stimulation in patients with chronic reflex sympathetic dystrophy. N Engl J Med 2000;343:618–624.
20. Silvers J, Campbell JN, North RB. Neurosurgical Modalities for Pain Management. In MA Ashburn, LJ Rice (eds), The Management of Pain. New York: Churchill Livingstone, 1998;519–525.
21. Paramore LC. Use of alternative therapies: estimates from the 1994 Robert Wood Johnson Foundation National Access to Care Survey. J Pain Symptom Manage 1997;13:83–89.

Suggested Readings

Besson JM. The neurobiology of pain. Lancet 1999;353:1610–1615.

Block A, Kremer E, Fernandez E (eds). Handbook of Pain Syndromes. New Jersey: Lawrence Erlbaum Associates, 1999.

Gatchel RJ, Turk DC (eds). Psychological Approaches to Pain Management: A Practitioner's Handbook. New York: The Guilford Press, 1996.

Gatchel RJ, Turk DC (eds). Psychosocial Factors in Pain: Critical Perspective. New York: The Guilford Press, 1999.

Psychological Components of Musculoskeletal Pain

Mary J. Wells

Since the beginning of mankind, individuals have attempted to understand and manage the role of pain in human life. Philosophers since Aristotle have pondered the question of whether pain resides in the body or in the mind. The traditional medical view has consistently held that pain is a sensory phenomenon with an organic cause. Modern medicine has based most of its pain treatment on the concept that pain has as its origin a specific underlying cause, and can be treated by modifying physiologic processes through either pharmacologic or surgical interventions. This assumption becomes more difficult to maintain when faced with a number of patients who complain of pain without clear underlying tissue pathology. Today, professionals who treat pain are recognizing that it is not linearly related to tissue pathology and that there are other, nonorganic factors contributing to the pain experience. Pain is not exclusively a physical experience. It is intrinsically connected to the emotional and cognitive realms as well.[1-3]

Psychological Pain Experience

To fully understand the psychological pain experience, there are a few concepts that need to be defined. Fordyce[4] differentiated the role of pain, suffering, and legal disability with regard to the treatment of low back pain. Drawing on conceptual formulations developed by Loeser,[5] Fordyce introduced four basic pain dimensions: nociception, pain, suffering, and pain behavior.

Nociception is defined as the mechanical, thermal, and chemical events acting on specific nerve endings that activate the pain fibers that signal the central nervous system that an aversive event is occurring. Essentially, nociception is the activity that occurs within specific peripheral nerve fibers and their synaptic connections.

Pain is defined as the sensation arising from nociception. This definition includes central pain states and phantom limb pain. It is important to note that a specific linkage between peripheral nociception and the sensation of pain is not always present.

Suffering is defined as the affective or emotional component of the central nervous system that is triggered by nociception, pain, or other emotionally aversive events. These could include such things as the loss of a loved one, threat, or fear.

Pain behavior is defined as the specific set of activities and behaviors that an individual engages in to show others that he or she is in pain. Keefe and Block[6] operationally identified a number of behaviors, including guarding, bracing, and grimacing, as pain behaviors often seen in conjunction with complaints of low back pain. Pain behavior has been conceptualized as a response to the pain experience, an output system, or a way of communicating to others the extent of distress experienced.

Of these four dimensions of pain, only nociception can be objectively verified in some cases. We believe that a patient is experiencing nociception when tissue abnormalities are detected, be this a tumor or a herniated disk. However, we still can't verify nociception on a cellular or microscopic level. Pain and suffering are personal and subjective experiences that can only be observed indirectly. Pain behavior, of course, is easily observed and sometimes that much harder to trust.

When an individual initially experiences musculoskeletal pain due to illness or injury, a complex series of psychological and biochemical events are set in motion. The physiologic component of pain, nociception, starts the process. The brain immediately interprets the nociceptive information as pain based on both the event itself and on previous experiences and beliefs about pain. Thus, even from the onset of a pain experience, cognitive factors play a large role in both the understanding of and the response to pain.

Following the injury or illness, changes in behavior are initiated by the sufferer. An individual experiencing pain is likely to decrease physical activity. Bed rest may be recommended. The patient may be told not to engage in activities that increase pain. This leads to a decrease in frequency or even the total cessation of a number of normal activities, including work, activities of daily living, household chores, and leisure activities. The pain itself acts as an aversive consequence of a number of normally pleasant activities. A person's life can be quickly altered.

In a typical acute pain episode, the aversive events are short-lived. The pain resolves and the individual quickly resumes normal activities. The pain is at best a minor annoyance, and at worst something to maneuver around. For some individuals however, this does not occur. The pain continues relentlessly. Normal activities are not resumed, and as the individual remains immobilized for longer and longer periods of time, negative physical cycles begin to set in. Muscle guarding results in an increased demand on muscles that often lack the flexibility and ability to manage the increased demands. Deconditioning sets in very quickly following an injury. Deconditioned muscles are unable to manage normal demands of daily living, thus resulting in increased experience of pain and a tendency to decrease activity even more.

Chronic pain has been linked to numerous antecedent factors, including early childhood deprivation and trauma, pain models in the family, and other family maladjustment and personality disorders.[7,8] However, because of flawed methodology, the conclusions drawn from a number of studies are questionable. Most studies now suggest that pain is consistently associated with current emotional disturbance and not with previous life functioning.[9–12] Overall, emotional disturbances, particularly depression, are more likely to be consequences than causes of pain.

Psychological Problems Associated with Persistent Pain

There are a number of psychological symptoms and problems associated with persistent or chronic pain. These include affective, behavioral, and vegetative changes as well as a number of cognitive factors associated with belief systems regarding health and health behavior.

Vegetative Signs

One of the most common complaints associated with chronic pain is sleep disturbance. Pain disrupts both sleep onset and sleep maintenance. It is not unusual to experience non-restorative sleep. The difficulties begin because an individual has difficulty finding a comfortable position. With position changes and restless sleep, pain reawakens individuals throughout the night. Chronic fatigue decreases pain tolerance and results in even minor injuries being perceived as traumatic events.

Appetite, another vegetative symptom, is often affected. Some individuals experience significant weight loss. More commonly, however, weight gain is reported. Individuals spend more time at home and less time engaged in other activities. They find themselves restlessly snacking throughout the day. This, combined with a decrease in physical activity, leads to an increase in weight. Self-esteem then becomes affected because individuals become uncomfortable with their weight gain and their physical appearance.

Vegetative problems of sleep disturbance and appetite disturbance are also frequently accompanied by changes in sexual desire or libido. Individuals who experience chronic pain often note difficulty in performance of the sexual act. Particularly for the individual suffering from low back pain, sexual activity can be almost intolerable. As an individual becomes more and more uncomfortable participating in a sexual relationship with his or her partner, he or she becomes more withdrawn and often notices a decrease in desire as well as difficulty with performance.

Affective Symptoms

Depressed mood is a common side effect of persistent pain. Patients often complain of feelings of helplessness or hopelessness related to pain control. As the pain continues over time, it is not unusual to hear patients complain of a loss of interest in activities that previously brought pleasure (anhedonia) or feelings of uselessness in the role of breadwinner or active family member. Suicidal thoughts, although rarely acted on, are common.[13]

A number of studies have noted the frequency with which depression accompanies a chronic pain problem. From 30% to 80% of all chronic pain sufferers have been reported in the literature as experiencing depression.[14] Depression has become known as the "handmaiden" of chronic pain. Although it is clear that many pain patients suffer from a variety of depressive symptoms, true clinical depression is probably over-diagnosed in chronic pain sufferers.[15,16]

Patients can also become anxious in response to pain. Fear of re-injury can play a central role in the development of a dysfunctional lifestyle due to pain.[17] A patient may worry that the underlying cause of the pain has not been found or adequately explained and may fear that it is life-threatening or that it will be made worse by activity. A slight increase in pain with activity sets off an extreme response, which only compounds the problem.

Another common psychological problem associated with chronic pain is that of irritability. Individuals (or their families) frequently complain of short temper, increased irritability, and loss of control over anger. To control their outbursts, individuals often withdraw from others. This withdrawal leads to increased isolation and an increased focus on the pain. The effort required to interact pleasantly with others seems overwhelming, even though pain patients are often lonely and would like to have others to talk to.[18]

Behavioral Changes

Patients often present with a number of behavioral symptoms during clinical examination and in the presence of others who express doubt about the seriousness of the pain problem. Pain behaviors are present in a large number of pain patients and vary in expression and intensity. They can and often do reflect genuine discomfort, but are also ways of communicating emotional distress to others. Waddell and colleagues[19,20] have demonstrated a number of methods of measuring emotional overlay through careful observation of pain behavior and its relation to anatomical structures. Their methods are an invaluable tool to quantify and somewhat objectively identify magnification of the pain problem. Table 22.1 lists a number of commonly observed pain behaviors.

Cognitions, Beliefs, and Expectations

Florence[21] describes the chronic pain syndrome as a perceptual illness. The chronic pain syndrome likely develops as a result of inappropriate perceptions regarding the meaning of pain and the value of various treatment options. Beliefs and expectations about pain and outcome play an essential role in the

TABLE 22.1   Pain behaviors

Behavior	Definition
Sighing	Obvious exaggerated exhalation of breath
Grimacing	Obvious facial expression of pain
Rubbing	Touching, holding, massaging affected area
Bracing	Stationary position in which fully extended limb supports and maintains abnormal weight distribution
Guarding	Abnormally stiff or rigid movement while shifting from one position to another

SOURCE: *Adapted from FJ Keefe, AR Block. Development of an observation method for assessing pain behavior in chronic low back pain patients. Behav Res Ther 1982;13:363–375.*

process of evaluating and treating musculoskeletal pain. *Cognitions* are defined as the set of attitudes, beliefs, and expectations developed by the individual over time, based on experience and social learning. Cognitions are thought to link external events and emotional response.[22,23]

It has been determined that a cognitive-behavioral mediation model is useful for understanding the relationship between pain and depression.[24] Results suggest that treatment success in a multidisciplinary pain clinic is moderated less by depression than by the cognitive appraisals (thoughts) and preferred coping strategies of patients. The presence of depression alone does not predict whether an individual will respond to cognitive-behavioral and interdisciplinary treatment strategies. Rather, influencing the style of coping and using active and skill-oriented activities are more likely to achieve a positive outcome.[25,26]

One study[27] evaluated coping strategies and pain beliefs. There were three distinct pain belief subgroups in a sample of chronic pain patients. They differed significantly in their use of and perceived effectiveness of pain coping strategies. The vast majority of these patients (70% of total sample) believed that their pain would be enduring and was of a mysterious nature. The authors characterize this subset of patients as individuals who are convinced that their pain will persist and that there is no adequate explanation regarding their pain. Patients in this subgroup rated their ability to use pain control strategies to be lower than patients in the other subgroups. They tended to use a more catastrophic response with less re-interpretation of pain sensations when coping.

Disability and Return to Work

One of the difficulties with the treatment of chronic low back (and other) pain patients is facilitating return to work. In one study, only 35–45% of chronic low back pain patients who had undergone treatment were managing a job 1 year after treatment. Epidemiologic data suggests that a person who is out on sick leave for more than 3 consecutive months for low back pain has virtually no chance of return to work. Absenteeism for back disorders accounts for approximately 25% of all sick leave[28] and chronic pain accounts for 70–87% of compensation benefits for workers.[29] In some areas of the United States, up to two-thirds of total compensation benefits are paid out for low back injuries.[30] In as many as 85% of these cases, no specific diagnosis can be made.[31,32]

Psychosocial and psychological factors tend to be underemphasized when assessing pain, especially early on. Despite considerable evidence from a wide body of literature suggesting that nonbiological factors contribute as much to the experience of pain and suffering as tissue pathology, efforts to assess and quantify psychosocial and psychological factors are not usually made until after the patient has already developed a chronic pain problem. The compensation system itself presents a number of disincentives to return to work. For compensable injuries on the job, the tax-free income can provide an incentive to remain at home. Employers are also less likely to rehire an injured worker or to provide him with "light duty." Individuals end up being frightened and confused by the "system"—they hear clear messages that they are unemployable in their previous setting and therefore need to stay on continued disability compensation.

The medical system reinforces disability by the continual search for a biological or physiologic cause of the pain. When it isn't found, the patient becomes anxious about occult disease and loses faith in the medical profession. Because medicine is so heavily based in a disease model, the psychosocial factors are often overlooked.

Effective vocational rehabilitation is very difficult to find. Vocational rehabilitation specialists are usually not part of the pain treatment team and often lack the sophisticated knowledge necessary to assist chronic pain patients with their specific needs. Because of their lack of understanding of the chronic pain process, they respond to pain problems as acute and send the patient back to the primary physician until such time as the pain is "cured." This inadvertently perpetuates a disability model.[33]

If an individual is unable to return to work for more than 6 months, there becomes less and less incentive to return to work at all. It is therefore essential to recognize early chronicity and to treat it effectively before the onset of total vocational disability.[29,31,33]

Malingering

Malingerers fraudulently present themselves as having nonexistent symptoms to obtain some kind of gain, usually financial. They differ from patients with psychological overlay or symptom magnification because they are consciously manipulating the system. The majority of chronic pain patients are not malingerers. They may exaggerate their symptoms to get attention (often subconsciously), but most should not be judged too harshly for this. They have simply been conditioned that this is the only way to get attention. The old saying that the squeaky wheel gets the grease is not without merit.

Treatment Strategies

There has been a gradually building body of evidence suggesting that the adjunctive use of psychological techniques to treat chronic pain is more effective than physical therapy or medications alone.[34-37] Psychological treatment strategies can include assessment and evaluation, individual and group psychotherapy, and interdisciplinary approaches such as relaxation training and biofeedback.

Assessment and Evaluation

Most physicians refer patients to psychologists when physical findings are insufficient to explain the extent of pain being reported by the patient. Physicians are traditionally trained in a model that assumes a direct correlation between the extent of tissue damage and the report of pain. Pain reports in the absence of specific physical pathology are assumed to be the result of psychological factors. This is the definition of *psychogenic pain*. The psychological evaluation is often requested when functional disability greatly exceeds that expected based on physical findings or when a patient is exhibiting significant

TABLE 22.2 Appropriate and inappropriate uses of psychological assessment

Appropriate uses

   To determine specific psychological and behavioral contributors to a patient's pain and concomitant behaviors, disability, and suffering

   To determine appropriate treatment strategies

   To provide essential information on particular aspects of a patient's psychosocial background and current situation that may be impacting the pain problem

Inappropriate uses

   To determine if pain is organic or functional (i.e., real or psychogenic)

   To catch malingerers

   To justify dumping of more difficult patients

SOURCE: *Adapted from DC Turk. Psychological assessment of patients with persistent pain: traditional views. Pain Management 1990(May/June):165–172.*

psychological distress such as depression or anxiety. Physicians often wait until a patient has become problematic or overly demanding before considering a psychological evaluation. Often the physician is fed up or frustrated with the patient's complaints.

Regardless of whether there is a clear organic basis for pain, factors including depression, beliefs and expectations, familial reinforcement of pain behaviors, anxiety, and stress response can all contribute to the maintenance and exacerbation of pain and suffering. A psychological evaluation can identify the psychosocial and behavioral factors that influence a patient's report of pain. If ignored, psychological factors frequently impede the recovery process and interfere with response to treatment and rehabilitation.[38] Table 22.2 delineates appropriate and inappropriate uses for psychological assessment.

Individual and Group Psychotherapy

Psychological treatment, whether offered in a group or individual format, should include specific content areas. Education regarding pain and function as well as some of the theoretical underpinnings of pain can increase a patient's understanding of pain responses. Cognitive strategies to alter belief systems and to decrease stress responses should also be standard aspects of treatment, along with strategies to combat depression and related helplessness and hopelessness. Behavioral techniques to modify specific behavior patterns related to movement and exercise can also be employed. Finally, instruction and practice in relaxation techniques should be included.

In an individual treatment format, the therapist has the luxury of fully exploring the relationship between the patient's personality and pain-coping strategies as well as gathering information on previous life experiences that impact the patient's level of distress. Patients with psychiatric illness in conjunction with their pain often respond better to the individual format, at least until good therapeutic rapport has been developed and the psychiatric problem has stabilized.[39]

TABLE 22.3 Clinical advantages to group treatment format

Credible feedback and confrontation from peers

Amelioration of sense of social isolation and alienation

Avoid patient dependency on therapist

More efficient use of therapist's time

SOURCE: *Adapted from WD Gentry, D Owens. Pain Groups. In AD Holzman, DC Turk (eds), Pain Management, A Handbook of Psychological Treatment Approaches. New York: Pergamon Press, 1986;100–112.*

Group psychotherapy provides a number of advantages over the traditional individual approach, although it is not appropriate for all patients.[40] Table 22.3 lists clinically relevant reasons for considering group psychotherapy as the primary or preferred treatment for pain patients.[41]

The strength of a group experience includes cost effectiveness as well as specific therapeutic factors of universality, cohesion, and instillation of hope.[42] Patients suffering with pain often feel hopeless, confused, and overwhelmed by their pain. The group experience can counteract those feelings and encourage patients to try out new behaviors that they might otherwise resist. More important, however, the patients can work together in a group to provide each other with support and encouragement and to decrease the sense of isolation and uniqueness so common to the chronic pain sufferer.[43]

Interdisciplinary Treatment Approaches

The current trend in treatment of the chronic pain patient (and concomitant vocational disability) is to provide an interdisciplinary approach.[35,37] These programs combine standard physical therapy with behavioral and psychological approaches consisting of education about pain, relaxation training, and cognitive-behavioral techniques, as well as more nontraditional techniques such as yoga and acupuncture. Such programs have been found to improve patients in terms of functional impairment, use of active coping strategy techniques, decreased medication use, and more effective self-efficacy beliefs.[35,37,39] In one study,[44] these changes were upheld over a 6-month follow-up with continued use of active coping strategies at a greater level than subjects in a controlled condition. Cognitive and behavioral treatments substantially augment effective physical therapy and traditional teaching.

Referral

It is clear that the way in which physicians convey perceptions of chronic pain treatment impacts the way in which individuals respond, both in the short- and long-term. The process of psychological consultation or evaluation requires the cooperation of patients. The patients' approach to this treatment is influenced by the way in which a psychological assessment or treatment is presented. If they feel comfortable and confident, they are much more likely to be open in describing their difficulties. If on the other hand, they are feeling angry, weary,

TABLE 22.4   Guidelines for psychological services referral

Clearly identify nonmedical consultants

Acknowledge problem is legitimate

Provide a positive rationale for referral

Inform other staff of rationale

Avoid making cynical comments about referral

Let patient know if referral is routine

Personalize the referral

Inform patient that referral doesn't imply transfer

SOURCE: *Adapted from R Cameron, LF Shepel. The Process of Psychological Consultation in Pain Management. In AD Holzman, DC Turk (eds), Pain Management: A Handbook of Psychological Treatment Approaches. New York: Pergamon Press, 1986;240–256.*

or apprehensive, they are much more likely to be guarded and suspicious of the evaluation process. In some cases, they may refuse a referral or not follow up on a referral. They may feel that the referring physician thinks they are "crazy" or that the pain is not real because they are being sent to the psychologist. Table 22.4 presents guidelines for making a good referral to psychological services.[45]

Early Warning Signs

The treating physician should constantly monitor patients for early warning signs of potential long-term problems with pain. Any pain that lasts longer that expected, given tissue-healing processes, should be considered as potentially problematic. Other early indicators may include an overreliance on the treating physician or physical therapist (i.e., frequent calls, multiple appointments on an emergency basis with no significant change in medical status), a passive approach to recovery, frequent or increasing reliance on narcotic analgesics, significant decrease in activity, or lack of return to normal activities. Complaints of pain with any or all activity may also suggest that a patient is at risk for chronic pain.

Points of Summary

1. The psychological pain experience is composed of four components: nociception, pain, suffering, and pain behavior.
2. A patient's beliefs and expectations about pain, its causes, and its treatment have a profound impact on the outcome of treatment.
3. It is essential to foster self-responsibility for treatment and outcome in the pain patient.
4. Depression and anxiety are most frequently consequences of pain, not causes.

5. Very few pain patients are true malingerers, although many do display pain amplification in their attempts to get their pain taken seriously.
6. Interdisciplinary treatment strategies, which include education, exercise, relaxation, and stress management, are the treatment strategies of choice for the chronic pain patient and may be beneficial in the subacute patient as well.

References

1. Turk DC, Holzman AD. Chronic Pain: Interfaces among Physical, Psychological, and Social Parameters. In AD Holzman, DC Turk (eds), Pain Management: A Handbook of Psychological Treatment Approaches. New York: Pergamon Press, 1986;1–9.
2. Turk DC. Biophysical perspective on chronic pain. In RJ Gatchel, DC Turk (eds), Psychological Approaches to Pain Management: A Practitioner's Handbook. New York: Guilford Press, 1996;3–32.
3. Eccleston C. Role of psychology in pain management. Br J Anaesth 2001;87(1):144–152.
4. Fordyce WE. Pain and suffering: a reappraisal. Am Psychol 1988;43(4):276–283.
5. Loeser JD. Perspectives on Pain. In Proceedings of the First World Conference on Clinical Pharmacology and Therapeutics. London: Macmillan, 1980;313–316.
6. Keefe FJ, Block AR. Development of an observation method for assessing pain behavior in chronic low back pain patients. Behav Res Ther 1982; 13:363–375.
7. Gatchel RJ. Psychological Disorders and Chronic Pain. In RJ Gatchel, DC Turk (eds), Psychological Approaches to Pain Management: A Practitioner's Handbook. New York: Guilford Press, 1996;33–52.
8. Crauford DIO, Creed F, Jayson MIV. Life events and psychological disturbance in patients with low-back pain. Spine 1990;15(6):490–494.
9. Gamsa, A. Is emotional disturbance a precipitator or a consequence of chronic pain? Pain 1990;42:183–195.
10. Roy R, Thomas M, Matas M. Chronic pain and depression: a review. Compr Psychiatry 1984;25(1):96–105.
11. Gamsa A, Vikis-Freibergs V. Psychological events are both risk factors in, and consequences of, chronic pain. Pain 1991;44:271–277.
12. Krishnan KRR, France RD, Houpt JL. Chronic low back pain and depression. Psychosomatics 1985;26:299–302.
13. Dworkin RH, Gitlin, MJ. Clinical aspects of depression in chronic pain patients. Clin J Pain 1991;7(2):79–94.
14. Romano JM, Turner JA. Chronic pain and depression: does the evidence support a relationship? Psychol Bull 1985;97(1):18–34.
15. Haythornthwaite JA, Seiber WJ, Kerns RD. Depression and the chronic pain experience. Pain 1991;46:177–184.
16. Wilson KG, Mikail SF, D'Eon JL, Minns JE. Alternative diagnostic criteria for major depressive disorder in patients with chronic pain. Pain 2001; 91(3):227–234.

17. Papciak AS, Feuerstein M. Fear of pain and distress in pain-related work disability. Paper presented at the 98th Annual Meeting for the American Psychological Association, Boston, Aug 1990.
18. Merskey H, Lau CL, Russell ES, et al. Screening for psychiatric morbidity. The pattern of psychological illness and premorbid characteristics in four chronic pain populations. Pain 1987;30:141–157.
19. Waddell G, Main CJ, Morris EW, et al. Chronic low back pain psycho-logic distress and illness behavior. Spine 1984;9(2):209–213.
20. Waddell G. A new perspective to the treatment of low back pain. Spine 1987;12:6–32.
21. Florence, DW. The chronic pain syndrome: a physical and psychologic challenge. Postgrad Med 1981;70(5):217–228.
22. Beck AT, Rush AJ, Shaw BF, et al. Cognitive therapy in the emotional dis-orders. New York: International Universities Press, 1976.
23. Beck AT. Cognitive therapy of depression. New York: Guilford Press, 1979.
24. Kleinke CL. How chronic pain patients cope with depression: relation to treatment outcome in a multidisciplinary pain clinic. Rehabil Psychol 1991;36(4),207–218.
25. Jenson MP, Turner JA, Romano JM. Changes in beliefs, catastrophizing, and coping are associated with improvement in multidisciplinary pain treatment. J Clin Consult Clin Psychol 2001;69(4):655–662.
26. Pincus T, Morley S. Cognitive-processing bias in chronic pain: a review and integration. Psychol Bull 2001;127(5):599–617.
27. Williams DA, Keefe, FJ. Pain beliefs and the use of cognitive-behavioral strategies. Pain 1991;46:185–190.
28. Linton SJ, Bradley LA, Jensen I, et al. The secondary prevention of low back pain: a controlled study with follow-up. Pain 1989;36:197–207.
29. Rucker K, Metzler H, Wehman P, et al. Pain literature and social security policy. J Back Musculoskel Rehabil 1991;1(3):67–73.
30. Dworkin RH, Handlin DS, Richlin DM, et al. Unraveling the effects of compensation, litigation and employment on treatment response and chronic pain. Pain 1985;23:49–59.
31. Feuerstein M, Zastowny TR. Occupational Rehabilitation: Multidisci-plinary Management of Work-Related Musculoskeletal Pain and Disabil-ity. In RJ Gatchel, DC Turk (eds), Psychological Approaches to Pain Management: A Practitioner's Handbook. New York: Guilford Press, 1996;458–485.
32. Frymoyer JW. Back pain and sciatica. N Engl J Med 1988;318(5):291–300.
33. Brena SF, Turk DC. Vocational Disability: A Challenge to Pain Rehabilita-tion Programs. In GM Aronoff (ed), Pain Centers: A Revolution in Health-care. New York: Raven Press, 1987;167–180.
34. Sternbach RA. Mastering Pain: A Twelve-Step Program for Coping with Chronic Pain. New York: Ballantine Books, 1987.
35. Mayer TG, Gatchel RJ, Mayer H, et al. The prospective two-year study of functional restoration in industrial low-back injury: an objective assess-ment procedure. JAMA 1987;258(13):1763–1767.
36. Gonzales VA, Martelli MF, Baker JM. Psychological assessment of per-sons with chronic pain. Neurorehabilitation 2000;14(2):69–83.

37. Newman RI, Seres J. The Interdisciplinary Pain Center: An Approach to the Management of Chronic Pain. In AD Holzman, DC Turk (eds), Pain Management: A Handbook of Psychological Treatment Approaches. New York: Pergamon Press, 1986;71–85.
38. Turk DC. Psychological assessment of patients with persistent pain: traditional views. Pain Management 1990(May/June):165–172.
39. Grzesiak RC. Toward a psychotherapy for chronic pain patients: some directions. Paper presented at the 12th Annual Meeting of the Society for Behavioral Medicine, Washington, DC, March 22, 1991.
40. Ettin MF, Heiman ML, Kopel SA. Group building: developing protocols for the psychoeducational groups. Group 1988;12(4):205–225.
41. Gentry WD, Owens D. Pain Groups. In AD Holzman, DC Turk (eds), Pain Management, A Handbook of Psychological Treatment Approaches. New York: Pergamon Press, 1986;100–112.
42. Yalom I. The Theory and Practice of Group Psychotherapy. New York: Basic Books, 1975.
43. Keefe FJ, Beaupre PM, Gil KM. Group Therapy for Patients with Chronic Pain. In RJ Gatchel, DC Turk (eds), Psychological Approaches to Pain Management: A Practitioner's Handbook. New York: Guilford Press, 1996;259–282.
44. Nicholas MK, Wilson PH, Goyen J. Comparison of cognitive-behavioral group treatment and an alternative non-psychological treatment for chronic low back pain. Pain 1992;48:339–347.
45. Cameron R, Shepel LF. The Process of Psychological Consultation in Pain Management. In AD Holzman, DC Turk (eds), Pain Management, A Handbook of Psychological Treatment Approaches. New York: Pergamon Press, 1986;240–256.

Suggested Readings

Brena SF, Turk DC. Vocational Disability: A Challenge to Pain Rehabilitation Programs. In GM Aronoff (ed), Pain Centers: A Revolution in Healthcare. New York: Raven Press, 1987;167–180.

Gatchel RJ, Turk DC (eds). Psychological Approaches to Pain Management: A Practitioner's Handbook. New York: Guilford Press, 1996.

Mayer TG, Gatchel RJ, Mayer H, et al. The prospective two-year study of functional restoration in industrial low-back injury: an objective assessment procedure. JAMA 1987;258(13):1763–1767.

Sternbach RA. Mastering Pain: A Twelve-Step Program for Coping with Chronic Pain. New York: Ballantine Books, 1987.

Turk DC. Psychological assessment of patients with persistent pain: traditional views. Pain Management 1990(May/June):165–172.

23   Fitness for Life: The Role of Exercise in Treating and Preventing Illness

David R. O'Brien, Jr., and Van Evanoff, Jr.

Sedentary lifestyles are common. With an abundance of food, entertainment, television, computers, and the Internet, physical activity is not a significant part of many peoples' lives. However, evidence clearly indicates that regular exercise and physical activity can protect against the development and progression of several chronic diseases. The goal of this chapter is to make the reader more aware of the beneficial effects of regular exercise on health, well-being, disease processes, and illness.

Cardiovascular Disease

Hypertension

Hypertension is a common risk factor for atherosclerotic and cardiovascular disease, including myocardial infarction and stroke. It often goes undetected, as there are few symptoms associated with mild to moderate elevations in blood pressure. Routine blood pressure screening is recommended.

Two basic types of hypertension exist: essential (or idiopathic), and hypertension due to a discernable cause such as renal artery stenosis or pheochromocytoma. The majority of people have essential hypertension, and in most cases it is mild.

In persons with a specific condition causing hypertension, the treatment obviously is to remove the cause. In those with essential hypertension, exercise can be useful. Endurance exercise at moderate intensity is believed to benefit individuals with mild to moderate essential hypertension.[1-4] These people can sometimes decrease their systolic and diastolic blood pressures, perhaps by approximately 10 mm Hg, with such moderate exercise.

A review of randomized, well-controlled exercise intervention studies indicates that mild to moderate aerobic exercise can significantly reduce blood pressure in patients with essential hypertension.[4] Additionally, regression of left ventricular hypertrophy may be achieved in these patients, even after reductions in their antihypertensive medications. Exercise also attenuates an exaggerated blood pressure response to physical exertion. All of these effects can lead to a reduction in cardiovascular problems and a reduction in the need for medications.

When one is diagnosed as having mild hypertension, the first line of treatment is conservative and non-pharmacologic. An aerobic exercise program is prescribed along with other lifestyle changes, including weight loss (if needed), behavioral modification, cessation of smoking, reduction of alcohol intake, and diet changes. If this fails, then pharmacologic treatment may be instituted. In moderate hypertension, medication is usually prescribed in addition to the modifications noted above, including exercise. Exercise may, in some cases, allow a reduction or discontinuation of the medication at a future date. Severe hypertension usually requires medical as well as behavioral and exercise changes.

The American College of Sports Medicine recommends that aerobic exercise at 60–90% of maximal heart rate be performed three to five times a week for 20–60 minutes in normotensive adults.[5] There is some evidence that exercise near the upper limit of this range of heart rate may actually worsen hypertension[6]; exercise of moderate intensity is probably most beneficial in the hypertensive patient. Also, isometric exercise, to which heavy weight lifting is similar, sometimes causes marked increases in blood pressure during the exercise, and may cause a sustained rise in pressure as well. It is thus usually not recommended in the hypertensive patient. Lighter weight/higher repetition and circuit weight training may be safer in hypertensive individuals who wish to pursue some strength training.

The mechanism by which moderate intensity endurance exercise lowers blood pressure is not yet fully understood, although some believe that it acts by lowering serum catecholamine levels. The antihypertensive effect of exercise is independent of weight loss or change in body composition.[7]

When medications are used to treat hypertension, it is important to consider some of their potential side effects, such as dehydration, potassium imbalance, and altered heart rate response to exercise.

Hyperlipidemia

Regular aerobic exercise improves serum lipid profiles. This benefit is demonstrated as a decrease in total serum triglycerides and very-low-density lipoproteins and as an increase in high-density lipoproteins.[8] A review of 95 studies in a meta-analysis suggests that reductions in cholesterol and low-density lipoprotein cholesterol levels are greatest when exercise training is combined with weight loss.[9] In patients with a history of hyperlipidemia, exercise stress testing should be performed before initiating an exercise program.

Atherosclerosis and Ischemic Heart Disease

Atherosclerotic cardiovascular disease (ASCD) is a major cause of morbidity and mortality. Formation of atherosclerotic plaques leads to ischemic disease that can adversely affect the heart, brain, and limbs, resulting in cardiac disease, stroke, and peripheral vascular disease. Regular exercise and physical activity is a lifestyle choice that can assist in the prevention of the onset and progression of ASCD.

Along with the direct benefits that occur to the cardiovascular system, various risk factors for ASCD can be reduced or eliminated with physical activity. These include hypertension, hyperlipidemia, abnormal glucose metabolism, and obesity. Additional lifestyle changes such as cessation of smoking and dietary modifications can augment the benefits of exercise.

For men who exercise regularly, the overall risk of cardiac arrest is significantly lower than in sedentary men. Epidemiologic studies consistently show lower all-cause death rates in physically active individuals and favorable risk ratios for active lifestyles.

Regular preoperative exercise in patients awaiting coronary artery bypass grafting has been shown to decrease postoperative length of hospitalization and time required in intensive care. During the preoperative period, exercising patients have a better quality of life than controls, and this effect continues for up to 6 months after surgery.[10]

Physical activity has been shown to be associated with a reduced risk of stroke in both men and women. Exercise does not need to be vigorous to achieve results.[11]

Regular exercise also results in significant improvements in patients with stable intermittent claudication, with a 150% average increase in walking time and distance in persons who were previously limited by leg pain.[12]

The mechanism of action by which exercise helps prevent atherosclerosis is still not completely elucidated, although when an exercise program is undertaken, there are predictable changes seen in the heart and vascular system as well as in muscle. Aerobic exercise increases the body's maximum ability to take up oxygen, $\dot{V}O_2$max. This is due to an increase in cardiac output and an increased ability of skeletal muscle to extract oxygen. In high-intensity aerobic exercise there is an increase in left ventricular chamber size, which allows for an increase in stroke volume.[13] There also appears to be an increase in myocardial blood supply due to an increase in coronary artery diameter. An increase in myocardial capillary density has been found in exercising animals.[14] Another adaptation to exercise is a lowering of the resting heart rate. This is thought to be due to increased parasympathetic nervous system activity.

Diabetes

There are two basic types of diabetes: type I, also known as *insulin-dependent diabetes mellitus* (IDDM) and type II, or *non–insulin-dependent diabetes mellitus* (NIDDM). Both are metabolic disorders in which blood glucose levels are not properly controlled. In type I there is an absolute deficiency of insulin. This almost always occurs in children, and necessitates supplementation with insulin in all cases. Type II diabetes occurs most often in adults. In these patients, insulin levels are often elevated and peripheral cell insulin receptors are thought to be insensitive to the circulating insulin. These receptors are found on cells including adipocytes, muscle cells, and liver cells. Type II diabetics usually have a strong family history of NIDDM and are often obese.

They can mostly be treated with oral hypoglycemic medication to reduce blood glucose levels. In this chapter we focus on type II diabetes and the role of exercise in its prevention and treatment. Exercise has little effect on type I diabetes except that by burning calories it may decrease insulin requirements.

Regular aerobic exercise can improve serum glucose levels and insulin sensitivity. A single episode of exercise can increase insulin sensitivity for at least 16 hours in healthy adults with NIDDM.[15] Insulin requirements are reduced due to increased sensitivity of skeletal and adipose tissue to insulin during and after exercise.[16] Regular exercise has been shown to decrease insulin requirements and improve glucose control in patients with NIDDM.[17]

A prospective, controlled study of patients with impaired glucose tolerance demonstrated that increasing physical activity, combined with weight loss and dietary modification, resulted in a 58% reduction in the development of NIDDM.[18]

Careful serum glucose monitoring needs to be performed and medications adjusted to prevent exercise-induced hypoglycemia in exercising diabetics. A thorough cardiac evaluation should also be considered before initiating an exercise program.

Obesity

When dieting, the body's basal metabolic rate decreases. This reduces baseline energy consumption and is one reason why sustained weight loss is difficult to achieve with dieting alone. Exercise, on the other hand, tends to have a sustained effect of raising the basal metabolic rate. This, in addition to the calories burned by the exercise itself, helps bring about a slow, steady weight loss.

As an individual exercises, changes in body composition occur. Exercise tends to favor a loss of body fat while increasing lean body mass. Because lean body mass is more metabolically active than fatty tissue, it tends to increase baseline energy consumption even further. However, to maintain this new composition, physical activity must be continued.

Dieting alone has been shown to be largely ineffective in maintaining initial weight loss. Regular exercise has been shown to be one of the best predictors of successful weight maintenance,[19] and studies have indicated that improved fitness through regular exercise reduces cardiovascular morbidity and mortality for overweight or obese individuals, even if they remain overweight.[20]

Exercises that minimize joint stress and weight bearing are usually better tolerated in obese patients, at least initially. Cycling, rowing, stair climbing, and aquatic exercises serve this purpose. Early on, the exercise program should focus on establishing an exercise routine. This is best done with low-intensity, low-impact exercises of relatively long duration. More rigorous exercise can be added later.

A study of young, healthy women who were mildly to moderately obese and wanted to lose weight showed that walking and cycling decreased weight, but swimming did not.[21] Although it may be an excellent form of exercise, swimming is not recommended as a particularly good weight-loss program. In the obese, however, any exercise is most likely a good start.

Osteoporosis

Osteoporosis is a common disease found primarily in postmenopausal white and Asian women. It is associated with considerable morbidity and mortality and is a major health issue among the elderly. The greatest complication of osteoporosis is bone fracture, the most common of which are vertebral, radial (Colles'), and hip fractures. Osteoporosis can be caused by medical diseases such as hyperthyroidism, chronic obstructive pulmonary disease, Cushing's disease, or malabsorption syndrome. It may also be caused by drugs such as anticonvulsants, glucocorticoids, or heparin. However, in most people, osteoporosis has no known cause. This section discusses the role of exercise in prevention and treatment of such osteoporosis. Adequate calcium intake, hormone replacement therapy, and other medication may augment the beneficial effects of regular weight-bearing exercises in preventing and treating osteoporosis.

Osteoporosis is defined as a decrease in absolute density of normal bone matrix and mineral. With this decrease comes an increased fragility of bone with associated susceptibility to fracture. The bone loss is primarily from trabecular bone, and must be fairly advanced to be detectable on routine radiographs.

Bone density peaks between the ages of 30 and 35. Thereafter, there is a slow, steady decline in density. In females the decline becomes more rapid once menopause is reached and estrogen levels drop.

Risk factors for osteoporosis include gender (female), ethnicity (white or Asian), lean body build, alcohol ingestion, cigarette smoking, nulliparity, prolonged amenorrhea, low calcium intake, and possibly, excessive caffeine ingestion.

Stressing bone, usually by weight-bearing activity but also by some other activities, improves skeletal health. Bone is constantly remodeling itself to be better able to tolerate stress. Inactivity, as found in the bedridden patient or with casting or weightlessness in astronauts, results in a loss of bone mass. Activity, on the other hand, increases bone mass, usually in the bones involved in bearing the body's weight but also sometimes in other bones that are stressed (such as in a tennis player's arm) or in bones that are far removed from the stressor.[22–24] Intermittent bone compression, not static loading, appears to be necessary to increase bone mass.[23]

A review of 21 randomized, controlled trials suggested that regular exercise can reduce the risk of osteoporosis and may even delay decreases in bone density.[25] Studies in older women indicate that there is a reduced risk for hip fracture in those who are regularly physically active.[26] Exercise early in life appears to reduce the incidence of osteoporosis in older age.[27] Weight-bearing exercises appear to be most useful in increasing bone mass, as a study of postmenopausal women with bone loss indicates that water aerobics does not help to increase bone density, although it does improve overall fitness.[28]

Although regular exercise may result in minimizing osteoporosis, indirect benefits such as increased coordination, balance, endurance, and muscle strength can also occur. These improvements appear to lower the risk of falls, thereby potentially decreasing the risk for fracture.[29]

Young women who exercise very vigorously may develop amenorrhea or a hypoestrogenic state. This can negate the beneficial effects of exercise, and must be evaluated.

Sense of Well-Being

Exercise has been shown to have a moderate effect on reducing anxiety and can improve physical self-perception and self-esteem. Good evidence exists that aerobic and resistive exercises enhance mood and that exercise should be considered as an adjunct method of treating depression and anxiety, as well as improving overall sense of well-being.[30]

Smoking Cessation

Smoking is the largest preventable cause of death in the United States. Health care providers are obligated to strongly urge smokers to quit. A list of programs or available handouts from the American Cancer Institute or the American Lung Association can be helpful, along with encouragement and support. Various medications and psychological interventions may aid in smoking cessation. Exercise may also help.[31]

Points of Summary

1. Moderate-intensity aerobic exercise may help control mild to moderate essential hypertension.
2. Intense exercise and heavy weight lifting may be contraindicated in hypertensive patients.
3. Exercise improves the high-density lipoprotein–low-density lipoprotein ratio to one more favorable to prevent coronary artery disease.
4. Aerobic exercise may help to control non–insulin-dependent diabetes (NIDDM), probably by increasing the sensitivity of cell receptors to insulin.
5. Aerobic exercise increases the basal metabolic rate and favors a loss of body fat.
6. Regular weight-bearing exercise may help in preventing and treating osteoporosis.
7. Regular exercise leads to an improved sense of well-being.

References

1. Hagberg JM, Seals DR. Exercise training and hypertension. Acta Orthop Scand Suppl 1986;711:131–136.
2. Tipton CM, Matthes RD, Marcus KD, et al. Influences of exercise intensity, age, and medication on resting systolic blood pressure of SHR populations. J Appl Physiol 1983;55(4):1305–1310.
3. Gordon NF, Scott CB. Exercise and mild hypertension. Prim Care 1991;18:683–694.
4. Kokkinos PF, Papademetriou V. Exercise and hypertension. Coron Artery Dis 2000;11:99–102.
5. American College of Sports Medicine. Guidelines for Exercise Testing and Prescription (6th ed). Philadelphia: Lea and Febiger, 2000.

6. Tanji JL. Hypertension part I: how exercise helps. Phys Sports Med 1990;18(7):77–82.
7. Gordon NF, Scott CB, et al. Exercise and mild essential hypertension: recommendation for adults. Sports Med 1990;10:390–404.
8. Mendoza SG, Carrasco H, Zerpa A, et al. Effect of physical training on lipids, lipoproteins, apolipoproteins, lipases, and endogenous sex hormones in men with premature myocardial infarction. Metabolism 1991;40:368–377.
9. Tran ZV, Weltman A. Differential effects of exercise on serum lipid and lipoprotein levels seen with changes in body weight. A meta-analysis. JAMA 1985;254:919–924.
10. Arthur HM. Effect of a preoperative intervention on preoperative and postoperative outcomes in low risk patients awaiting elective coronary artery bypass graft surgery. A randomized, controlled trial. Ann Intern Med 2000;133:253–262.
11. Wannamethee SG, Sharper AG. Physical activity and the prevention of stroke. J Cardiovasc Risk 1999;6:213–216.
12. Leng GC, Fowler B, Ernst E. Exercise for intermittent claudication. Cochrane Database Syst Rev 2000;2:CD000990.
13. Maron BJ. Structural features of the athletic heart as defined by echocardiography. J Am Coll Cardiol 1986;7:190–203.
14. Ljungqvist A, Unge G. Capillary proliferative activity in myocardium and skeletal muscle of exercised rats. J Appl Physiol 1977;43(2):306–307.
15. Borghouts LB, Keizer HA. Exercise and insulin sensitivity: a review. Int J Sports Med 2000;21:1–12.
16. Ruderman N, Apelian AZ, Schneider SH. Exercise in therapy and prevention of type II diabetes. Diabetes Care 1990;13:1163–1168.
17. Zinker BA. Nutrition and exercise in individuals with diabetes. Clin Sports Med 1999;18:585–606.
18. Tuomilehto J, Lindstrom J, Eriksson JG, et al. Prevention of type 2 diabetes mellitus by changes in lifestyle among subjects with impaired glucose tolerance. N Eng J Med 2001;344:1343–1350.
19. American College of Sports Medicine. Guidelines for Exercise Testing and Prescription (4th ed). Philadelphia: Lea and Febiger, 1991:195–196.
20. McInnis KJ. Exercise and obesity. Coron Artery Dis 2000;11:111–116.
21. Gwinup G. Weight loss without dietary restriction: efficacy of different forms of aerobic exercise. Am J Sports Med 1987;15(3):275–279.
22. Jones HH, Priest JD, Hayes WC, et al. Humeral hypertrophy in response to exercise. J Bone Joint Surg 1977;59A(2):204–208.
23. Dalen N, Olsson E. Bone mineral content and physical activity. Acta Orthop Scand 1974;45:170–174.
24. Camay A, Tschantz P. Mechanical influences in bone remodeling. Experimental research on Wolff's law. J Biomech 1972;5:173–180.
25. Ernst E. Exercise for female osteoporosis. A systematic review of randomized clinical trials. Sports Med 1998;25:359–368.
26. Gregg EW, Cauley JA, Seeley DG, et al. Physical activity and osteoporotic fracture risk in older women. Ann Intern Med 1998;129:81–88.
27. Bischoff HA, Conzelmann M, Lindemann D, et al. Self-reported exercise before age 40: influence on quantitative skeletal ultrasound and fall risk in the elderly. Arch Phys Med Rehabil 2001;82:801–806.

28. Bravo G, Gauthier P, Roy PM, et al. A weight-bearing, water-based exercise program for osteopenic women: its impact on bone, functional fitness, and well-being. Arch Phys Med Rehabil 1997;78:1375–1380.
29. Gardner MM, Robertson MC, Cambell AJ. Exercise in preventing falls and fall related injuries in older people: a review of randomized controlled trials. Br J Sports Med 2000;34:7–17.
30. Fox KR. The influence of physical activity on mental well-being. Public Health Nutr 1999;2:411–418.
31. Ussher MH, Taylor AH, West R, et al. Does exercise aid in smoking cessation? A systematic review. Addiction 2000;95:199–208.

Suggested Readings

American College of Sports Medicine. Guidelines for Exercise Testing and Prescription (6th ed). Philadelphia: Lea and Febiger, 2000.

Borghouts LB, Keizer HA. Exercise and insulin sensitivity: a review. Int J Sports Med 2000;21:1–12.

Ernst E. Exercise for female osteoporosis. A systematic review of randomized clinical trials. Sports Med 1998;25:359–368.

Kokkinos PF, Papademetriou V. Exercise and hypertension. Coron Artery Dis 2000;11:99–102.

Wannamethee SG, Sharper AG. Physical activity and the prevention of stroke. J Cardiovasc Risk 1999;6:213–216.

Index

Page numbers followed by *f* refer to figures; those followed by *t* refer to tables.

waveforms in, 40
Electromyography. *See* Electrodiagnostic studies
Elevation in RICE protocol, 9, 242
Endurance exercise, 28–29, 34
  cardiovascular and respiratory response in, 29, 29t, 34, 34f
  of elderly, 313–314
  fuel use in, 28f, 28–29
  heart rate in, 29, 29t, 34, 34f
  in hypertension, 364
  physiologic response to, 28–29
  of women, 326, 328
Energy sources and utilization in endurance exercise, 28f, 28–29
Epicondyles of humerus, 141, 148, 149
  apophysitis of, 158, 302
  inflammation of, 152–154, 156. *See also* Epicondylitis
Epicondylitis
  lateral, 152–154
    examination in, 148, 149f, 153
    treatment of, 153–154
  medial, 156
    examination in, 149, 156
    treatment in, 156
Epiphysis, slipped capital femoral, 303–304
Erythema ab igne, 16
Evoked potentials, somatosensory, 42
Exercise, 27–37
  in activity-specific training, 36–37
    in elbow injuries, 150–151
  aerobic, 28f, 28–29, 34
    in atherosclerosis, 365
    in hypertension, 364
  anaerobic, 29
  in atherosclerosis, 364–365
  cardiovascular response to. *See* Cardiovascular response to exercise
  in diabetes mellitus, 366
  of elderly, 313–314
  endurance, 28–29, 34. *See also* Endurance exercise
  female athlete triad in, 330
  for fitness, 9–10, 34
    benefits of, 363–368
  for flexibility, 30, 35–36
  heart rate in. *See* Heart rate during exercise
  in hyperlipidemia, 364
  in hypertension, 363–364
  isokinetic, 33
    in complex regional pain syndrome, 282
  isometric. *See* Isometric exercise

  isotonic, 32–33
    in complex regional pain syndrome, 282
  kinetic chain in, 36, 238
  in menstrual cycle, 329–330
  in obesity, 366
  in osteoporosis, 107, 367
  overload principle in, 27
  physiologic response to, 27–30
    in women, 326, 328
  postpartum, 329
  in pregnancy, 328–329
  prescription of, 30, 31t
  in prevention and treatment of illness, 363–368
  proprioceptive, 9, 35
    in ankle injuries, 9, 36, 244, 244f
    in knee injuries, 215
  respiratory response to, 9–10, 29, 29t
    in women, 326, 328
  and self-esteem, 368
  strengthening, 10, 27–28, 32–34. *See also* Strengthening exercises
  stretching, 30, 35–36. *See also* Stretching exercises
  types of, 27–30, 31t
Expectations and beliefs about pain, 354–355, 357
Extensor mechanism rupture of knee, 214, 223
Extensor tendinosis of wrist in wheelchair use, 335–336

Faber test, 190, 190f
Facet joint pain, 108
Failed back syndrome, 107–108
Fajersztajn test, 96
Falls of elderly, 320
Fascia, plantar, 232
  in gait cycle, 235
  inflammation of, 246–247, 320
Fasciitis, plantar, 246–247, 320
Femoral nerve, stretch test of, 96
Femur
  anatomy of
    at hip, 185
    at knee, 203, 204, 205
  osteonecrosis of head, 303
  slipped capital epiphysis of, 303–304
Fibromyalgia, 291–295, 328
  diagnostic criteria in, 293, 294t
  etiology of, 291–293
  tender points in, 291, 292f, 293, 294t
  treatment of, 293–295
Fibula, anatomy of, 229, 230f, 230–231

Fingers. *See* Hand
Finkelstein's test, 169, 170f, 177
Fitness exercise, 9–10, 34
    benefits of, 363–368
Flat foot, 251–252
Flexibility, 30, 35–36
    in heat therapy, 19, 35
    neural factors in, 30, 35
    of piriformis muscle, testing of, 191, 191f
    in progression of rehabilitation, 10
    stretching exercises for. *See* Stretching
        exercises
Flexor digitorum profundus
    anatomy of, 165, 166f
    avulsion injury of, 182
    testing of, 168, 169f
Flexor digitorum superficialis
    anatomy of, 165, 166f
    testing of, 168–169, 169f
Foot, 229–253
    alignment with lower leg, 237, 237f
    anatomy of, 229–232
    bones in, 229–230, 231f–232f
    in children, 309
    in elderly, 319–320
    examination and testing of, 237–240
        subtalar joint position in, 238
    flat, 251–252
    in gait cycle, 233–236
    in hallux valgus and rigidus, 250, 320
    metatarsalgia of, 249, 320
    Morton's neuroma of, 249–250
    osteoarthritis of, 320
    in pes planus and cavus, 251–252, 320
    plantar fasciitis of, 246–247, 320
    pronation of, 233
        in pes planus, 251–252
        signs of hyperpronation, 237
    stress fractures of, 248
    supination of, 234
    turf toe of, 251
    in women, 327
Footwear. *See* Shoes and footwear
Forearm, 141–161
    anatomy of, 141–146
    bones of, 141–142, 142f
    carrying angle of, 147, 148f
    compartment syndrome of, 160–161
    muscles of, 144–145, 145f
    neurovascular structures in, 145–146
    overuse injuries of, 148, 156
    range of motion, 147
Fractures, 7
    in falls of elderly, 320

of hip, 319
metacarpal and phalangeal, 181–182
in osteoporosis
    of hip, 319
    in spinal cord injuries, 338
    of spine, 106–107, 317
of radius, distal, 180
of scaphoid, 181
of spine, 105, 106–107, 317
stress, 7
    of foot and lower leg, 248
    of olecranon, 160
of wrist, 181
    reflex sympathetic dystrophy and vita-
        min C in, 285–286
Froment's sign, 168, 174
Fuel use in endurance exercise, 28f, 28–
    29
Functional capacity evaluation in work-
    related injuries, 264–265, 265t

Gaenslen's test, modified, 192
Gait, 60–62
    in elderly, 314
    foot in, 233–236
    in hip disorders, 61, 61f, 187
    muscles used in, 61t
        hip abductor, 61, 61f, 187
    normal cycle in, 60, 60f
    observation of, 237
    in sesamoiditis, 251
    stride and step length in, 60, 60f
    Trendelenburg, 61, 61f, 192
Gamekeeper's thumb, 182
Ganglion cysts of wrist and hand, 178–179
Gastrocnemius muscle, 240
Gate control theory on pain, 342
Genetic factors in complex regional pain
    syndrome, 275
Genu
    recurvatum, 60
    valgum, 305–306
    varum, 305–306
Geriatric disorders, 313–322
    drug-induced, 320–322
        in corticosteroid therapy, 318, 319,
            321
    in falls, 320
    of foot, 319–320
    of hip, 319
    of knee and leg, 316, 319
    of neck and back, 316–318
    in osteoarthritis, 315–317
    of shoulder, 318

in wheelchair use, 334–335
Oxford isotonic exercise technique, 33
Oxygen consumption in exercise, 29, 29t, 34
in women, 326, 328

Pain, 9–10
    acupuncture in, 285, 295, 347
    in back, 94–109. *See also* Back, pain in
    behavioral symptoms in, 352, 354, 354t
        in chronic pain syndrome, 343
        and treatment strategies, 357, 358
    beliefs and expectations in, 354–355, 357, 358
    in chest, in costochondritis, 136
    chronic, 341–347, 352–353
        in back, 107–108
        compared to chronic pain syndrome, 341
        etiology of, 342–343
        symptoms and problems associated with, 353–354
        treatment of, 344–347
    chronic pain syndrome in, 341, 354–355
        anxiety and avoidance behavior in, 343
        drug therapy in, 345
    clinical assessment of, 344
    complex regional syndrome, 269–286. *See also* Complex regional pain syndrome
    cryotherapy in, 14t, 21
    definition of, 351–352
    disability and return to work in, 355–356
    drug therapy in, 345, 346t
        in complex regional pain syndrome, 283
        in elderly, 321
    early warning signs in, 359
    in elbow, 146–160
    electrical nerve stimulation in, transcutaneous, 23
    epidemiology of, 342
    in fibromyalgia, 291–295
    in forearm compartment syndrome, 160–161
    gate control theory of, 342
    in groin, 198, 199
    heating modalities in, 14t
    in hip and pelvis, 188–199
        locations of, 188
        myofascial, 197–198
    injection techniques in, 45–47, 297, 345

interdisciplinary approach to, 341–342, 358
invasive treatment procedures in, 347
in knee, 206–223
myofascial, 295–297. *See also* Myofascial pain
in neck, 75–84
    myofascial, 74, 76–78
nerve pathways in, 342, 351
in phantom limb, 342
psychogenic, 356
psychological factors in, 351–360
    assessment of, 344, 356–357, 357t
    in chronic pain, 341, 343–344, 352–353
    in complex regional pain syndrome, 277
    referral in, 358–359, 359t
radiating, 58
radicular, 58
referred, 58
    in myofascial pain, 296
in shoulder, 128–138
suffering in, 352
sympathetically independent, 277
sympathetically maintained, 277
in thigh, 223–225
Waddell criteria in, 96–97, 97t, 344
    in work-related injuries, 264, 264t
Palpation, 55
of elbow, 147, 148
of hip and pelvis, 189
of knee and thigh, 208
of lower leg and foot, 237
of shoulder, 119
Panner's disease, 302
Paraspinal muscles, 90
Parsonage-Turner syndrome, 138
Patella, 204
    alta, 208, 218
    apprehension test of, 211, 218
    baja, 208
    grind test of, 212
    inspection of, 208, 218
    instability of, 217–219
        examination and testing in, 208, 211–212, 218
Patellar tendonitis, 214, 220
Patellofemoral joint
    anatomy of, 203, 204
    dysfunction of, 208, 219–220
        diagnosis of, 214, 219
        in disabled population, 337
        quadriceps angle in, 212, 213t, 219

Quadriceps femoris muscles, 186
  anatomy of, 205, 205f
  contusion of, 223–224
  delayed onset soreness of, 224
  diagnosis of disorders, 214
  imbalance in, 219
  strain of, 224
  tendonitis of, 214, 220

Radial artery, Allen's test of, 171
Radial nerve anatomy in hand and wrist, 165
Radiculopathy
  cervical, 79–82
    Spurling's maneuver in, 72, 73f
  electromyography in, 41–42
  lumbar, 100–103
  in spinal stenosis of elderly, 318
  traction in, 24
Radiocapitellar chondromalacia, 155
Radiocarpal joint, 163, 164f
Radiocarpal ligaments, 163
Radiography, 43
  of back, 97
  in complex regional pain syndrome, 271, 273f, 279
  of elbow, 149
  of hand and wrist, 171
  of hip and pelvis, 193
  of knee and thigh, 212
  of lower leg, ankle, and foot, 240
  of neck, 74
  of shoulder, 127, 127t
Radionuclide scans of bone, 49
  in complex regional pain syndrome, 279
  in knee and thigh disorders, 214
Radius
  anatomy of
    at elbow, 142
    at wrist, 163
  fracture of, distal, 180
Range of motion, 58–60
  in complex regional pain syndrome, 282
  of elbow, 147
  of hand and wrist, 168
  of hip and pelvis, 189, 190
  of knee, 208, 209
  in progression of rehabilitation, 10
  of shoulder, 120, 120f
    in adhesive capsulitis, 134
Raynaud's disease, 179–180
Reactivation techniques in complex regional pain syndrome, 280

Rectal examination
  in back pain, 96
  in hip and pelvic pain, 192–193
Referral
  for psychological services, 358–359, 359t
  in work-related injuries, 260
Reflex sympathetic dystrophy, 269–286
  diagnostic criteria in, 270–271
  diagnostic tests in, 278–280
  epidemiology and triggering conditions in, 271–275, 274t
  pathophysiology in, 275–278
  treatment of, 280–286
    clodronate in, 285
    spinal cord stimulation in, 284–285
    vitamin C in, 285–286
Reflex testing, 58, 58t
Regional pain syndrome, complex, 269–286
Reiter's syndrome, sacroiliac joint dysfunction in, 194
Remodeling stage in healing process, 4
  in bone injury, 7
Repair stage in healing process, 4–5
Repetitive use injuries, 3, 4. *See also* Overuse injuries
Respiratory response to exercise, 29, 29t
  and modified activities for maintenance of fitness, 9–10
  in women, 326, 328
Rest
  relative, 9
  in RICE protocol, 9, 242
Retrolisthesis, 105
Rheumatoid arthritis, 6
  of hand, 175–177
    diagnosis of, 175, 176f
    treatment of, 176–177
  of knee, Baker's cyst in, 223
  of neck, 83
RICE protocol, 9
  in ankle sprains, 242
Rotator cuff, 115, 117t
  anatomy of, 115, 116f
  drop arm test of, 124, 129
  impingement of, 128–130
    examination in, 122–124, 123f, 124f, 129
    in wheelchair use, 334–335
  infraspinatus muscle in, 115, 116f, 130
  strength testing of, 122, 124–126, 126f
  strengthening exercises for, 130
  subscapularis muscle in, 115, 116f, 130

osteoarthritis of, 135–136, 318
pediatric disorders of, 301–302
rotator cuff of. *See* Rotator cuff
Sprengel's deformity of, 302
strength testing of, 121–122, 123f
   of supraspinatus, 124–126, 126f
strengthening exercises for, 130, 133–134
wheelchair use affecting, 334–335
Sinding-Larsen-Johansson syndrome, 305
Sinuvertebral nerves, 69, 90
Skier's thumb, 182
Skin disorders in disabled population, 338
Skin response test in complex regional pain
   syndrome, 279
Sleep disorders
in chronic pain, 353
in fibromyalgia, 293
history of, 55
Sling in acromioclavicular sprain, 135
Smoking cessation, 368
Snuffbox, anatomic, 181, 181f
Soleus muscle, 240
Somatosensory evoked potentials, 42
Spasms
of back, 99
cryotherapy in, 21
electrical stimulation in, 23
Speed's test in bicipital tendonitis, 124,
   125f, 129
Spinal accessory nerve trauma, 138
Spinal canal, 69, 90–91
stenosis of, 102, 103–105
   cervical, 78, 317
   in elderly, 317–318
Spinal cord, 69, 90–91
myelopathy of, 102
   cervical, 80, 81–82
stimulation techniques
   in chronic pain, 347
   in complex regional pain syndrome,
   284–285
trauma of, 338
   in elderly, 318
   osteoporosis and fractures in, 338
   skin care in, 338
Spinal nerves, 87, 88f
anesthetic block of, 47f
cervical, 69
   radiculopathy of, 72, 73f, 79–82
in dermatomes, 58, 59f
lumbar, 90
   radiculopathy of, 100–103
in myotomes, 56, 57t
thoracic, 90

Spine
anatomy of, 87–90, 88f, 89f, 90f
   cervical, 65–68, 66f, 67f
cervical, 65–68. *See also* Cervical spine
fractures of, 105
   in osteoporosis, 106–107, 317
geriatric disorders of, 316–318
intervertebral disks in. *See* Disk, intervertebral
lumbar, 87, 88f. *See also* Lumbar spine
motions of, 92–94
   cervical, 70, 71, 71f
osteoarthritis of, 103f, 103–105
   cervical, 78–79
   in elderly, 316–317
osteoporosis of, 103, 106–107, 317
pediatric disorders of, 307–309
physical examination of, 94–97
   cervical, 70–74
Scheuermann's disease of, 308
scoliosis of, 307–308
spondylolisthesis of, 105–106
   in children, 308–309
   in elderly, 317
stenosis of, 102, 103–105
   cervical, 78, 317
   in elderly, 317–318
thoracic, 87, 92, 308
traction of, 24
Spinous vertebral process, 87
cervical, 66, 66f
Splints for hand and wrist
in carpal tunnel syndrome, 174
in complex regional pain syndrome,
   282
in rheumatoid arthritis, 176, 177
Spondylitis, ankylosing
cervical, 83–84
sacroiliac joint dysfunction in, 194
Spondylolisthesis, 105–106
in children, 308–309
in elderly, 317
isthmic, 105, 317
Spondylolysis, 105–106, 308, 317
Spondylosis, 103
cervical, 78–79
Sports hernia. *See* Hernia in sports injuries
Sports medicine approach to rehabilitation,
   8–10
Sprain
of acromioclavicular joint, 135
of ankle, 9, 36, 240–244
of back, 98–100
cervical, 75–76

Weber's two-point discrimination test, 168
Wheelchair use
    epidemiology of musculoskeletal injuries
        in, 333
    myofascial pain in, 338
    skin problems in, 338
    upper extremity injuries in, 334–336
Whiplash injuries of neck, 75–76
Windlass mechanism, 236
Women, 325–331
    anatomy and physiology issues concern-
        ing, 325–326
    athlete triad in, 330
    back pain in, 328
    breast disorders in, 330–331
    carpal tunnel syndrome in, 327–328
    fibromyalgia in, 328
    foot injuries in, 327
    knee injuries in, 325–326, 327
    menstruation and athletic performance
        of, 329–330
    osteoporosis in, 325, 331
        in athlete triad, 330
    training and exercise of, 326, 328–329
        postpartum, 329
        in pregnancy, 328–329
Work-related injuries, 257–267
    claims processing in, 258–259, 262–
        263
    definitions of terms in, 258
    functional capacity evaluation in, 264–
        265, 265t
    historical aspects of, 257
    history-taking in, 261–262, 262t

malingering and symptom magnification
    in, 263, 356
maximum medical improvement in, 265
permanent partial impairment in, 259,
    265–267, 266t
recovery time in, 260, 261t, 355–356
return to work in, 355–356
    work conditioning and work harden-
        ing in, 260–261
treatment approach in, 260–267
unique features of, 258–260
Wrist, 163–183
    anatomy of, 163–166
    examination of, 168–171
    extensor tendinosis in wheelchair use,
        335–336
    ganglion cysts of, 178–179
    median nerve compression at, 173–174,
        327–328, 336
    tendonitis of, 178
    tenosynovitis of, DeQuervain's, 177–
        178
    trauma of, 180–181
    reflex sympathetic dystrophy and vitamin
        C therapy in, 285–
        286
    ulnar neuropathy at, 174–175

Yergason's test in bicipital tendonitis, 124,
    125f, 129

Zygapophyseal joints
    cervical, 65
    lumbar and thoracic, 87